SUPERANTIGENS

SUPERANTIGENS

Molecular Basis for Their Role in Human Diseases

Edited by

Malak Kotb
and John D. Fraser

ASM
PRESS

Washington, D.C.

Cover illustration: A hypothesized functional complex of SEB, MHC-II, and TCR (see Chapter 6 and Color Plate 6) (courtesy of Vickery Arcus).

Address editorial correspondence to ASM Press, 1752 N St., N.W., Washington, DC 20036-2904, USA

Send orders to ASM Press, P.O. Box 605, Herndon, VA 20172, USA
Phone: 800-546-2416; 703-661-1593
Fax: 703-661-1501
E-mail: books@asmusa.org
Online : http://estore.asm.org

Copyright © 2007   ASM Press
                     American Society for Microbiology
                     1752 N St., N.W.
                     Washington, DC 20036-2904

Library of Congress Cataloging-in-Publication Data

Superantigens: molecular basis for their role in human diseases / edited by Malak Kotb and John
    D. Fraser.
        p. ; cm.
    Includes bibliographical references and index.
    ISBN-13: 978-1-55581-424-3 (hardcover : alk. paper)
    ISBN-10: 1-55581-424-7 (hardcover : alk. paper)
    1. Superantigens.   I. Kotb, Malak.   II. Fraser, John D.   III. American Society for
Microbiology.
    [DNLM: 1. Superantigens—physiology.   2. Bacteria—immunology.   3. Virulence Factors.
    QW 573 S9594 2007]

    QR186.6.S94S875 2007
    616.07'92—dc22

                                                                                    2007013806

10 9 8 7 6 5 4 3 2 1

This book is dedicated to the memory of Edwin H. Beachey,
a great scientist, mentor, and friend

CONTENTS

**V. THERAPEUTIC INTERVENTIONS IN SUPERANTIGEN-MEDIATED
    DISEASES**

CONTRIBUTORS

K. Ravi Acharya • Department of Biology and Biochemistry, University of Bath, Building 4 South, Room 0.29, Claverton Down, Bath BA2 7AY, United Kingdom

Gila Arad • Department of Molecular Virology, The Hebrew University-Hadassah Medical School, 91120 Jerusalem, Israel

Vickery L. Arcus • AgResearch Protein Engineering Laboratory, Department of Biological Sciences, University of Waikato, Private Bag 3105, Hamilton, New Zealand

Edward N. Baker • Centre for Molecular Biodiscovery, School of Biological Sciences, University of Auckland, Private Bag 92-019, Auckland, New Zealand

Matthew D. Baker • Department of Biology and Biochemistry, University of Bath, Building 4 South, Room 0.29, Claverton Down, Bath BA2 7AY, United Kingdom

Gregory A. Bohach • Department of Microbiology, Molecular Biology, and Biochemistry, University of Idaho, Moscow, ID 83846

Sang-Hyun Cho • Department of Dermatology, The Catholic University of Korea, Seoul, Korea 403-720

Barry C. Cole • Division of Rheumatology, University of Utah School of Medicine, Salt Lake City, UT 84132

Alexander Emmer • Neurology Hospital, Martin Luther University, D-06097 Halle-Wittenberg, Germany

John D. Fraser • School of Medical Sciences, University of Auckland, Private Bag 92019, 85 Park Rd., Grafton, Auckland, New Zealand

Kristina Gerlach • Neurology Hospital, Martin Luther University, D-06097 Halle-Wittenberg, Germany

Goutam Gupta • Los Alamos National Laboratory, Bioscience Division, Los Alamos, NM 87545

Dalia Hillman • Department of Molecular Virology, The Hebrew University-Hadassah Medical School, 91120 Jerusalem, Israel

Brigitte T. Huber • Department of Pathology, Tufts University School of Medicine, 150 Harrison Ave., Boston, MA 02111

Raymond Kaempfer • Department of Molecular Virology, The Hebrew University-Hadassah Medical School, 91120 Jerusalem, Israel

Malte E. Kornhuber • Neurology Hospital, Martin Luther University, D-06097 Halle-Wittenberg, Germany

Malak Kotb • University of Tennessee Health Science Center, 930 Madison, Suite 468, Memphis, TN 38163

Teresa Krakauer   •   Department of Immunology, Integrated Toxicology Division, United States Army Medical Research Institute of Infectious Diseases, Fort Detrick, Frederick, MD 21702-5011

Meghan Kunkel   •   Los Alamos National Laboratory, Bioscience Division, Los Alamos, NM 87545

Donald Y. M. Leung   •   Department of Pediatrics, National Jewish Medical and Research Center, Denver, CO 80206, and University of Colorado Health Sciences Center, Denver, CO 80262

Revital Levy   •   Department of Molecular Virology, The Hebrew University-Hadassah Medical School, 91120 Jerusalem, Israel

Donald E. Low   •   Department of Microbiology, Mount Sinai Hospital, University of Toronto, Toronto, Ontario M5G 1X5, Canada

Eva Medina   •   Department of Microbial Pathogenesis and Vaccine Research, Infection Immunology Research Group, GBF-German Research Center for Biotechnology, Mascheroder Weg 1, D-38124 Braunschweig, Germany

Tohru Miyoshi-Akiyama   •   Department of Infectious Disease, International Medical Center of Japan, Tokyo 162-8655, Japan

Hong-Hua Mu   •   Division of Rheumatology, University of Utah School of Medicine, Salt Lake City, UT 84132

Iris Nasie   •   Department of Molecular Virology, The Hebrew University-Hadassah Medical School, 91120 Jerusalem, Israel

Anna Norrby-Teglund   •   Karolinska Institutet, Center for Infectious Medicine, Karolinska University Hospital, Huddinge, S-141 86 Stockholm, Sweden

Thomas Proft   •   School of Medical Sciences, University of Auckland, Private Bag 92019, 85 Park Rd., Grafton, Auckland, New Zealand

Patrick M. Schlievert   •   Department of Microbiology, University of Minnesota Medical School, 420 Delaware Street S.E., Minneapolis, MN 55455

M. S. Staege   •   Children's Cancer Research Center, Division of Pediatric Hematology and Oncology, Martin Luther University, D-06097 Halle-Wittenberg, Germany

Albert K. Tai   •   Department of Pathology, Tufts University School of Medicine, Boston, MA 02111

Andrej Tarkowski   •   Department of Rheumatology and Inflammation Research, Göteborg University, Guldhedsgatan 10, S-413 46 Göteborg, Sweden

Takehiko Uchiyama   •   Department of Microbiology and Immunology, Department of Infectious Diseases, Institute of Laboratory Animals, School of Medicine, Tokyo Women's Medical University, Tokyo 162-8666, Japan

Hidehiro Ueshiba   •   Institute of Laboratory Animals, Tokyo Women's Medical University, Tokyo 162-8666, Japan

Björn Walse   •   SARomics AB, Scheelevägen 22, SE-220 07 Lund, Sweden

PREFACE

Microbial superantigens are fascinating proteins that have structurally evolved to interact in a unique manner with host immune defense systems. These molecules are unusual in the sense that they can simultaneously activate cells involved in innate immunity as well as T cells, which normally mediate acquired immune responses. As a result of this unusual mode of interaction, superantigens have the capacity to stimulate large numbers of immune cells to release inflammatory mediators that, if uncontrolled, can inflict serious damage upon the host and may even cause death. Through our studies of the various superantigens, we have learned so much about immune system activation and regulation and about the various mechanisms by which different cells of the immune system interact and exchange biochemical signals that program their response and function.

Years prior to their designation as superantigens and the discovery of the mechanism by which they function, several laboratories had been studying these proteins and noticing the unconventional way by which they elicit immune activation. The massive proliferative response they elicit in resting leukocytes resembled that of polyclonal mitogens, yet the requirement for cells expressing HLA class II molecules to induce leukocyte activation resembled antigenic responses. Unlike conventional antigens, however, these molecules required no processing by antigen-presenting cells and their presentation to T cells was MHC unrestricted. These seemingly perplexing properties were resolved when it became evident that the superantigens interact in a unique manner with HLA class II as well as with specific elements within the variable region of the β chain of the αβ T cell receptor (TCR). Furthermore, it was found that superantigens use these receptors as a means to bring different types of cells closer, forcing them to interact and exchange activation signals that trigger biochemical cascades, resulting in the elaboration of potent inflammatory cytokine responses and massive T cell proliferation.

Shortly after their discovery, it was believed that all superantigens were alike, that they interact in the same way with immune cells, and that they cause similar diseases, namely toxic shock, serious skin infections, and food poisoning. A common remark was "if you've studied one superantigen, you've studied them all." We now know that nothing could have been further from the reality of these molecules. The fact that bacteria like *Streptococcus pyogenes* have over twelve different superantigens suggested that these microbial proteins are functionally nonredundant.

Thousands of articles have been published on superantigens, with a marked increase in the past two years, underscoring the fact that the field has been advancing considerably. This, we believe, is a result of the advent of sophisticated technologies and bioinformatics tools that unraveled new structure-function information and considerable differences in the way that distinct superantigens interact with HLA class II and/or TCR molecules. These new discoveries provided an impetus for more in-depth studies of molecular features underlying differences in the biological function of superantigens, their tissue specificity and capacity to cause or exacerbate different diseases.

Although several outstanding books on superantigens have been published, we wanted this book to highlight several new and exciting findings. We assembled an outstanding team of scientists with highly diverse expertise but a common interest in superantigen structure, function, and biology. These authors brilliantly captured some of the latest advances in the field, presenting information on newly discovered superantigens in bacteria and viruses, demonstrating how some superantigens interact with receptors other than, or in addition to, HLA class II and TCR molecules, and proposing novel mechanisms for the association of certain superantigens with various types of acute and chronic diseases, including autoimmune diseases. Exciting developments in therapeutic modalities for super-antigen-mediated diseases are also highlighted in this book. This latter aspect has been given some priority in recent years, particularly since certain superantigens, in the aerosolized form, have potential for use as biological weapons and in bioterrorism.

More importantly, we wanted the readers of this book to develop a better appreciation for how newly discovered structural variations among superantigens affect the mode by which they interact with immune cells. We hope that the readers will have a better understanding of how these structure/function differences may explain why different superantigens contribute to the initiation and/or exacerbation of distinct diseases, why certain ones are effective in some tissues but not others, and how the host's genetic makeup can grossly alter the course of superantigen-mediated diseases. We also hope that the readers of this book will appreciate how this new information has informed the design and development of novel intervention strategies or suggested the use of existing modalities to ameliorate or modulate superantigen responses in severe acute infections or certain chronic illnesses.

On the flip side, however, the powerful immune-stimulating potential of certain super-antigens may be exploited to modulate and direct the type of inflammatory responses in a way that increases the host's efficiency in overcoming certain chronic diseases and infections. These new insights may provide information on disease mechanism and thereby focus efforts to develop effective therapeutics and intervention measures for superantigen-mediated illnesses.

Malak Kotb
John D. Fraser

Section I

SUPERANTIGENS: WHAT IS NEW?

Superantigens: Molecular Basis for Their Role in Human Diseases
Edited by Malak Kotb and John D. Fraser
© 2007 ASM Press, Washington, D.C.

Chapter 1

The Streptococcal Superantigens

John D. Fraser and Thomas Proft

INTRODUCTION

Streptococcus pyogenes (Group A Lancefield type) is a gram-positive bacterium that colonizes the throat and upper respiratory tract of 5 to 15% of humans. Most individuals experience no ill effects, but in some, an infection can cause acute pharyngitis and tonsillitis. Left untreated, it can develop into the serious sequelae of acute rheumatic fever (ARF), rheumatic heart disease (RHD), and poststreptococcal glomerulonephritis (15, 53). Group A *Streptococcus* (GAS) also causes scarlet fever (SF) and invasive disease such as deep wound infection leading to cellulitis, myositis, necrotizing fasciitis, and the acute condition streptococcal toxic shock syndrome (STSS) (79, 86, 87).

Streptococcal epidemics were very common prior to World War II, with outbreaks of SF and ARF a common occurrence in Europe, North America, and Australasia. The widespread use of penicillin and improved hygiene and housing has seen the rates of SF and ARF plummet. They are now exclusive to the overcrowded communities of the poor. The decline in SF and ARF has been countered by an alarming increase in the frequency and severity of invasive GAS disease such as STSS. STSS has a 30 to 60% mortality; it was first recognized in 1983 (97) but has since been observed worldwide (52, 85–87). STSS is characterized by the rapid onset of hypotension, fever, rash, vomiting, diarrhea, multiple organ failure, systemic shock, and multisystem collapse (98). It is caused by a sudden release of one or more streptococcal superantigens into the blood. The conditions that result in this sudden production of toxin remain one of the major questions in the study and treatment of invasive streptococcal disease.

THE PYROGENIC EXOTOXINS FROM GROUP A STREPTOCOCCI

The application of streptococcal exotoxins in medicine dates back to the late 1800s and a leading New York surgeon, William B. Coley, M.D. (1862 to 1936). Dr. Coley discovered that a patient with advanced cancer who had failed conventional treatment made a complete recovery after two attacks of erysipelas, a severe skin infection involving lymph

John D. Fraser and Thomas Proft • The School of Medical Sciences and the Centre for Molecular Biodiscovery, University of Auckland, Auckland, New Zealand.

nodes, caused by *S. pyogenes*. Dr. Coley subsequently attempted to produce similar responses in patients with late-stage cancer by injecting cultures of *S. pyogenes*. Using a particularly potent streptococcal culture obtained from the bacteriologist Robert Koch, he succeeded in inducing tumor regression and published his first paper on this treatment in 1893. Over the next 43 years, Dr. Coley treated nearly 900 patients with "Coley Toxins" and achieved remarkable success, in particular, with advanced solid tumors. His observations were that certain streptococcal strains were more effective and that the active substance(s) were secreted into the culture supernatants. Dr. Coley is now widely recognized as the father of cancer immunotherapy and many have since assigned these remarkable clinical results to the action of the pyrogenic exotoxins or superantigens in triggering the immune system to produce antitumor cytokines such as tumor necrosis factor alpha (TNF-α). With the advent of radiotherapy and chemotherapy, Dr. Coley's treatments fell into disrepute but the science behind these remarkable results has since been validated and studied in considerable detail (60).

In 1924, culture filtrates of GAS were injected subcutaneously into individuals and produced the classic "scarlatina" rash (17). This reaction, known as the "Dick reaction," was believed to be caused by an erythrogenic toxin subsequently named "scarlet fever toxin" or toxin A.

Pyrogenic toxin B was identified by Hooker and Follensby in 1934 (30) and first purified and characterized by Stock and Lynn in 1969 (88). A third toxin, C, which was immunologically different from A and B, was isolated in 1960 from the culture filtrate of a scarlet fever-causing strain (94).

Streptococcal pyrogenic exotoxin (SPE) A, B, and C had three activities: T-cell blastogenesis, pyrogenicity in rabbits, and enhanced susceptibility to lethal endotoxin shock in rabbits. Pyrogenicity was for many years believed to be their principal function, hence their name, but they are indeed three manifestations of the one activity—stimulating lymphocytes (41).

The 756-bp gene coding for a 232-amino-acid SPE-A was first cloned in 1986 and found located on the bacteriophage T12 (95). T-cell mitogenicity of SPE-A was demonstrated by Schlievert and Gray (76) and shortly thereafter shown to bind to major histocompatibility class II (MHC II)-dependent and T-cell receptor (TcR) Vβ-specific mode in a fashion similar to the staphylococcal superantigens (34).

The *speB* gene was cloned from a serotype M12 GAS strain (10) and shown to be identical to streptococcal cysteine protease (SCP), confirming earlier results (23). SPE-B induced T-cell proliferation (1), but this was later shown to be due to contamination from an unknown superantigen called SPE-X (11, 25), later defined as streptococcal mitogenic exotoxin Z (SMEZ).

The gene coding for SPE-C was cloned from an *S. pyogenes* strain T18P (25) and also shown to be an MHC II, TcR Vβ-dependent superantigen (45).

The *ssa* gene was isolated from an M3 serotype strain of *S. pyogenes* (56).

SMEZ was first detected as a potent hVβ4 and 8 stimulating superantigen from *S. pyogenes* serotype M1/T1 strain (37). An allelic variant of this toxin was later purified from large volumes of a streptococcal culture harboring the T12 phage and designated SPE-X/SMEZ3 (22). The gene for SMEZ-2 was finally cloned in 1999 (68) and later shown to exist in numerous allelic variants (67).

IDENTIFICATION OF STREPTOCOCCAL
SUPERANTIGENS BY GENOME SCANNING

The availability of streptococcal genomes has simplified the effort of identifying new superantigens. There are two strongly conserved regions among superantigens designated by the PROSITE signatures STAPH_STREP_TOXIN motifs Y-G-G-[LIV]-T-X(4)-N (PROSITE entry PS00277) and K-X(2)-[LIVF]-X(4)-[LIVF]-D-X(3)-R-X(2)-L-X(5)-[LIV]-Y (PS00278). These motifs were used to identify *speG*, *speH*, *speI*, and *speJ* from published genomes (67, 68). SPE-J induced fever in rabbits and was lethal in two rabbit models of STSS (52).

The *speL* gene was identified on the temperate phage ΦNIH1.1 in the serotype M3 strain (33). The same gene was independently identified in a separate study and named *speK* (7), even though the name had already been assigned to a pseudogene on the *S. pyogenes* M1 genome (21). Henceforth, this superantigen (SAg) will be referred to as SPE-K/L. Given their ease of identification, naming of new SAgs has reached a confusing stage where the same sequence has received multiple names. The *speK/L* gene was found on a New Zealand serotype M89 strain and named *speL* in accordance with the Japanese designation (70). *speM* was cloned from a serotype M80 strain using a similar strategy (70). Another study of a serotype M18 strain yielded two novel *sag* genes, named *speL* and *speM*, although different from the *speL* and *speM* already identified (80). *speL* (M18) is identical to *speM* (M80 strain) and will henceforth be referred to as *speL/M*, while *speM* (M18 strain) was novel. Recombinant forms of SPE-K/L and SPE-L/M stimulated T cells in a Vβ-specific and MHC II-dependent mode (70, 80).

STREPTOCOCCAL SUPERANTIGEN GENES

The GAS superantigen genes have been found both on the chromosome and more commonly on integrated bacteriophage regions, which is the mechanism for their horizontal transfer. Evidence of the transmissibility of a superantigen gene was first provided by Zabriskie in 1964 (103), who showed that a nonlysogenic *speA*[−] strain T25[3] became *speA*[+] by infection with the φT12 phage from the *S. pyogenes* strain T12g1. To date, six GAS genomes have been completed. These include the serotypes M1 (21), two M3 (7, 59), M6 (5), M18 (81), and M28 (27). Of the 11 known streptococcal superantigen genes, all but *smeZ*, *speG,* and *speJ* genes are phage encoded. Of 94 clinical GAS isolates from New Zealand, all were found to have the *smeZ* and *speG* genes in a stable chromosomal location (67). The *speJ* gene was not found in M3 and M18 isolates, suggesting that *speJ* might be located on a less stable part of the chromosome. With the discovery that large chromosomal regions have been extensively shuffled among *S. pyogenes* strains (20) the stable retention and location of the *smeZ* and *speG* gene close to the *emm* locus that codes for the classic M protein surface antigen suggests that these two genes play an important and nonredundant role in defense of the organisms (20).

Fifty GAS isolates comprising 29 M types and 3 nontypeable strains have shown the following relative frequencies; *smeZ* >90%, *speJ* >90%, *speA* 30%, *speC* 36%, *speH* 22%, *speI* 2%, *ssa* 26%, *speK/L* 28%, and *speL/M* 4% (70). Only 12% of the isolates contained both *speI* and *speH* (located in tandem orientation on phage 370.2 [M1]), while 10%

of the isolates contained *speH* only. None of the isolates carried the *speI* gene without the *speH* gene. In all the temperate phage analyzed, the superantigen genes were located at the distal end of the integrated phage genome (with respect to the integrase gene) suggesting that these genes may have been acquired or lost through some aberrant excision of host genomic material from phage integration (20). A study by Ikebe et al. (33) showed that none of ten M3 isolates recovered before 1974 carried the *speL/K* gene, while all of 18 M3 isolates collected during or after 1992 contained *speL/K*, reflecting a recent integration event.

VARIATION IN STREPTOCOCCAL SUPERANTIGEN GENES

Minor allelic variation has been found for SPE-A and SPE-C. SPE-A1, SPE-A2, and SPE-A3 differ by a single amino acid (G110S in SPE-A2 and V106I in SPE-A3). SPE-A4 differs from SPE-A1 by approximately 11% and was reported to be frequent in serotype M6 (5, 61).

speA5 differs from *speA4* by four synonymous and one nonsynonymous mutation, while *speA6* differs from *speA1* by a single synonymous mutation. This indicates that *speA* arose from two phylogenetic lineages designated lineage I (*speA1*, *speA2*, *speA3*, *speA6*) and lineage II (*speA4*, *speA5*) (8).

The *speC2* allele differs from *speC1* by two silent A/G transitions (38), while *speC3* and *speC4* differ from *speC2* by one base pair, resulting in nonsynonymous amino acid changes (62).

The *smeZ* gene uniquely has much greater variation. The amino acid sequence of SMEZ-2 isolated from strain 2035 (M5) (68) differed by 17 amino acids (8.1%) from the very first published SMEZ protein, now named SMEZ-1. The greatest difference in SMEZ alleles is a pentapeptide sequence 96-EEPMS-100 to 96-KTSIP-100 in SMEZ-2. This represents a potential B-cell epitope. Twenty-two further *smeZ* alleles (including three pseudogenes) were identified from 37 GAS isolates (67). The *smeZ* gene is in linkage equilibrium with the M/*emm* gene. Comparison of the amino acid sequences of all the SMEZ sequences reveals a mosaic structure that could only have arisen through homologous recombination events rather than random point mutations. Despite wide allelic differences, the MHC class II and Vβ specificity was the same while serum-neutralizing responses of healthy donors to individual alleles varied substantially. This clearly suggests that the allelic polymorphism has arisen to produce escape variants to antibody selection. Most of the variable amino acids have side chains that are surface exposed and occur in positions around the SMEZ surface except for the MHC class II-binding site and TcR-binding site (90).

Vβ SPECIFICITY OF THE STREPTOCOCCAL SUPERANTIGENS

The potency of SAgs is measured by the amount required to stimulate human T cells at 50% of their maximum activity (P_{50}). The P_{50} values for the streptococcal SAgs range from a very low 0.02 pg/ml (SMEZ-2) to 50 pg/ml (SPE-H). SMEZ-2 is the most potent of all known SAgs with proliferative activity on human peripheral blood lymphocytes (PBLs) still detectable at <0.1 fg/ml (68). Streptococcal SAgs stimulate T cells across many species including rabbits and mice, but the P_{50} values are usually substantially lower. SPE-C is completely inactive in mice even though it binds murine I-E molecules (47).

The human genome has 50 different V-region gene segments in the β-chain region forming approximately 24 families, yet surprisingly, the streptococcal SAgs target only a fraction of the available Vβs. The most common TcR is Vβ2 which is targeted by SPE-C, SPE-G, and SPE-J, and to a lesser extent by SPE-A, SPE-H, and SMEZ (Table 1). T cells bearing Vβ1 are primarily stimulated by SPE-K/L, SPE-M/L, and SPE-M (70, 80), and less frequently by SSA. SMEZ is unique and strongly stimulates Vβ4- and Vβ8-bearing cells.

GENE REGULATION

Acute streptococcal toxic sequelae in humans have been attributed to the strain's ability to suddenly produce large amounts of one or more superantigenic toxins. The production of SPE-A and SPE-C in GAS cell culture differs significantly between individual isolates. Eleven strains from various M/T serotypes were shown to produce between 0.03 and 16 μg/ml, while the amounts of SPE-C produced by three different strains were 0.9, 1.2, and 1 μg/ml (24). Higher amounts of toxin were produced by 26 isolates from patients with STSS with average concentrations of 3.2 μg/ml of SPE-A and 0.6 μg/ml of SPE-C (44). In contrast, many strains isolated from patients with STSS in France, Sweden, and Chile produced very low or no detectable amounts of either SPE-A or SPE-C (71). It has been suggested that *speA* expression varies in a clonal manner with respect to the M serotype (40). However, several recently conducted experiments suggest that *sag* gene expression is tightly controlled and unknown host factors may up-regulate superantigen gene transcription during infection.

Table 1. Functional properties of streptococcal superantigens

SAg[a]	MW (kDa)	Organism	Crystal structure solved	Zinc binding	MHC II binding α/β-chain	Human TcR Vβ specificity	P_{50} (h)[b] (pg/ml)
SPE-A	26.0	*S. pyogenes*	+	+	+/−	2.1, 12.2, 14.1, 15.1	?
SPE-C	24.4	*S. pyogenes*	+	+	−/+	2.1, 3.2, 12.5, 15.1	0.1
SPE-G	24.6	*S. pyogenes*	−	+	−/+	2.1, 4.1, 6.9, 9.1, 12.3	2
SPE-H	23.6	*S. pyogenes*	+	+	−/+	2.1, 7.3, 9.1, 23.1	50
SPE-I	26.0	*S. pyogenes*	−	+	−/+	6.9, 9.1, 18.1, 22	0.1
SPE-J	24.6	*S. pyogenes*	+	+	−/+	2.1	0.1
SPE-K/L	27.4	*S. pyogenes*	−	+	−/+	1.1, 5.1, 23.1	1
SPE-L/M	26.2	*S. pyogenes*	−	+	−/+	1.1, 5.1, 23.1	10
SPE-M	25.3	*S. pyogenes*	−	+	?	1.1, 5.1, 23.1	?
SSA	26.9	*S. pyogenes*	−	−	+/−	1.1, 3, 15	?
SMEZ-1	24.3	*S. pyogenes*	−	+	−/+	2.1, 4.1, 7.3, 8.1	0.08
SMEZ-2	24.1	*S. pyogenes*	+	+	−/+	4.1, 8.1	0.02
SePE-H	23.6	*S. equi*	−	+	−/+	?	?
SePE-I	25.7	*S. equi*	−	+	−/+	?	?
SPE-L$_{Se}$	27.4	*S. equi*	−	+	−/+	?	?
SPE-M$_{Se}$	26.2	*S. equi*	−	+	−/+	?	?
SPE-G^{dys}	24.4	*S. dysgalactiae*	−	+	−/+	?	?
SDM	25.4	*S. dysgalactiae*	−	+	−/+	1.1, 23	?

[a]List of all currently known streptococcal SAgs. The major T-cell receptor Vβ targets are underlined.
[b]P_{50} (h), concentration needed for half-maximum proliferation of human T cells.

Broudy et al. (12) reported the up-regulation of SPE-C in GAS by cocultured human pharyngeal cells. This led to the induction of the $speC^+$ bacteriophage by a soluble factor produced by the pharyngeal cells. Coculture of strain MGAS315 with Detroit 562 (D562) human epithelial pharyngeal cells induced the prophage-encoding $speK/L$ (ϕ315.4). However, no significant production of SPE-K/L was observed (5). The production of SPE-A increased during coculture of GAS with D562 cells despite the lack of induction of the prophage-encoding $speA$ (ϕ315.5).

Control of the $speA$ gene has been studied using micropore Teflon diffusion chambers housing a clonal MT1 strain implanted subcutaneously in BALB/c mice. No SPE-A was detectable until 7 days when SPE-A was detected in the chamber fluid of all animals tested. Isolates recovered from the chamber and grown in vitro continued to produce SPE-A even after 21 passages, suggesting a stable switch of the $speA$ gene (39).

The recent completion of several GAS genome projects combined with DNA microarray-based transcription analysis provided a genome-wide perspective of those genes regulated by host factors. When serotype M1 strain was grown in human blood, $speG$, $speJ$, and $smeZ$ were up-regulated after 30 min (62-fold, 264-fold, and 52-fold, respectively), but expression was reduced after 60 min. $speA$ was up-regulated continuously, showing a 483-fold increase after 30 min and a remarkable 2,139-fold increase of mRNA after 90 min (26). Serotype M1 strain was also examined during an 86-day infection protocol in 20 cynomolgus macaques. This revealed differences in sag expression in distinct disease phases (93). Expression of $speA$, $speJ$, and $smeZ$ increased during the colonization phase, but $speJ$ expression started at early infection stage and correlated with low GAS cell densities, while $speA$ and $smeZ$ genes responded at a later stage at higher cell densities. $smeZ$ expression correlated with peak levels of C-reactive protein, a sensitive indicator of inflammation. Furthermore, $smeZ$ was the most dominant acute-phase-correlated proinflammatory gene, but expression did not correlate with peak increases of pharyngitis or tonsillitis.

The molecular mechanisms of sag gene regulation are not well understood, but a recent study suggests that they are under the control of the Nra transcription regulator, a member of the RofA-like protein (RALP) family (65). Nra represses the expression of several virulence genes, including $speA$. Maximum expression of Nra occurs in the early-stationary-growth phase.

SUPERANTIGENS FROM OTHER STREPTOCOCCI

An increasing number of reports have implicated group C streptococcus (GCS) and group G streptococcus (GGS) with severe invasive infections, such as necrotizing fasciitis and toxic shock syndrome (63). The first report of a superantigen from GCS came from Timoney's group, who identified two superantigens from *Streptococcus equi*, which causes strangles in horses but can also infect humans. The *S. equi* pyrogenic exotoxins (SePE-H and -I) are highly homologous to their *S. pyogenes* counterparts SPE-H and SPE-I (>98% amino acid sequence identities), indicating horizontal gene transfer from *S. pyogenes* to *S. equi* or vice versa (3). Neither gene was found in the closely related *Streptococcus zooepidemicus*. The acquisition of the sag genes might be an important event in the formation of a more virulent *S. equi* strain from its putative *S. zooepidemicus* ancestor (3). SePE-I and SePE-H both elicited strong mitogenic responses from horse peripheral blood mononuclear cells (PBMCs) and both were pyrogenic in rabbits, but only SePE-I was pyrogenic in ponies. Horses recovered from strangles or immunized with SePE-I were seropositive and resistant to the pyrogenic effects of SePE-I, suggesting a potential role for this toxin in strangles.

Another two *sag* genes were identified from the *S. equi* genome at the Sanger Centre and named *speL_Se* and *speM_Se* because of the homology to their *S. pyogenes* counterparts *speL* and *speM* (here described as *speK/L* and *speL/M*) with 99% and 98.1% nucleotide identities, respectively (70). Both genes were not detected in eight genetically different *S. equi* isolates, suggesting that they are also rare in GCS isolates.

Four SAgs have been identified from *Streptococcus dysgalactiae* subsp. *equisimilis*. All are highly similar to their GAS counterparts SPE-A, SPE-C, SPE-G, and SPE-M. *S. dysgalactiae*-derived mitogen (SDM) is 99% similar to SPE-M (55), and SPE-G^dys is 86% similar to SPE-G (36, 74). Oster and Bisno (63) analyzed 34 genetically distinct group C/G streptococci and found the *speA* gene in three isolates and *speC* in one isolate. The *speA* alleles from two isolates were identical to GAS alleles, *speA*2 and *speA*4, respectively, while the third *speA* allele is characterized by two unique nucleotide substitutions that are not observed among *speA* alleles from GAS. This was designated *speA*7. However, the translated protein is 100% identical with the SPE-A5 variant of GAS. The *speC* allele was found to be identical to *speC*1 of GAS.

In all non-GAS toxins, amino acid exchanges are outside the MHC class II and TcR-binding sites suggesting that the GAS toxins and the non-GAS toxins are orthologues with identical functions.

BIOCHEMICAL PROPERTIES OF THE STREPTOCOCCAL SUPERANTIGENS

To ensure they concentrate onto the surface of antigen-presenting cells at the immunological synapse, superantigens have developed several ways of binding MHC class II. These can be divided into three distinct modes: MHC class II β-chain binding, MHC class II α-chain binding, or dual β-chain and α-chain binding. All streptococcal SAgs except SPE-A and SSA, bind to the MHC class II β-chain using a coordinated zinc atom at the center of the interface (32). SPE-C binding to MHC class II is completely abolished by EDTA and restored by excess of Zn^{2+} (47). Three residues in the C-terminal domain of SPE-C— His167, His201, and Asp203—are analogous to the zinc-binding residues of SEA (73). The cocrystallization of SPE-C with HLA-DR2 bearing a peptide derived from myelin basic protein (MBP) confirmed the zinc complex, but also revealed extensive interaction of the superantigen with bound peptide accounting for approximately one-third of the surface area of the MHC class II molecule buried in the complex (48, 64). SPE-C also makes several interactions with backbone atoms of the peptide. However, other interactions involve unique interactions with peptide side chains, suggesting that there must be a wide range of affinities for MHC class II that are governed by particular peptides in the groove. This finding suggested that affinity and thus sensitivity and pathogenicity are in part governed by bound peptide as well as toxin level, MHC haplotype, or seroconversion.

From primary amino acid sequence, SPE-G, SPE-H, SPE-I, SPE-J, SPE-K/L, SPE-L/M, SPE-M, and SMEZ were all predicted to possess a zinc-binding site in the C-terminal domain similar to SPE-C. Binding of recombinant toxins to MHC class II bearing cells was completely abolished by EDTA and restored by excess Zn^{2+} for all these SAgs (66, 68).

These SAgs lack the generic MHC class II α-chain-binding motif (a hydrophobic loop region in the N-terminal domain) and thus did not compete with SEB and TSST for MHC class II binding (66, 68, 69). These SAgs were only marginally competitive for MHC class II binding among each other and followed a hierarchy ((SPE-C, SMEZ-1) > SMEZ-2 > SPE-H > SPE-G). SPE-G did not compete with any other toxin suggesting that the first (SPE-C and SMEZ) had broad binding specificity less affected by peptide, while SPE-G had a very restricted specificity for only a small number of MHC class II molecules.

DIMER FORMATION OF STREPTOCOCCAL SUPERANTIGENS

SPE-C was found to exist in both monomeric and dimeric forms at neutral or alkaline pH (47). The SPE-C crystal structure was also a dimer formed through the outer face of the OB-fold that in many other superantigens is the α-chain-binding site (73). The biological function of SPE-C dimer formation is unknown, but it has been suggested that it might lead to cross-linking of MHC class II molecules on the surface of antigen-presenting cells and that this may have a stimulatory effect on the antigen-presenting cells (73). Such an effect has been demonstrated previously for SEA (91). MHC class II cross-linking by SEA (staphylococcal SAg that binds to both MHC class II chains) resulted in rapid induction of homotypic B-cell aggregation, tyrosine kinase activation, and proinflammatory cytokine gene expression. Homotypic B-cell aggregation has also been demonstrated for SPE-C (47) and SPE-J (66).

The crystal structure of SPE-J revealed a different mode of homodimerization through the proposed TcR-binding face (4) implying two possible functions—normal MHC class II and TcR binding or in dimer mode, cross-linking of two MHC class II molecules.

Monomeric and dimeric forms of SSA were found in supernatants of GAS cultures (16). Dimer formation occurred via an intermolecular cysteine bridge involving Cys26 and probably prevents TcR interaction. The role of these dimer forms in functions other than T-cell mitogenicity remains to be clarified.

CELL RECEPTOR BINDING OF STREPTOCOCCAL SUPERANTIGENS

Human T-cell receptor Vβ repertoire responses to individual superantigens have been determined by quantitative analysis of Vβ cDNA in stimulated cultures of PBL (Table 1).

Two cocrystal structures of streptococcal superantigens bound to soluble TcR reveal how SPE-A interacts with murineVβ8.2 and SPE-C interacts with human Vβ2.1 complexes (89). The TcR-binding site is a shallow groove between the two globular domains of the SPE-A molecule created by residues from the α2-helix, the β2-β3-loop, the β4-strand, the β4-β5-loop, the β5-strand, and the α5-helix. In the murine TcR Vβ8.2 molecule, residues from the complementarity-determining region 2 (CDR2), framework region 2 (FR2), and, to a lesser extent, the hypervariable region 4 (HV4) and FR3 bind SPE-A. Comparison between the SPE-C/mVβ8.2 and SPE-C/hVβ2 structures reveals several hydrogen bonds between side-chain atoms of SPE-A and mVβ8.2 that are absent in the hVβ2 complex. Instead SPE-C residues primarily contact main-chain atoms in the hVβ2 complex (46).

The interaction between SPE-C and hVβ2.1 differs from other SAg/TcR complexes by including a substantially larger buried-surface area. The intermolecular contacts are more numerous than in SPE-A/mVβ8.2 and include the highly variable CDR3 loop, which is not coded for by the β-chain but is instead hypervariable. SPE-C is very specific for hVβ2 and it has been proposed that this specificity derives from two single amino acid insertions, one each in CDR1 and CDR2, and an extended CDR3 loop. The CDR1 insertion shifts this loop toward the SPE-C molecule, resulting in additional intermolecular contacts involving hydrogen bonds with SPE-C residues Arg45, Tyr49, and Asn79, while the CDR2 insertion produces a noncanonical CDR2 loop that positions the inserted residue for optimal contact with SPE-C. The CDR2 contact region includes hydrogen bonds with SPE-C residues Tyr15, Glu178, and Arg181. Mutational analysis confirmed the crucial role of Tyr15 in SPE-C. A single Y15A mutant was 10,000-fold less active than wild-type SPE-C (99).

The crystal structure of SPE-J reveals it is most closely related to SPE-C, consistent with its also targeting hVβ 2.1 (4). Mutation of SPE-J at Tyr14 and Arg181 (corresponding to SPE-C residues Tyr15 and Arg181) reduced activity of SPE-J by 10,000-fold.

Based on structural observations, three categories of SAg-TcR complexes have been proposed: (i) highly promiscuous, including SEB and SEC3, that bind many TcR β-chains in a simple conformation-dependent manner and interact only with CDR2; (ii) moderately promiscuous such as SPE-A, that form direct side-chain/side-chain contacts that additionally involve the CDR1 loop as well as the CDR2 loop; and (iii) highly selective T-cell activators, such as SPE-C (and probably SPE-J), that bind limited numbers of TcRVβ by contacting all three CDR loops, including CDR3 which, unlike CDR1 and CDR2, is subject to somatic hypervariability (i.e., not hard encoded in the Vβ germ line) (90).

PYROGENICITY OF SUPERANTIGENS AND SYNERGY WITH ENDOTOXINS

Rabbits injected with either SPE-A or SPE-C purified from cultures of *S. pyogenes* develop elevated temperature for periods of 4 to 5 h (78). The minimal pyrogenic dose of SPE-A and SPE-C ranged between 0.1 and 0.7 μg/kg. Pyrogenicity in rabbits has also been reported for recombinant SPE-J and SMEZ (51, 58). The mechanism for superantigen-induced pyrogenicity in rabbits has been attributed to the release of the proinflammatory cytokines interleukin-1 (IL-1) and tumor necrosis factor alpha (TNF-α) by T cells and macrophages and their subsequent effects on the hypothalamus (19), but the true mechanism remains to be established. These studies are plagued by possible endotoxin contamination that arises from the gram-negative host that the recombinant protein is produced in, or other contaminants that might be ligands for the Toll-like receptors such as CpG DNA. More importantly, streptococcal superantigens when combined with small doses of endotoxin such as lipopolysaccharide (LPS) are lethal in rabbits. In one early study, rabbits receiving SPE-C alone had only mild fever, but those given a combination of SPE-C and LPS also developed fever but rapidly became hypothermic, exhibited respiratory distress, diarrhea, vascular collapse, and finally death (77). Death occurred within 9 h. Lethality of the endotoxin was enhanced by as much as 50,000-fold. It has long been postulated that toxic shock syndrome is actually a combination of both gram-positive superantigen and gram-negative endotoxin producing a "double-hit" through simultaneously triggering the adaptive immune system via the TcR and the innate immune system via the Toll-like receptors responsible for recognition of microbial molecular patterns or PAMPs. This could occur in the absence of any obvious bacterial infection if the production of both superantigen and endotoxin were sufficient (49).

CYTOKINE INDUCTION

Streptococcal superantigens are potent inducers of cytokines and the T cell is the main source. Toxin-mediated activation of T cells results in a rapid systemic release of TNF-α and TNF-β, followed sequentially by IL-2, IL-6, IL-1, and gamma interferon (IFN-γ) (9, 28, 35, 54). In particular, TNF-α increases dramatically within the first few hours of SAg stimulation (54). TNF-α induces the production of IL-1 and IL-6 and acts synergistically with IL-1 to cause fever and shock. Besides these proinflammatory cytokines, the release of anti-inflammatory cytokines, such as IL-4, IL-5, and IL-10, and the production of hematopoietic cytokines, such as IL-3 and granulocyte macrophage colony-stimulating factor (GM-CSF) after stimulation with SPE-A or SPE-C, have also been reported (57, 72). A comparative study with SPE-A and SMEZ revealed that both produce substantial amounts of pro- and anti-inflammatory, chemotactic, and hematopoietic cytokines, but SMEZ was approximately 10-fold better than SPE-A (58). The importance of SMEZ as a major contributor of cytokine production by streptococcal isolates was revealed by a study that selectively disrupted the *smeZ* gene in an M89 GAS strain. This abrogated the immunoactive properties of the strain completely even though it produced several other superantigens. Culture supernatant from the *smeZ* mutant was unable to stimulate any IFN-γ, TNF-α, TNF-β, IL-1β, or IL-8 from PBMCs, thus confirming that SMEZ was the major immunoactive superantigen produced by GAS (92).

INVASIVE GAS DISEASE AND STREPTOCOCCAL TOXIC SHOCK SYNDROME

Invasive GAS causes cellulitis, myositis, and necrotizing fasciitis (or flesh-eating disease) (reviewed in references 52 and 87). The most severe form of invasive GAS disease is STSS, with mortality rates ranging from 30 to 70%. The clinical symptoms of STSS are very similar to those of staphylococcal toxic shock, but STSS is often associated with bacteremia, myositis, or necrotizing fasciitis (87) and can occur in patients with no outward signs of bacterial infection. STSS is characterized by a rash, hypotension, respiratory distress, and finally multiple organ failure.

Epidemiological Studies

Yu and Ferretti (102) found that 65 of 146 isolates (45%) from scarlet fever patients were *speA*$^+$, compared with 15% of isolates from patients with unrelated conditions. For STSS, 29 of 34 (85%) of GAS isolates from STSS patients were *speA*$^+$ (29). A similar study conducted by Reichardt et al. (71) found *speA* and *speC* in 64% and 28% of STSS-related strains isolated in Europe and Chile. STSS is most commonly associated with serotypes M1 and M3 and both strains frequently produce the superantigens SPE-A and SPE-C. The *speA* gene has been found in 40 to 90% of GAS isolates from the United States associated with invasive GAS disease and STSS but in only 15 to 20% of noninvasive disease isolates, such as pharyngitis (102). An 80% frequency of *speA*$^+$ isolates was observed in STSS cases collected in Australia (13). A more recent study by Hsueh et al. (31) showed no significant difference in *speA*$^+$ frequency between invasive and noninvasive GAS isolates collected in Taiwan (39% for invasive and 36% for noninvasive). The focus on *speA* without knowledge of other more potent streptococcal superantigens such as SMEZ and SPE-J tends to reduce the significance of these earlier studies by adding the potential for two or more SAgs to contribute to toxicity.

Effects of Streptococcal Superantigens on Primates

Stevens et al. (85) showed that intravenous infusion of an SPE-A-producing serotype M3 strain into baboons resulted in profound hypotension, leukopenia, metabolic acidosis, renal impairment, thrombocytopenia, and disseminated coagulopathy within 3 h. Serum TNF-α peaked at 3 h and anti-TNF-α antibodies markedly improved arterial pressure and survival, indicating the important role for TNF-α in STSS.

Experiments with isogenic GAS strains lacking the *speA* gene administered into rabbits showed that only the wild-type strain caused STSS, while the *speA* mutant knockout strain did not (75). An isogenic *speA* mutant strain was used to evaluate the role of SPE-A in a murine model of bacteremia and streptococcal muscle infection (82). Surprisingly, disruption of *speA* was not associated with attenuation of virulence and paradoxically the *speA* mutant led to increased bacteremia and a reduction of neutrophils at the site of primary muscle infection. A possible explanation for this outcome is that SAgs are significantly less active in mice (68), probably because of inefficient binding to murine MHC class II. Indeed, different results were obtained in studies with HLA-DQ transgenic mice (84, 96). Expression of HLA-DQ rendered the mice susceptible to SPE-A-induced lethal shock that was accompanied by massive cytokine production. Immune activation during GAS infection was manifested by Vβ-specific T-cell repertoire changes and widespread lymphoblastic tissue infiltration. In contrast, lymphoid activation was undetectable in transgenic mice infected with an isogenic *speA* mutant strain demonstrating the pivotal role of a single SAg in pathogenesis of invasive GAS disease (84).

In vivo experiments using an i.p. model of infection demonstrated that SMEZ did not contribute to mortality or impede bacterial clearance in HLA-DQ transgenic mice, but led to a rise of Vβ11 T cells in the spleen (92). Infection with an isogenic M89 *smez* mutant strain failed to elicit significant cytokine production compared with the parent strain, but resulted in a clear rise in murine Vβ4 T cells, suggesting a role for SMEZ as a repressor of cognate antistreptococcal response.

Clinical Studies Revealing the Consequence of Superantigen Intoxication

Few studies have attempted to observe the course of a seriously ill STSS patient relative to the expression of one or more SAgs. SPE-A has been detected by ELISA in the sera of STSS patients and its presence was associated with elevated levels of TNF-β providing some evidence of SPE-A-induced T-cell activation (83). In a more recent study, mitogenic activity due to circulating SAg was readily detected in the serum of two patients with STSS, one of whom died. Although the infecting GAS strains carried *speA*, *speC*, *speG*, *speJ*, and *smeZ* genes, the mitogenic activity was wholly attributed to SMEZ, with a small contribution of SPE-J (69). During the acute phase, the quantity of circulating unbound SMEZ in the serum of the patient that died was calculated to be 100 pg/ml. The surviving patient rapidly developed neutralizing antibodies against SMEZ during convalescence. This study provided direct evidence for the significance of SMEZ in STSS. Considering that the majority of SMEZ would be bound to and concentrated in lymphoid organs such as the spleen, this study was the first to show the very high levels of SMEZ that must be produced from the infection causing the shock. The lack of neutralizing antibodies against SMEZ was most likely to be the most significant risk factor for these patients. In a recent case study, a novel *smeZ* allele (*smeZ-34*) was identified in an *emm118* strain isolated from a patient with STSS. SMEZ-34 is closely related to the extremely potent SMEZ-2 variant. When grown in vitro, the *emm118* isolate produced SMEZ as the major mitogenic toxin. The patient's acute serum lacked protective antibodies against SMEZ-2, but seroconverted during convalescence (100). Eriksson et al. (18) reported that anti-SPE-A neutralization was totally absent in sera from patients with STSS and low in sera from patients with uncomplicated bacteremia compared with levels in sera from uncomplicated erysipelas. Another study showed that the levels of neutralizing anti-SPE-A antibodies in plasma samples from severe and nonsevere invasive GAS infections were significantly lower than in age- and geographically matched healthy controls (6).

Influence of the Host Genetic Background

HLA polymorphism may influence susceptibility to GAS-invasive infection. Kotb and coworkers found that SPE-A triggered significantly higher proliferative responses when presented by HLA-DQ than HLA-DR1, -DR4, or -DR5 alleles, whereas SPE-C was preferentially presented by HLA-DR4 (62). Patients with the DRB1*1501/DQB1*0602 haplotype mounted reduced responses to streptococcal SAgs and were found to be less likely to develop severe systemic disease than individuals with risk or neutral haplotypes (43). The dependence of SPE-A on HLA-DQ α-chain polymorphism was demonstrated (50). SPE-A bound better to HLA-DQA1*01 than to HLA-DQA1*03/05, which resulted in quantitative and qualitative differences in T-cell proliferation, cytokine production, and Vβ-specific changes in the T-cell repertoire.

ACUTE RHEUMATIC FEVER (ARF)

ARF is a postinfection sequela and remains a leading cause of preventable pediatric heart disease. It usually occurs in school-age children and young adults following a pharyngeal infection with *S. pyogenes*. ARF is believed to result from the development of a cross-reactive antibody response between streptococcal antigens and the host's cardiac tissue and it has been proposed that the process might be driven by SAgs. Recently, several novel streptococcal SAgs have been identified from ARF-associated serotypes. The genes for SPE-K/L were found in high frequencies on serotypes M3 (United States and Japan) (7, 33) and on M89 (New Zealand) (70), while SPE-L/M and SPE-M were found in M18 (United States) (80). It was shown that antibodies against SPE-L/M and SPE-M were more common in convalescent sera from ARF patients than in patients with pharyngitis (81). A common target of the SAgs SPE-K/L, SPE-L/M, and SPE-M are T cells bearing the TcRs with Vβ1.1.

KAWASAKI DISEASE (KD)

KD is an acute multisystem vasculitis of unknown etiology that affects mostly young children and is now recognized as the leading cause of acquired heart disease in children in the developed world. Although KD has been reported in most countries, it is overrepresented among Asian populations, especially Japanese (14).

KD is associated with marked activation of T cells and monocytes and there is a remarkable similarity among KD, staphylococcal toxic shock, STSS, and scarlet fever in the clinical symptoms. Intravenous immunoglobulin therapy is an effective treatment if given early, suggesting that the causative agent is a toxin. Several investigators have reported the selective expansion of T cells bearing the Vβ2.1 TcR, which points toward a SAg involvement in the disease (2, 42). Elevated plasma levels of IL-1β, IL-2, IL-6, IL-8, IL-10, IFN-γ, and TNF-α were observed in the acute phase of KD and levels of anti-SPE-C antibodies were significantly higher in patients with acute and convalescent KD than in age-matched controls (101).

CONCLUSION

The streptococcal superantigens are a family of secreted toxins similar to their staphylococcal cousins, but with some unique features, in particular with regard to expression and potency. It is clear that the superantigen genes originated in staphylococci, and the fact that most are encoded in mobile phage suggests that they confer a significant advantage to the organism. Despite all we know about their structure and mechanism of action as well as their associations or even direct involvement in acute bacterial disease, we understand very little about how they enhance survival of the organism. Their ability to cause acute toxicity is very likely a secondary effect of toxin overproduction; the real role of superantigens is to modify the local site of infection by altering the capacity of T cells to drive an effective inflammatory response.

REFERENCES

1. **Abe, J., J. Forrester, T. Nakahara, J. Lafferty, B. Kotzin, and D. Leung.** 1991. Selective stimulation of human T cells with streptococcal erythrogenic toxins A and B. *J. Immunol.* **146**:3747–3750.
2. **Abe, J., B. L. Kotzin, K. Jujo, M. E. Melish, M. P. Glode, et al.** 1992. Selective expansion of T cells expressing T-cell receptor variable regions V beta 2 and V beta 8 in Kawasaki disease. *Proc. Natl. Acad. Sci. USA* **89**:4066–4070.
3. **Artiushin, S. C., J. F. Timoney, A. S. Sheoran, and S. K. Muthupalani.** 2002. Characterization and immunogenicity of pyrogenic mitogens SePE-H and SePE-I of *Streptococcus equi*. *Microb. Pathog.* **32**:71–85.
4. **Baker, H., T. Proft, P. Webb, V. Arcus, J. Fraser, and E. Baker.** 2004. Crystallographic and mutational data show that the streptococcal pyrogenic exotoxin J can use a common binding surface for T cell receptor binding and dimerization. *J. Biol. Chem.* **279**:38571–38576.
5. **Banks, D., B. Lei, and J. Musser.** 2003. Prophage induction and expression of prophage-encoded virulence factors in group A Streptococcus serotype M3 strain MGAS315. *Infect. Immun.* **71**:7079–7086.
6. **Basma, H., A. Norrby-Teglund, Y. Guedez, A. McGeer, D. E. Low, et al.** 1999. Risk factors in the pathogenesis of invasive group A streptococcal infections: role of protective humoral immunity. *Infect. Immun.* **67**:1871–1877.
7. **Beres, S. B., G. L. Sylva, K. D. Barbian, B. Lei, J. S. Hoff, et al.** 2002. Genome sequence of a serotype M3 strain of group A *Streptococcus*: phage-encoded toxins, the high-virulence phenotype, and clone emergence. *Proc. Natl. Acad. Sci. USA* **99**:10078–10083.
8. **Bessen, D. E., M. W. Izzo, T. R. Fiorentino, R. M. Caringal, S. K. Hollingshead, and B. Beall.** 1999. Genetic linkage of exotoxin alleles and emm gene markers for tissue tropism in group A streptococci. *J. Infect. Dis.* **179**:627–636.
9. **Bette, M., M. K. Schafer, N. van Rooijen, E. Weihe, and B. Fleischer.** 1993. Distribution and kinetics of superantigen-induced cytokine gene expression in mouse spleen. *J. Exp. Med.* **178**:1531–1539.
10. **Bohach, G., A. Hauser, and P. Schlievert.** 1988. Cloning of the gene, *speB*, for streptococcal pyrogenic exotoxin type B in *Escherichia coli*. *Infect. Immun.* **56**:1665–1667.

11. **Braun, M. A., D. Gerlach, U. F. Hartwig, J. H. Ozegowski, F. Romagne, et al.** 1993. Stimulation of human T cells by streptococcal "superantigen" erythrogenic toxins (scarlet fever toxins). *J. Immunol.* **150**:2457–2466.

12. **Broudy, T. B., V. Pancholi, and V. A. Fischetti.** 2001. Induction of lysogenic bacteriophage and phage-associated toxin from group A streptococci during coculture with human pharyngeal cells. *Infect. Immun.* **69**:1440–1443.

13. **Carapetis, J., R. Robins-Browne, D. Martin, T. Shelby-James, and G. Hogg.** 1995. Increasing severity of invasive group A streptococcal disease in Australia: clinical and molecular epidemiological features and identification of a new virulent M-nontypeable clone. *Clin. Infect. Dis.* **21**:1220–1227.

14. **Cimaz, R., and F. Falcini.** 2003. An update on Kawasaki disease. *Autoimmun. Rev.* **2**:258–263.

15. **Cunningham, M.** 2000. Pathogenesis of group A Streptococcal Infections. *Clin. Microbiol. Rev.* **13**:470–511.

16. **De Marzi, M. C., M. M. Fernandez, E. J. Sundberg, L. Molinero, N. W. Zwirner, et al.** 2004. Cloning, expression and interaction of human T-cell receptors with the bacterial superantigen SSA. *Eur. J. Biochem.* **271**:4075–4083.

17. **Dick, G., and G. Dick.** 1983. Landmark article Jan 26, 1924: the etiology of scarlet fever. By George F. Dick and Gladys Henry Dick. *JAMA* **250**:3096.

18. **Eriksson, B. K. G., J. Andersson, S. E. Holm, and M. Norgren.** 1999. Invasive Group A Streptococcal infections: T1M1 isolates expressing pyrogenic exotoxins A and B in combination with selective lack of toxin-neutralizing antibodies are associated with increased risk of streptococcal toxic shock syndrome. *J. Infect. Dis.* **180**:410–418.

19. **Fast, D. J., P. M. Schlievert, and R. D. Nelson.** 1989. Toxic shock syndrome-associated staphylococcal and streptococcal pyrogenic toxins are potent inducers of tumor necrosis factor production. *Infect. Immun.* **57**:291–294.

20. **Ferretti, J. J., D. Ajdic, and W. M. McShan.** 2004. Comparative genomics of streptococcal species. *Indian J. Med. Res.* **119**(Suppl):1–6.

21. **Ferretti, J. J., W. M. Mcshan, D. Ajdic, D. J. Savic, G. Savic, et al.** 2001. Complete genome sequence of an M1 strain of *Streptococcus pyogenes*. *Proc. Natl. Acad. Sci. USA* **98**:4658–4663.

22. **Gerlach, D., B. Fleischer, M. Wagner, K. Schmidt, S. Vettermann, and W. Reichardt.** 2000. Purification and biochemical characterization of a basic superantigen (SPEX/SMEZ3) from *Streptococcus pyogenes*. *FEMS Microbiol. Lett.* **188**:153–163.

23. **Gerlach, D., H. Knoll, W. Köhler, J. Ozegowski, and V. Hribalova.** 1983. Isolation and characterization of erythrogenic toxins. V. Communication: identity of erythrogenic toxin type B and streptococcal proteinase precursor. *Zentralbl. Bakteriol. Mikrobiol. Hyg. [A]* **255**:221–233.

24. **Gerlach, D., H. Knoll, W. Kohler, and J. H. Ozegowski.** 1981. Isolation and characterization of erythrogenic toxins of Streptococcus pyogenes. 3. Communication: comparative studies of type A erythrogenic toxins. *Zentralbl. Bakteriol. Mikrobiol. Hyg. [A]* **250**:277–286. (In German.)

25. **Gerlach, D., W. Reichardt, B. Fleischer, and K. Schmidt.** 1994. Separation of mitogenic and pyrogenic activities from so-called erythrogenic toxin type B (Streptococcal proteinase). *Zentralbl. Bakteriol.* **280**:507–514.

26. **Graham, M., K. Virtaneva, S. Porcella, W. Barry, B. Gowen, et al.** 2005. Group A Streptococcus transcriptome dynamics during growth in human blood reveals bacterial adaptive and survival strategies. *Am. J. Pathol.* **166**:455–465.

27. **Green, N. M., S. Zhang, S. F. Porcella, M. J. Nagiec, K. D. Barbian, et al.** 2005. Genome sequence of a serotype M28 strain of group A streptococcus: potential new insights into puerperal sepsis and bacterial disease specificity. *J. Infect. Dis.* **192**:760–770.

28. **Hackett, S. P., and D. L. Stevens.** 1992. Streptococcal toxic shock syndrome: synthesis of tumor necrosis factor and interleukin-1 by monocytes stimulated with pyrogenic exotoxin-A and streptolysin-O. *J. Infect. Dis.* **165**:879–885.

29. **Hauser, A., D. Stevens, E. Kaplan, and P. Schlievert.** 1991. Molecular analysis of pyrogenic exotoxins from *Streptococcus pyogenes* isolates associated with toxic shock-like syndrome. *J. Clin. Microbiol.* **29**:1562–1567.

30. **Hooker, S., and E. Follensby.** 1934. Studies on scarlet fever. II. Different toxins produced by hemolytic streptococci of scarlatinal origin. *J. Immunol.* **27**:177–193.

31. **Hsueh, P., J. Wu, P. Tsai, J. Liu, Y. Chuang, and K. Luh.** 1998. Invasive group A streptococcal disease in Taiwan is not associated with the presence of streptococcal pyrogenic exotoxin genes. *Clin. Infect. Dis.* **26**:584–589.

32. **Hudson, K. R., R. E. Tiedemann, R. G. Urban, S. C. Lowe, J. L. Strominger, and J. D. Fraser.** 1995. Staphylococcal enterotoxin A has two cooperative binding sites on major histocompatibility complex class II. *J. Exp. Med.* **182:**711–720.

33. **Ikebe, T., A. Wada, Y. Inagaki, K. Sugama, R. Suzuki, et al.** 2002. Dissemination of the phage-associated novel superantigen gene speL in recent invasive and noninvasive *Streptococcus pyogenes* M3/T3 isolates in Japan. *Infect. Immun.* **70:**3227–3233.

34. **Imanishi, K., H. Igarashi, and T. Uchiyama.** 1990. Activation of murine T cells by streptococcal pyrogenic exotoxin type A. Requirement for MHC class II molecules on accessory cells and identification of V beta elements in T cell receptor of toxin-reactive T cells. *J. Immunol.* **145:**3170–3176.

35. **Jupin, C., S. Anderson, C. Damais, J. E. Alouf, and M. Parant.** 1988. Toxic shock syndrome toxin as an inducer of human tumor necrosis factors and γ-interferon. *J. Exp. Med.* **167:**752–761.

36. **Kalia, A., M. C. Enright, B. G. Spratt, and D. E. Bessen.** 2001. Directional gene movement from human-pathogenic to commensal-like streptococci. *Infect. Immun.* **69:**4858–4869.

37. **Kamezawa, Y., T. Nakahara, S. Nakano, Y. Abe, J. Nozaki-Renard, and T. Isono.** 1997. Streptococcal mitogenic exotoxin Z, a novel acidic superantigenic toxin produced by a T1 strain of Streptococcus pyogenes. *Infect. Immun.* **65:**3828–3833.

38. **Kapur, V., K. Nelson, P. M. Schlievert, R. K. Selander, and J. M. Musser.** 1992. Molecular population genetic evidence of horizontal spread of two alleles of the pyrogenic exotoxin C gene (speC) among pathogenic clones of Streptococcus pyogenes. *Infect. Immun.* **60:**3513–3517.

39. **Kazmi, S. U., R. Kansal, R. K. Aziz, M. Hooshdaran, A. Norrby-Teglund, et al.** 2001. Reciprocal, temporal expression of SpeA and SpeB by invasive M1T1 group a streptococcal isolates *in vivo. Infect. Immun.* **69:**4988–4995.

40. **Kim, M. H., and P. M. Schlievert.** 1997. Molecular genetics, structure, and immunobiology of streptococcal pyrogenic exotoxin A and C, p. 257–279. *In* D. Y. M. Leung, B. T. Huber, and P. M. Schlievert (ed.), *Superantigens. Molecular Biology, Immunobiology and Relevance to Human Disease.* Marcel Dekker, New York, N.Y.

41. **Kim, Y., and D. Watson.** 1970. A purified group A streptococcal pyrogenic exotoxin. Physiochemical and biological properties, including the enhancement of susceptibility to endotoxin lethal shock. *J. Exp. Med.* **131:**611–622.

42. **Konishi, N., K. Baba, J. Abe, T. Maruko, K. Waki, et al.** 1996. A case of Kawasaki disease with coronary artery aneurysms documenting *Yersinia pseudotuberculosis* infection. *Acta Paediatr.* **86:**661–664.

43. **Kotb, M., A. Norrby-Teglund, A. McGeer, H. El-Sherbini, M. Dorak, et al.** 2002. An immunogenetic and molecular basis for differences in outcomes of invasive group A streptococcal infections. *Nature Med.* **8:**1398–1404.

44. **Lee, P. K., and P. M. Schlievert.** 1989. Quantification and toxicity of group A streptococcal pyrogenic exotoxins in an animal model of toxic shock syndrome-like illness. *J. Clin. Microbiol.* **27:**1890–1892.

45. **Leonard, B., P. Lee, M. Jenkins, and P. M. Schlievert.** 1991. Cell and receptor requirements for streptococcal pyrogenic exotoxin T cell mitogenicity. *Infect. Immun.* **59:**1210–1214.

46. **Li, H., A. Llera, D. Tsuchiya, L. Leder, X. Ysern, et al.** 1998. Three-dimensional structure of the complex between a T cell receptor beta chain and the superantigen staphylococcal enterotoxin B. *Immunity* **9:**807–816.

47. **Li, P. L., R. E. Tiedemann, S. L. Moffat, and J. D. Fraser.** 1997. The superantigen streptococcal pyrogenic exotoxin C (SPE-C) exhibits a novel mode of action. *J. Exp. Med.* **186:**375–383.

48. **Li, Y., H. Li, N. Dimasi, J. K. McCormick, R. Martin, et al.** 2001. Crystal structure of a superantigen bound to the high-affinity, zinc-dependent site on MHC Class II. *Immunity* **14:**93–104.

49. **Llewelyn, M., and J. Cohen.** 2002. Superantigens: microbial agents that corrupt immunity. *Lancet Infect. Dis.* **2:**156–162.

50. **Llewelyn, M., S. Sriskandan, M. Peakman, D. Ambrozak, D. Douek, et al.** 2004. HLA class II polymorphisms determine responses to bacterial superantigens. *J. Immunol.* **172:**1719–1726.

51. **McCormick, J., A. Pragman, J. Stolpa, D. Leung, and P Schlievert.** 2001. Functional characterization of streptococcal pyrogenic exotoxin J, a novel superantigen. *Infect. Immun.* **69:**1381–1388.

52. **McCormick, J. K., J. M. Yarwood, and P. M. Schlievert.** 2001. Toxic shock syndrome and bacterial superantigens: an update. *Annu. Rev. Microbiol.* **55:**77–104.

53. **McDonald, M., B. Currie, and J. Carapetis.** 2004. Acute rheumatic fever: a chink in the chain that links the heart to the throat? *Lancet Infect. Dis.* **4:**240–245.

54. **Miethke, T., C. Wahl, K. Heeg, B. Echtenacher, P. H. Krammer, and H. Wagner.** 1992. T cell-mediated lethal shock triggered in mice by the superantigen staphylococcal enterotoxin B: critical role of tumor necrosis factor. *J. Exp. Med.* **175:**91–98.

55. **Miyoshi-Akiyama, T., J. Zhao, H. Kato, K. Kikuchi, K. Totsuka, Y. Kataoka, M. Katsumi, and T. Uchiyama.** 2003. Streptococcus dysgalactiae-derived mitogen (SDM), a novel bacterial superantigen: characterization of its biological activity and predicted tertiary structure. *Mol. Microbiol.* **47:**1589–1599.

56. **Mollick, J. A., G. G. Miller, J. M. Musser, R. G. Cook, D. Grossman, and R. R. Rich.** 1993. A novel superantigen isolated from pathogenic strains of *Streptococcus pyogenes* with aminoterminal homology to staphylococcal enterotoxins B and C. *J. Clin. Invest.* **92:**710–719.

57. **Mueller-Alouf, H., J. E. Alouf, D. Gerlach, J. H. Ozegowski, C. Fitting, and J. M. Cavaillon.** 1996. Human pro- and anti-inflammatory cytokine patterns induced by *Streptococcus pyogenes* erythrogenic (pyrogenic) exotoxins A and C superantigens. *Infect. Immun.* **64:**1450–1453.

58. **Muller-Alouf, H., T. Proft, T. M. Zollner, D. Gerlach, E. Champagne, et al.** 2001. Pyrogenicity and cytokine-inducing properties of Streptococcus pyogenes superantigens: comparative study of streptococcal mitogenic exotoxin Z and pyrogenic exotoxin A. *Infect. Immun.* **69:**4141–4145.

59. **Nakagawa, I., K. Kurokawa, A. Yamashita, M. Nakata, Y. Tomiyasu, et al.** 2003. Genome sequence of an M3 strain of Streptococcus pyogenes reveals a large-scale genomic rearrangement in invasive strains and new insights into phage evolution. *Genome Res.* **13:**1042–1055.

60. **Nauts, H. C., and J. R. McLaren.** 1990. Coley toxins—the first century. *Adv. Exp. Med. Biol.* **267:**483–500.

61. **Nelson, K., P. M. Schlievert, R. K. Selander, and J. M. Musser.** 1991. Characterization and clonal distribution of four alleles of the speA gene encoding pyrogenic exotoxin A (scarlet fever toxin) in Streptococcus pyogenes. *J. Exp. Med.* **174:**1271–1274.

62. **Norrby-Teglund, A., G. T. Nepom, and M. Kotb.** 2002. Differential presentation of group A streptococcal superantigens by HLA class II DQ and DR alleles. *Eur. J. Immunol.* **32:**2570–2577.

63. **Oster, H., and A. Bisno.** 2000. Group C and G streptococcal infections: epidemiologic and clinical aspects, p. 184–190. *In* J. J. Fischetti, R. Novick, J. J. Ferretti, D. Portnoy, and J. Rood (ed.), *Gram-Positive Pathogens.* ASM Press, Washington, D.C.

64. **Petersson, K., M. Hakansson, H. Nilsson, G. Forsberg, L. A. Svensson, et al.** 2001. Crystal structure of a superantigen bound to MHC class II displays zinc and peptide dependence. *EMBO J.* **20:**3306–3312.

65. **Podbielski, A., M. Woischnik, B. A. Leonard, and K. H. Schmidt.** 1999. Characterization of nra, a global negative regulator gene in group A streptococci. *Mol. Microbiol.* **31:**1051–1064.

66. **Proft, T., V. Arcus, V. Handley, E. Baker, and J. Fraser.** 2001. Immunological and Biochemical Characterization of Streptococcal Pyrogenic Exotoxins I and J (SPE-I and SPE-J) from *Streptococcus pyogenes. J. Immun.* **166:**6711–6719.

67. **Proft, T., S. Moffatt, K. Weller, A. Paterson, D. Martin, and J. Fraser.** 2000. The streptococcal superantigen SMEZ exhibits wide allelic variation, mosaic structure, and significant antigenic variation. *J. Exp. Med.* **191:**1765–1776.

68. **Proft, T., S. L. Moffatt, C. J. Berkahn, and J. D. Fraser.** 1999. Identification and characterization of novel superantigens from *Streptococcus pyogenes. J. Exp. Med.* **189:**89–101.

69. **Proft, T., S. Sriskandan, L. Yang, and J. D. Fraser.** 2003. Superantigens and streptococcal toxic shock syndrome. *Emerg. Infect. Dis.* **9:**1211–1218.

70. **Proft, T., P. D. Webb, V. Handley, and J. D. Fraser.** 2003. Two Novel Superantigens Found in Both Group A and Group C *Streptococcus. Infect. Immun.* **71:**1361–1369.

71. **Reichardt, W., H. Müller-Alouf, J. Alouf, and W. Köhler.** 1992. Erythrogenic toxins A, B, and C: occurrence of the genes and exotoxin formation from clinical Streptococcus pyogenes strains associated with streptococcal toxic shock-like syndrome. *FEMS Microbiol. Lett.* **79:**313–322.

72. **Rink, L., J. Luhm, M. Koester, and H. Kirchner.** 1996. Induction of a cytokine network by superantigens with parallel TH1 and TH2 stimulation. *J. Interferon Cytokine Res.* **16:**41–47.

73. **Roussel, A., B. F. Anderson, H. M. Baker, J. D. Fraser, and E. N. Baker.** 1997. Crystal structure of the streptococcal superantigen SPE-C: dimerization and zinc binding suggest a novel mode of interaction with MHC class II molecules. *Nat. Struct. Biol.* **4:**635–643.

74. **Sachse, S., P. Seidel, D. Gerlach, E. Gunther, J. Rodel, et al.** 2002. Superantigen-like gene(s) in human pathogenic *Streptococcus dysgalactiae*, subsp. *equisimilis:* genomic localisation of the gene encoding streptococcal pyrogenic exotoxin G (speG(dys)). *FEMS Immunol. Med. Microbiol.* **34:**159–167.

75. **Schlievert, P., A. Assimacopoulos, and P. Cleary.** 1996. Severe invasive group A streptococcal disease: clinical description and mechanisms of pathogenesis. *J. Lab. Clin. Med.* **127:**13–22.

76. **Schlievert, P. M., and E. D. Gray.** 1989. Group A streptococcal pyrogenic exotoxin (scarlet fever toxin) type A and blastogen A are the same protein. *Infect. Immun.* **57:**1865–1867.

77. **Schlievert, P. M., and J. A. Kelly.** 1982. Staphylococcal pyrogenic exotoxin type C: further characterization. *Ann. Intern. Med.* **96:**982–986.

78. **Schuh, V., V. Hribalova, and E. Atkins.** 1970. The pyrogenic effect of scarlet fever toxin. IV. Pyrogenicity of strain C 203 U filtrate: comparison with some basic characteristics of the known types of scarlet fever toxin. *Yale J. Biol. Med.* **43:**31–42.

79. **Seal, D.** 2001. Necrotizing fasciitis. *Curr. Opin. Infect. Dis.* **14:**127–132.

80. **Smoot, J. C., K. D. Barbian, J. J. Van Gompel, L. M. Smoot, M. S. Chaussee, et al.** 2002. Genome sequence and comparative microarray analysis of serotype M18 group A *Streptococcus* strains associated with acute rheumatic fever outbreaks. *Proc. Natl. Acad. Sci. USA* **99:**4668–4673.

81. **Smoot, L. M., J. K. McCormick, J. C. Smoot, N. P. Hoe, I. Strickland, et al.** 2002. Characterization of two novel pyrogenic toxin superantigens made by an acute rheumatic fever clone of *Streptococcus pyogenes* associated with multiple disease outbreaks. *Infect. Immun.* **70:**7095–7104.

82. **Sriskandan, S., D. Moyes, L. Buttery, T. Krausz, T. Evans, et al.** 1996. Streptococcal pyrogenic exotoxin A release, distribution, and role in a murine model of fasciitis and multiorgan failure due to *Streptococcus pyogenes. J. Infect. Dis.* **173:**1399–1407.

83. **Sriskandan, S., D. Moyes, and J. Cohen.** 1996. Detection of circulating bacterial superantigen and lymphotoxin-a in patients with streptococcal toxic shock syndrome. *Lancet* **348:**1315–1316.

84. **Sriskandan, S., M. Unnikrishnan, T. Krausz, H. Dewchand, S. Van Noorden, et al.** 2001. Enhanced susceptibility to superantigen-associated streptococcal sepsis in human leukocyte antigen-DQ transgenic mice. *J. Infect. Dis.* **184:**166–173.

85. **Stevens, D., A. Bryant, S. Hackett, A. Chang, G. Peer, et al.** 1996. Group A streptococcal bacteremia: the role of tumor necrosis factor in shock and organ failure. *J. Infect. Dis.* **173:**619–626.

86. **Stevens, D. L.** 1992. Invasive group A streptococcus infections. *Clin. Infect. Dis.* **14:**2–13.

87. **Stevens, D. L.** 2000. Streptococcal toxic shock syndrome associated with necrotizing fasciitis. *Annu. Rev. Med.* **51:**271–288.

88. **Stock, A. H., and R. J. Lynn.** 1969. Extracellular esterases of streptococci and the distribution of specific antibodies in human sera of various age groups. *J. Immunol.* **102:**859–869.

89. **Sundberg, E. J., H. Li, A. S. Llera, J. K. McCormick, J. Tormo, et al.** 2002. Structures of two streptococcal superantigens bound to TCR β chains reveal diversity in the architecture of T cell signalling complex. *Structure* **10:**687–699.

90. **Sundberg, E. J., Y. Li, and R. A. Mariuzza.** 2002. So many ways of getting in the way: diversity in the molecular architecture of superantigen-dependent T cell signaling complexes. *Curr. Opin. Immunol.* **14:**36–44.

91. **Tiedemann, R. E., and J. D. Fraser.** 1996. Cross-linking of MHC class II molecules by staphylococcal enterotoxin A is essential for antigen-presenting cell and T cell activation. *J. Immunol.* **157:**3958–3966.

92. **Unnikrishnan, M., D. Altmann, T. Proft, F. Wahid, J. Cohen, et al.** 2002. The bacterial superantigen streptococcal mitogenic exotoxin Z is the major immunoactive agent of *Streptococcus pyogenes. J. Immunol.* **169:**2561–2569.

93. **Virtaneva, K., S. Porcella, M. Graham, R. Ireland, C. Johnson, et al.** 2005. Longitudinal analysis of the group A Streptococcus transcriptome in experimental pharyngitis in cynomolgus macaques. *Proc. Natl. Acad. Sci. USA* **102:**9014–9019.

94. **Watson, D.** 1960. Host-parasite factors in group A streptococcal infections. Pyrogenic and other effects of immunologic distinct exotoxins related to scarlet fever toxins. *J. Exp. Med.* **111:**255–284.

95. **Weeks, C. R., and J. J. Ferretti.** 1986. Nucleotide sequence of the type A streptococcal exotoxin (erythrogenic toxin) gene from Streptococcus pyogenes bacteriophage T12. *Infect. Immun.* **52:**144–150.

96. **Welcher, B., J. Carra, L. DaSilva, J. Hanson, C. David, et al.** 2002. Lethal shock induced by streptococcal pyrogenic exotoxin A in mice transgenic for human leukocyte antigen-DQ8 and human CD4 receptors: implications for development of vaccines and therapeutics. *J. Infect. Dis.* **186:**501–510.

97. **Willoughby, R., and R. N. Greenberg.** 1983. The toxic shock syndrome and streptococcal pyrogenic exotoxins. *Ann. Intern. Med.* **98:**559.

98. **Working Group on Severe Streptococcal Infections.** 1993. Defining the group A streptococcal toxic shock syndrome. Rationale and consensus definition. *JAMA* **269:**390–391.

99. **Yamaoka, J., E. Nakamura, Y. Takeda, S. Imamura, and N. Minato.** 1998. Mutational analysis of superantigen activity responsible for the induction of skin erythema by streptococcal pyrogenic exotoxin C. *Infect. Immun.* **66:**5020–5026.

100. **Yang, L., M. Thomas, A. Woodhouse, D. Martin, J. Fraser, and T. Proft.** 2005. Involvement of streptococcal mitogenic exotoxin Z in streptococcal toxic shock syndrome. *J. Clin. Microbiol.* **43:**3570–3573.

101. **Yoshioka, T., T. Matsutani, S. Iwagami, T. Toyosaki-Maeda, T. Yutsudo, et al.** 1999. Polyclonal expansion of TCRBV2- and TCRBV6-bearing T cells in patients with Kawasaki disease. *Immunology* **96:**465–472.

102. **Yu, C. E., and J. J. Ferretti.** 1989. Molecular epidemiologic analysis of the type A streptococcal exotoxin (erythrogenic toxin) gene (speA) in clinical *Streptococcus pyogenes* strains. *Infect. Immun.* **57:**3715–3719.

103. **Zabriskie, J. B.** 1964. The role of temperate bacteriophage in the production of erythrogenic toxin by group a streptococci. *J. Exp. Med.* **119:**761–780.

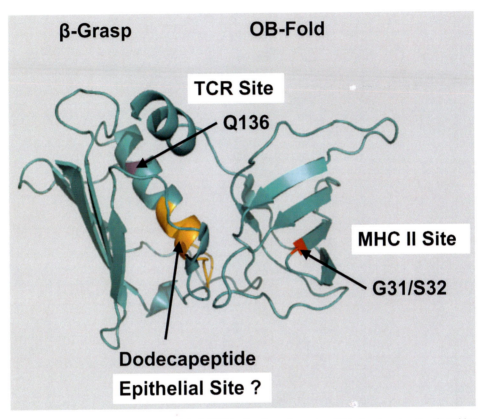

β-Grasp

OB-Fold

TCR Site

Q136

MHC II Site

G31/S32

Dodecapeptide

Epithelial Site ?

Color Plate 1 (Chapter 2). Cartoon model of TSST-1, showing eukaryotic cell binding domains. Purple residue (Q136) is involved in Vβ2-TCR binding; Red residues (G31/S32) are involved in α-chain MHC II binding; and orange residues (dodecapeptide) are hypothesized to be involved in epithelial cell binding. Residues 120 to 123 in the dodecapeptide region are dominant surface-exposed residues.

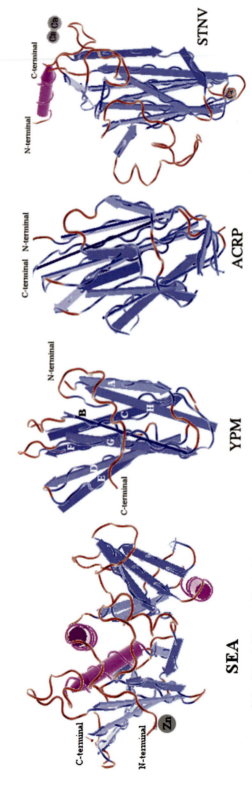

Color Plate 2 (Chapter 5). Tertiary structure of SEA, YPMa, the capsid protein of STNV, and ACRP. Structural data for SEA (accession number 1SXT), YPMa (accession number 1PM4), ACRP (accession number 1C28), and STNV (accession number 2STV) are depicted by Cn3D. α-Helices and β-sheets are presented as cylinders and arrows, respectively.

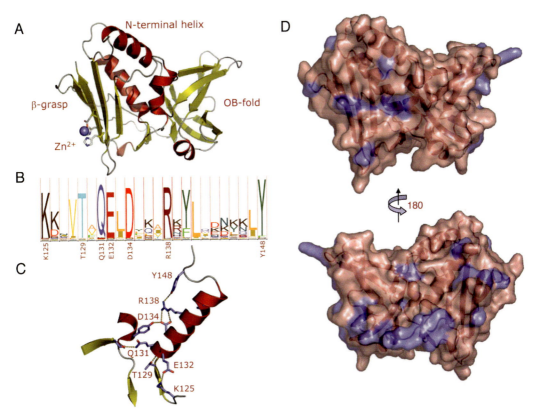

Color Plate 3 (Chapter 6). The structure of SMEZ-2. (A) Ribbon diagram showing the arrangement of secondary structure elements for SMEZ-2 (α-helices are red, β-sheets are green, and loops are grey) (6). The two domains and the N-terminal helix are labeled. A bound Zn²⁺ ion is shown as a blue sphere along with the three residues that ligate this ion (H162, H202, D204). This ion is a key contributor to the interaction between SMEZ-2 and MHC-II. (B) An "HMM Logo" representation (39) of the superantigen signature sequence showing the amino acid conservation in the region of the central α-helix. Numbers beneath the figure are those for SMEZ-2. (C) The position of the conserved residues in the structure of SMEZ-2 and their hydrogen-bonding patterns. Note that this figure is rotated 180° in the vertical axis in comparison to (A). (D) Allelic variation at the surface of SMEZ-2 is shown in blue. The molecules are rotated 180° in the vertical axis with respect to each other. This figure along with subsequent figures were drawn using the molecular graphics program PyMol (DeLano Scientific, http://www.pymol.org).

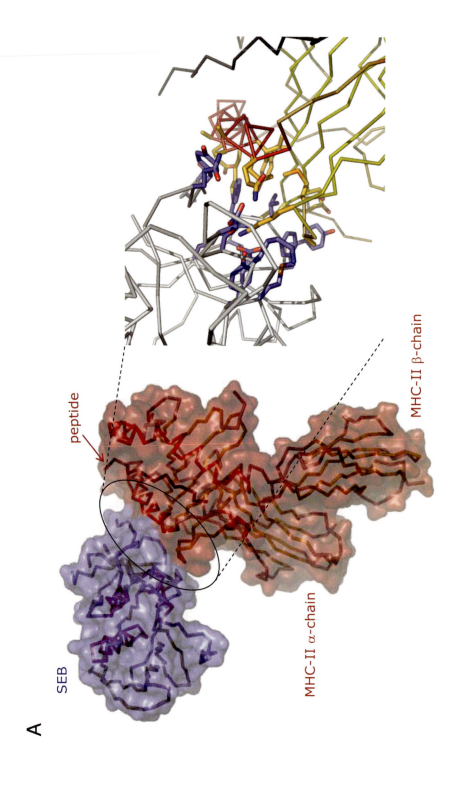

A

SEB

peptide

MHC-II α-chain

MHC-II β-chain

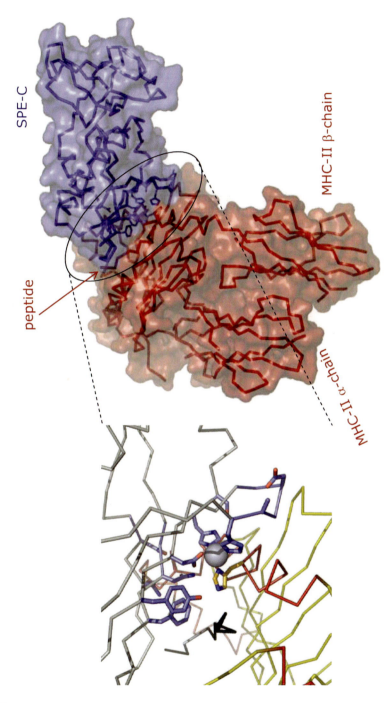

Color Plate 4 (Chapter 6). Superantigen binding to MHC-II. (A) SEB is shown binding to the α-chain of MHC-II. At left, the complex is shown as a surface with SEB in blue and MHC-II in red. The surface is semitransparent and the protein chains are shown as Cα traces beneath the surface. Details of the interacting residues are shown at the right of the figure. Residues at the interface from SEB are shown in blue and residues from MHC-II are orange. The principal α-chain helix for MHC-II is red and the bound peptide is black. The coordinates used to draw this figure have PDB code 1SEB (17). (B) SPE-C is shown binding to the β-chain of MHC-II. At right, the complex is shown as a surface with SPE-C in blue and MHC-II in red. The surface is semitransparent and the protein chains are shown as Cα traces. Details of the interacting residues are shown at the left of the figure. Residues at the interface from SPE-C are shown in blue and single Zn^{2+}-ligating histidine from MHC-II is orange. The Zn^{2+} ion at the protein-protein interface is shown as a light-blue sphere. The peptide bound to MHC-II is black. The coordinates used to draw this figure have PDB code 1HQR (24).

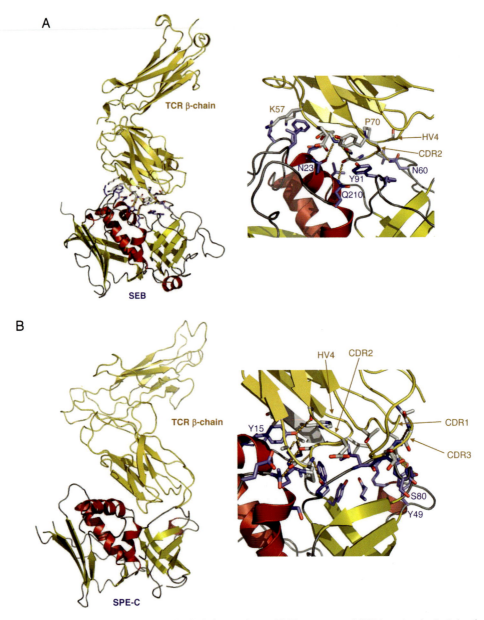

Color Plate 5 (Chapter 6). The SAg/TCR β-chain complexes. (A) The structure of SEB bound to the β-chain of the TCR (22). At left the TCR and SEB proteins are shown as ribbon diagrams and regions of the proteins that lie at the interface are shown as sticks. At right this region is expanded and the three hydrogen bonds at the interface are shown as gold broken lines. Residues from SEB are shown as blue sticks and residues from the TCR are shown as grey sticks. Some residues and loops are labeled for reference. (B) The structure of SPE-C bound to the TCR β-chain (41). As in (A), at left is a ribbon diagram of the complex with the two proteins labeled and at right is an expanded region showing the interacting side chains and loops. The nine hydrogen bonds are shown although some are obscured.

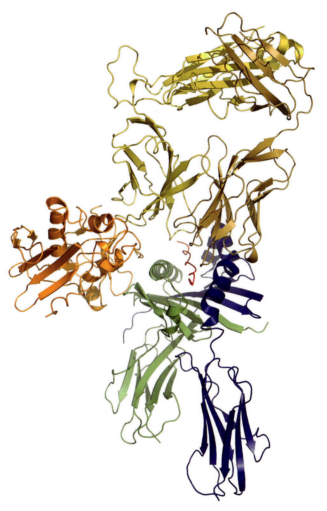

Color Plate 6 (Chapter 6). The putative MHC-II/SEB/TCR complex. A hypothesized functional complex of SEB, MHC-II, and TCR. This complex is modeled based on the binary complexes of SEB/MHC-II (PDB code 1SEB [17]), SPE-A/TCRβ (PDB code 1L0Y [41]), and TCRαβ (PDB code 1J8H [15]). The α-chain of MHC-II is shown in green and the β-chain is shown in blue. The bound peptide is red. SEB is orange and the TCR β-chain is yellow. The TCR α-chain is brown.

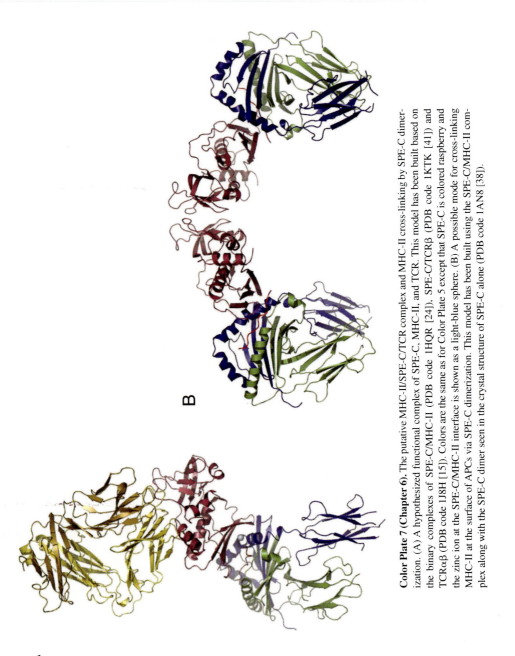

Color Plate 7 (Chapter 6). The putative MHC-II/SPE-C/TCR complex and MHC-II cross-linking by SPE-C dimerization. (A) A hypothesized functional complex of SPE-C, MHC-II, and TCR. This model has been built based on the binary complexes of SPE-C/MHC-II (PDB code 1HQR [24]), SPE-C/TCRβ (PDB code 1KTK [41]) and TCRαβ (PDB code 1J8H [15]). Colors are the same as for Color Plate 5 except that SPE-C is colored raspberry and the zinc ion at the SPE-C/MHC-II interface is shown as a light-blue sphere. (B) A possible mode for cross-linking MHC-II at the surface of APCs via SPE-C dimerization. This model has been built using the SPE-C/MHC-II complex along with the SPE-C dimer seen in the crystal structure of SPE-C alone (PDB code 1AN8 [38]).

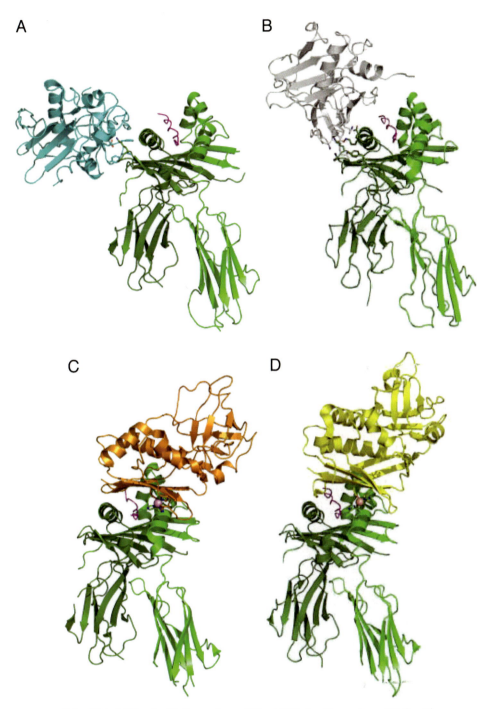

Color Plate 8 (Chapter 7). Comparison of SAg–MHC class II complexes. (A) Crystal structure of SEB (cyan) interacting with the α-chain of MHC class II (50). (B) Crystal structure of TSST-1 (white) interacting with the α-chain of MHC class II (55). (C) Crystal structure of SPE-C (orange) interacting with the β-chain of MHC class II (64). (D) Crystal structure of SEH (yellow) interacting with the β-chain of MHC class II (82). Residues involved in the SEB–MHC and TSST-1–MHC interactions and residues involved in zinc binding are shown as sticks. The α-chain and the β-chain of MHC class II are dark green and green, respectively. The molecular representations were generated with PyMOL (22).

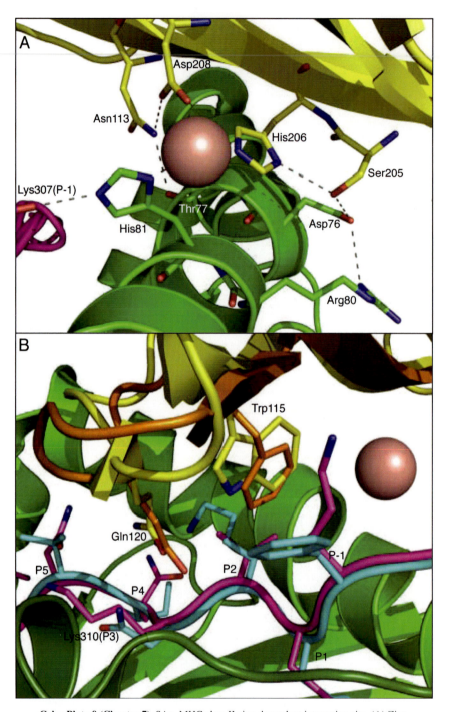

Color Plate 9 (Chapter 7). SAg–MHC class II zinc-dependent interaction site. (A) Zinc-coordination and hydrogen bond pattern in the SEH (yellow)–HLA-DR1 (green)–HA-peptide (magenta) complex (82). (B) Comparison between the SEH (yellow)–HLA-DR1 (green)–HA-peptide (magenta) complex (82) and the SPE-C (orange)–HLA-DR2a (not shown)–MBP-peptide (cyan) complex (64). The molecular representations were generated with PyMOL (22).

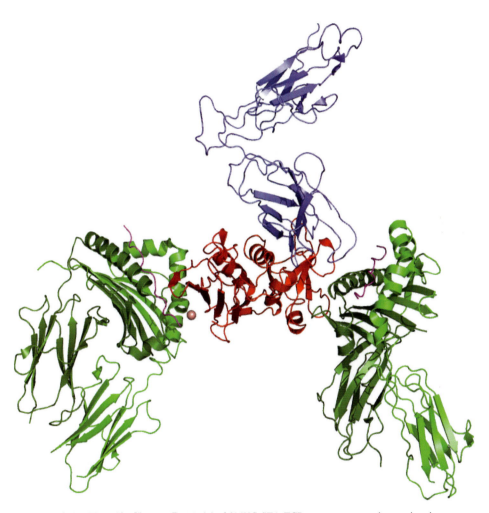

Color Plate 10 (Chapter 7). Model of 2MHC-SEA-TCR quaternary complex produced by superposition of the SEH–HLA-DR1 complex (82), the SEA–HLA-DR1 complex (84), and the SPE-C–TCR β-chain complex (99). The α-chain and the β-chain of HLA-DR1 are dark green and green, respectively, SEA is red and the TCR β-chain is blue. The molecular representation was generated with PyMOL (22).

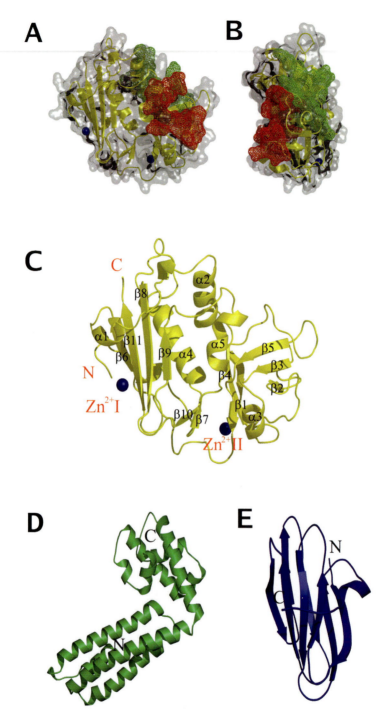

Color Plate 11 (Chapter 8). (A) Surface representation of a typical staphylococcal/strep-tococcal superantigen with TCR binding region (green) and MHC class II binding region (red) indicated (front view). (B) Side view of A giving a better picture of the size and position of the TCR binding site. (C) Ribbon diagram of SEA representative of the common structural features of the staphylococcal and streptococcal superantigen family. Blue spheres represent the positions of the two possible zinc sites. The cysteine residues that form the disulfide loop are shown in ball-and-stick representation. (D) The nonclassical superantigen MAM. (E) The nonclassical superantigen YPM.

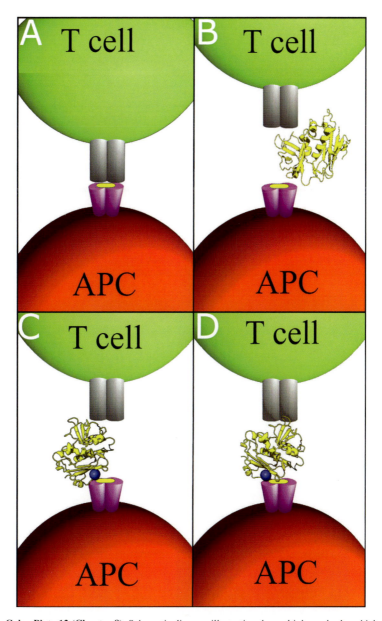

Color Plate 12 (Chapter 8). Schematic diagram illustrating the multiple modes by which superantigens can interact with MHC class II molecules. (A) Conventional peptide antigen. (B) Interaction with a single MHC class II molecule via the generic binding site on the α-chain (e.g., SEB and TSST-1). Interaction of a non-zinc-linked superantigen dimer with two separate MHC class II molecules via the α-chain generic site (e.g., MAM). (C) Interaction of a superantigen with MHC class II β-chain via a high-affinity zinc site and TCR $V_β$-chain (e.g., SEC2, SpeA1, and SpeC). (D) Interaction of a superantigen with MHC class II β-chain via a high-affinity zinc site and TCR $V_α$-chain (e.g., SEH).

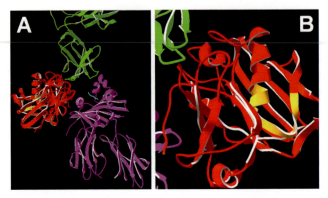

Color Plate 13 (Chapter 14). Superantigen in complex with TCR Vβ chain and MHC class II molecule. (A) Left view. Atomic coordinates of complexes of SEB (red ribbon) with the TCR β-chain (green ribbon) (23) and with HLA DR1 (magenta ribbon) (16) have been superimposed in SEB. (B) Right view and closeup. The antagonist domain in SEB is shown in yellow. Reprinted from *Molecular Diversity* (17) with permission of the publisher.

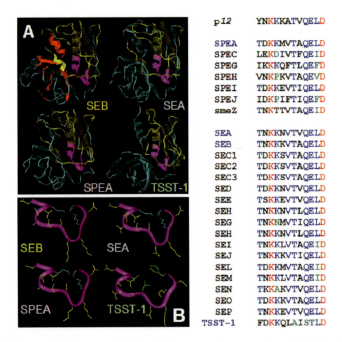

p12	YNKKKATVQELD
SPEA	TDKKMVTAQELD
SPEC	LEKDIVTFQEID
SPEG	IKKKQFTLQEFD
SPEH	VNKPKVTAQEVD
SPEI	TDKKEVTIQELD
SPEJ	IDKPIFTIQEFD
smeZ	TNKTTVTAQEID
SEA	TNKKNVTVQELD
SEB	TNKKKVTAQELD
SEC1	TDKKSVTAQELD
SEC2	TDKKSVTAQELD
SEC3	TDKKSVTAQELD
SED	TDKKNVTVQELD
SEE	TSKKEVTVQELD
SEH	TNKKNVTLQELD
SEG	TNKNMVTIQELD
SEH	TNKKNVTLQELD
SEI	TNKKLVTAQEID
SEJ	TNKKKVTIQELD
SEL	TDKKMVTAQEID
SEM	TNKKLVTAQEID
SEN	TKKAKVTVQELD
SEO	TDKKKVTAQELD
SEP	TNKKEVTVQELD
TSST-1	FDKKQLAISTLD

Color Plate 14 (Chapter 14). The antagonist domain is conserved in superantigens. (A) In backbone structures (PDB codes 1SEB, 1SEA, SPEA_STRPY, 1TSS), the domain corresponding to residues $SEB_{150-161}$ is shown as a magenta ribbon. In SEB, domains that interact with TCR, MHC-II, or both are shown as orange/yellow ribbons. The N-terminal 138 residues in SEB are shown as orange ribbons and cyan strands; corresponding regions in SEA, SPEA, and TSST-1 are cyan. (B) Detail of the 12-amino-acid β-strand/hinge/α-helix antagonist domains that show homology to superantigen antagonist peptide p12. On the right, sequence comparison of p12 with antagonist domains of streptococcal and staphylococcal superantigens is shown. Full amino acid conservation is designated in red, partial conservation in blue. Modified from *Nature Medicine* (3) with permission of the publisher.

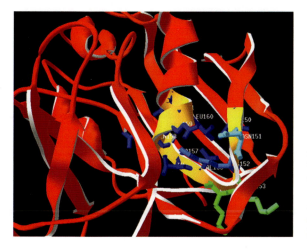

Color Plate 15 (Chapter 14). Accessibility of the antagonist domain in SEB. In the structure of SEB, side chains in the 150-161 β-strand/hinge/α-helix domain are color-coded according to surface accessibility. Dark blue, not exposed; light blue and green, exposed.

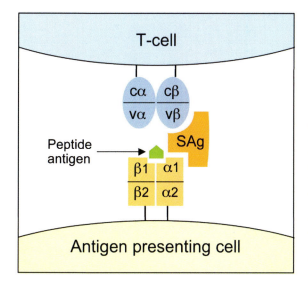

Color Plate 16 (Chapter 16). Schematic representation illustrating the differences between conventional peptide antigen presentation and superantigen presentation to MHC class II and TCRs. Conventional antigen is processed by the APC and displayed as discrete peptide fragments within the peptide-binding groove of MHC class II molecules. Superantigens bind to the solvent-exposed face of the MHC class II molecule (α1), forming a bridge between α1 and TCRVβ.

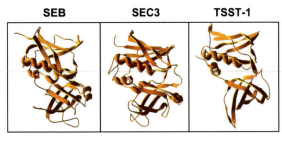

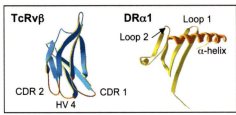

Color Plate 17 (Chapter 16). Upper panel shows a comparison of the structures of three *S. aureus* superantigens. Ribbon diagram of crystal structures of SEB (left), SEC3 (center), and TSST-1 (right). The lower panel shows the native folds of the major components of the chimeric proteins, with major SAg contact areas labeled. On the left is a ribbon diagram of the crystal structure of TCRVβ and on the right is a ribbon diagram of the crystal structure of MHC class II DRα1.

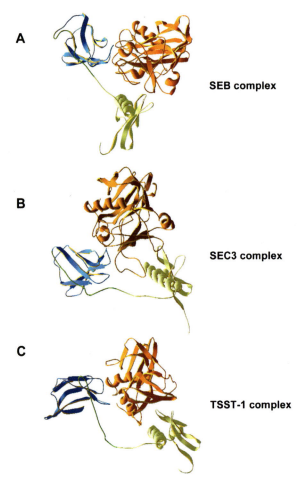

Color Plate 18 (Chapter 16). Comparison of the minimized average structures of the superantigen-chimera complexes. (A) SEB-chimera complex. (B) SEC3-chimera complex. (C) TSST-1-chimera complex. The superantigen is orange, the DRα1 is yellow, the TCRVβ is blue, and the linker is green.

Superantigens: Molecular Basis for Their Role in Human Diseases
Edited by Malak Kotb and John D. Fraser
© 2007 ASM Press, Washington, D.C.

Chapter 2

Staphylococcal and Streptococcal Superantigens: an Update

Patrick M. Schlievert and Gregory A. Bohach

INTRODUCTION

The term superantigen (SAg) was applied by Marrack and Kappler (67) in 1990 to describe a large family of exotoxins secreted primarily by *Staphylococcus aureus* and *Streptococcus pyogenes*. These exotoxins were previously known as pyrogenic toxins and scarlet fever toxins (17) and included staphylococcal enterotoxins (SEs), the causes of staphylococcal food poisoning and cases of nonmenstrual toxic shock syndrome (TSS) (13, 90, 99), toxic shock syndrome toxin-1 (TSST-1), the principal cause of menstrual and one-half of nonmenstrual TSS (14, 98), and streptococcal pyrogenic exotoxins (SPEs), the causes of scarlet fever and streptococcal TSS (22, 48, 93, 96, 106). Marrack and Kappler referred to the exotoxins as SAgs because of their novel mechanism of T-cell stimulation (67). SAgs interact with the variable part of the β-chain of certain T-cell receptors (Vβ-TCRs). The exotoxins also interact with relatively invariant regions of major histocompatibility complex class II (MHC II) molecules. In menstrual TSS, the cross-bridging of Vβ2-TCR (the only Vβ-TCR that TSST-1 binds) with MHC II molecules on macrophages results in stimulation of T-cell proliferation such that stimulated cells become 60 to 70% of the patient's T cells (referred to as T-cell skewing) instead of approximately 10% of T cells under usual conditions (18). This T-cell proliferation mechanism is greatly magnified compared with typical stimulation of T cells by antigenic peptide presented in the groove of MHC II on antigen-presenting cells, where only approximately 1/10,000 T cells is stimulated. The stimulation of both T cells and macrophages by SAgs leads to massive cytokine production by both cell types, including interleukin-2 (IL-2), interferon gamma (IFN-γ), and tumor necrosis factor β (TNF-β) by T cells and IL-1β and TNF-α by macrophages (49, 71, 96). This massive cytokine "storm" is thought to cause the clinical signs of TSS (Table 1).

Hundreds of publications have defined the mechanism of SAg stimulation of both T cells and macrophages. Many of these are discussed in detail in later chapters of this book.

Patrick M. Schlievert • Department of Microbiology, University of Minnesota Medical School, Minneapolis, MN 55455. *Gregory A. Bohach* • Department of Microbiology, Molecular Biology, and Biochemistry, University of Idaho, Moscow, ID 83846.

Table 1. Clinical definition of toxic shock syndrome

Staphylococcal TSS (27, 102, 111)[a]	Streptococcal TSS (5, 22, 106)
Fever	Isolation of group A streptococci from:
	1. A sterile site for a definitive case
	2. A nonsterile site for a probable case
Hypotension	Hypotension
Diffuse macular erythroderma	Two of the following symptoms:
Skin desquamation upon recovery	1. Renal dysfunction
Three of the following organ system changes:	2. Liver involvement
1. Liver	3. Erythematous macular rash
2. Blood	4. Coagulopathy
3. Renal	5. Soft tissue necrosis
4. Mucous membrane	6. Adult respiratory distress syndrome
5. Gastrointestinal	
6. Muscular	
7. Central nervous system	
If performed, negative serological tests for measles, leptospirosis, Rocky Mountain spotted fever, and negative cultures for other causative organisms except *S. aureus*	

[a]Probable staphylococcal TSS is defined as the same illness, except that one of the defining criteria (fever, hypotension, rash, desquamation, three multiorgan changes) is absent (85).

In addition, many studies have described the SAg causation of TSS and related illnesses. With typical exotoxins and their host cell interaction, this wealth of publications would have provided an adequate explanation for disease causation. However, SAgs do not fit the "usual" pattern of exotoxin interaction with host cells. For example, (i) there are large numbers of serologically distinct SAgs, many of which have interesting and important structural differences, leading to potential differences in illness associations; (ii) not all SAgs interact with Vβ-TCRs and MHC II molecules in the same way, which leads to differences in T-cell and macrophage stimulation; (iii) some SAgs are made in very high (1–100 μg/ml in planktonic cultures) concentrations, while others are made in very low (0.0001–0.001 μg/ml) concentrations, with some bacterial strains making only one serotype of SAg and other bacterial strains making as many as 16; and (iv) because of the scientific attention paid to understanding the interesting mechanism of superantigenicity, there have been important aspects of SAg biology that remain understudied.

The goal of this chapter is to provide an introduction to bacterial SAgs (examples i and ii above) and to present our current understanding of disease association and causation by SAgs, with the intent of identifying needed future research studies of SAgs (examples iii and iv above).

SAg DEFINITION

In the introduction, we provided some attributes of exotoxins that allow them to be categorized as SAgs, as defined by Marrack and Kappler (67). We will now provide a more formal definition. First, SAgs may be produced by any microorganism, and thus far have been demonstrated for certain bacteria, viruses, and yeasts. Bacterial SAgs include those produced by β-hemolytic streptococci (including *S. pyogenes*) (96), *S. aureus* and *S. intermedius* (36, 71), *Mycoplasma arthritidis* (19, 20), and certain species of *Yersinia* (107, 114). Viral SAgs include murine mammary tumor viruses and may include proteins from selected other viruses such as HIV (68, 87). Yeast SAgs have been suggested in *Candida albicans*.

SAgs may be defined as either T-cell or B-cell SAgs. For purposes of this chapter, however, we will consider only T-cell SAgs; definitions listed may be easily adapted to define B-cell SAgs. Table 2 provides the defining properties of T-cell SAgs. In response to SAgs, T cells are stimulated when the SAg interacts with the Vβ-TCR, leading to polyclonal stimulation. Thus, for a molecule to function as a SAg, the toxin should stimulate and skew T cells bearing certain Vβ-TCRs, and junctional diversity in the variable region of TCRs should be demonstrable. This latter aspect of the definition rules out particularly strong antigenic peptides that may stimulate T cells bearing a certain Vβ-TCR, but derived from a single T-cell clone rather than multiple clones. T-cell activation should depend on interaction of the SAg with MHC II molecules on antigen-presenting cells, α-chain, β-chain, or both α- and β-chains; this interaction should be with intact SAg in the absence of processing. Finally, both CD4+ and CD8+ T cells are stimulated to proliferate in response to SAgs, but CD4+ T-cell proliferation dominates. Note that this definition does not include any requirement for the dose of SAg required for activity.

When pyrogenic toxin SAgs were examined for activity, it was noted that these proteins are exceptionally active in T-cell stimulation. For example, TSST-1 is able to stimulate T-cell proliferation at concentrations as low as 10^{-5} μg/1 × 10^5 human T cells (98). Because of this exceptional activity, there has been an assumption that all SAgs must be comparably active to be called SAgs. This is not the case, however. SAgs such as SEA, SMEZ, and many others are active at doses approximately 100-fold lower than TSST-1 (10^{-7} μg/1 × 10^5 human T cells) (69). This greater activity results from the ability of these higher-activity SAgs to interact with the β-chain of MHC II or both α- and β-chains, rather than only the α-chain as with TSST-1. It is also possible that SAgs will be identified that have reduced activity as compared with the pyrogenic toxin SAgs. It has been suggested that certain proteases and nucleases are SAgs. Thus, researchers have suggested that SPE B, a cysteine protease (112), and exfoliative toxin A, a serine protease (115), may have superantigenic activity. Although not firmly established, it is possible that cleavage of certain Vβ-TCRs by these proteases leads to T-cell proliferation in a polyclonal and Vβ-TCR-dependent way. Similarly, SPE F (mitogenic factor) has been shown to have SAg activity; this molecule is a DNase (34, 41, 74, 105, 113, 116). One structural feature of all pyrogenic toxin SAgs in common with DNases is the presence of an oligosaccharide/oligonucleotide binding (OB) fold (83). Thus, it is not unreasonable to suggest that SPE F functions as a SAg. For these putative SAgs, ad-

Table 2. Defining properties of T-cell SAgs

---

1. Activation of T cells dependent on composition of the variable region of the β-chain of the T-cell receptor (Vβ-TCR)
2. Polyclonal activation of T cells, as demonstrated by variable region T-cell receptor junctional diversity (or another demonstration of polyclonal activation)
3. Requirement of antigen-presenting cell presentation of superantigen without superantigen processing

---

ditional studies are required to establish with certainty whether they are indeed T-cell SAgs. Incidentally, this domain of SAgs is present structurally also in many other exotoxins that bind host cells, including cholera toxin, heat-labile enterotoxin of *Escherichia coli*, shiga toxin, shiga-like toxin, and pertussis toxin (72).

In the remainder of this review, we will discuss only the large family of pyrogenic toxin SAgs, referring to them only as SAgs.

CATEGORIZATION OF SAgs

The pyrogenic toxin SAgs include the SEs, which are known to cause emesis when administered orally to monkeys, and thus are the causes of staphylococcal food poisoning (13). This is in addition to their ability to cause TSS. The SEs include serotypes A, B, C_n, D, E, G, and I. A large group of SE-like molecules either have not been tested for emetic activity (SEs H, J, M, N, O, and P) or have been tested and lack emetic activity (SEs K, L, and Q). These molecules should more correctly use the designation SE-like (61). A few undefined SE-like molecules that are essentially unstudied (SE-like R, S, and T) should be completely characterized for inclusion in the SAg family. TSST-1 is included in the SAg family as a stand-alone member because of its high association with menstrual TSS and its lack of primary sequence similarity to other SAgs (14, 16, 98). Finally, SPEs (erythrogenic toxins, scarlet fever toxins) now include the classic SPE A and C, but also serotypes G, H, I, J, K, L, M, streptococcal superantigen (SSA), and streptococcal mitogenic exotoxin Z_n (SMEZ) (69). SPE A and SSA are highly similar to SEs B and C, but at least SPE A lacks emetic activity (95). Related SPE SAgs have been demonstrated in groups C and G streptococci (11, 40, 84, 86).

Recently, McCormick et al. established a useful system of categorization of pyrogenic toxin SAgs, with use of structure–function characteristics (71). SAgs may be categorized into five subgroups, I–V (Table 3). TSST-1 is contained within group I and together with an ovine variant (TSST-ovine) (55) are the only members. These toxins have unique primary amino acid sequence, but fold into the prototypical pyrogenic toxin SAg structure (Color Plate 1) (2, 83). The TSST-1 structure consists of a short amino-terminal α-helix that progresses into the OB fold of amino acids. This structure is followed by a central diagonal α-helix, open on the back of the protein, and carboxy-terminal wall of β-strands that together form a β-grasp motif. TSST-1 interacts with the α-chain of the MHC II in the OB fold but does not bind the β-chain of MHC II (45). Group II SAgs (SEB-related SAgs) contain cystine loop structures above the OB fold, that contain 10 to 19 amino acids be-

Table 3. Categorization of pyrogenic toxin SAgs

| Group | Defining properties | |
	Structural feature	MHC II binding
I	Unique amino acid sequence	Low-affinity site
II	Variable length cystine loop	Low-affinity site
III	9-amino-acid length cystine loop	Low- and high-affinity sites
IV	No cystine loop	Low- and high-affinity sites
V	No cystine loop + 15-amino-acid insert	Low- and high-affinity sites

tween the two cysteines. It has been demonstrated previously that the cystine loop structure is important in the emetic activity of SEs. Indeed, SEs lacking one or both cysteine residues are either nonemetic or are weakly emetic (42). However, the loop alone may not be sufficient since SPE A falls in this group, has a cystine loop, but is not emetic (95). Recent data confirm the importance of the loop, but suggest the conformation induced by certain amino acids adjacent to the cysteines and within the loop is more important than the loop itself (39). These group II SAgs interact only with the MHC II α-chain on antigen-presenting cells in the OB fold, but not with MHC II β-chains. Group III SAgs, such as the prototype SEA, contain the cystine loop, but their loop is exactly 9 amino acids in length. The SEs within group III are emetic, like group II SEs, but unlike group II SAgs, group III proteins interact with both MHC II α- and β-chains in the OB fold and β-grasp domain, respectively. The ability of these SAgs to interact with the MHC II β-chain depends on interaction with the Zn^{2+} cation; this site is often referred to as the high-affinity MHC II site because it has higher affinity for the MHC II β-chain than the MHC II α-chain binding site in the OB fold (low-affinity site). Group IV SAgs, with SPE C as the prototypical toxin, lack the cystine loop structure but contain both the low- and high-affinity MHC II sites. Finally, the group V SAgs, with SE-like Q as prototype, differ from group IV SAgs in that group V SAgs have an extra 15-amino-acid loop at the top of the β-grasp domain; these toxins contain low- and high-affinity MHC II sites.

Structurally, another aspect of SAgs should be mentioned. SAgs typically interact with Vβ-TCRs in a groove at the top front of the SAgs (60, 65, 109). However, TSST-1 interacts with Vβ-TCR at the top back of the groove (70). Thus, when the trimolecular complex of SAgs with MHC II and Vβ-TCR is modeled, two different structural arrangements are seen: (i) the SAg appearing as a wedge on the side of the immune molecules, and (ii) the trimolecular complex appearing as three beads on a string. The group II SAgs, and those SAgs excluding TSST-1 that interact with the low-affinity MHC II site, act as wedges on the side of the trimolecular complexes. All other SAgs that interact through the high-affinity MHC II site and TSST-1 form a trimolecular complex in the beads on a string arrangement. The significance of these two differing patterns of interaction is unclear, except interaction through the high-affinity MHC II site makes those SAgs 100-fold more active than those that interact with the low-affinity MHC II site, regardless of trimolecular complex arrangement.

SAg ASSOCIATION WITH HUMAN DISEASE

The causation or association of pyrogenic toxin SAgs with human diseases is shown in Table 4. Classically, these SAgs induce TSS. Staphylococcal and streptococcal TSS are defined by criteria previously listed in Table 1. It is well recognized today that SAgs have the ability to cause TSS in humans and animal models. SAg amounts from 0.1 μg to 5 μg have been administered to humans, with their development of TSS clinical features (31, 71, 96). The TSS fever is most likely the result of IL-1β (endogenous pyrogen) effects on the hypothalamic fever response control center (91, 100). Hypotension appears to result from combinations of TNF-α and -β induction of capillary leak (28, 29, 49). Rash production may depend on both IL-2 and IFN-γ production by CD4+ T cells (93). Thus, prior encounter with SAgs, with possible recruitment of high numbers of CD4+ T cells, is likely to lead to rash production. The rash has previously been referred to as SAg-amplified hypersensitivity that is preexistent to SAg or other microbial factors (93). This rash can be duplicated in experimental animals

Table 4. Human disease causation/association with SAgs

Human disease (reference[s])	SAgs associated (reference[s])
Staphylococcal menstrual TSS (27, 102, 111)	TSST-1 (14, 98)
Staphylococcal nonmenstrual TSS	TSST-1 and any SE, but mainly SEB and SEC (90, 99)
1. Wound, boil, abscess (85)	
2. Postrespiratory viral (64)	
3. Purpura fulminans (50)	
4. Necrotizing pneumonia (6, 7)	
5. Recalcitrant erythematous desquamating in AIDS (21)	
6. Anaphylactic	
7. Kawasaki-like (57, 58)	
8. Scleroderma-like	
9. Acute-onset rheumatoid arthritis-like	
Streptococcal TSS (22, 48, 69, 106)	Any SPE
Staphylococcal food poisoning (13, 61)	Any SE
Guttate psoriasis (59)	Any SPE
Atopic dermatitis (37, 38)	TSST-1, SEs, SE-like
Asthma (35)	TSST-1, SEs, SE-like
Conjunctivitis	TSST-1, SEs, SE-like
Severe nasal polyposis (15)	TSST-1, SEs, SE-like
Sudden infant death syndrome (62, 73)	Any
Obsessive compulsive and other nervous system disorders (46)	SPEs, mainly SPE C, L, and M
Acute rheumatic fever (92, 104)	SPEs, mainly SPE C, L, and M
Perineal erythema (66)	TSST-1, SEs, SE-like

only when the animals have previously been exposed to SAgs. The multiorgan changes that occur in TSS have been only incompletely studied. Some of the changes seen are likely to result from cytokines, but for others, such as hypocalcemia, central nervous system changes, and vomiting and diarrhea, the role of cytokines is less certain. Studies are needed to clarify their origin. Later, we will address the origin of vomiting and diarrhea due to SEs, but it is unclear where these symptoms arise due to TSST-1-induced TSS, since this SAg lacks emetic activity.

In production of TSS, not all SAgs are of equal importance. This is most noticeable in staphylococcal TSS where defined subsets of illness are seen. Menstrual TSS is essentially all caused by TSST-1 (14, 98). Nonmenstrual TSS, of which there are many subsets of illness, may be 50% caused by TSST-1, but the remaining 50% is caused by SEs B and C (90, 99); occasionally, other staphylococcal SAgs cause TSS. This seems paradoxical since these three SAgs interact only with the MHC II low-affinity site, and thus are less active (100-fold) than those SAgs that interact with the MHC II high-affinity site. It is important to remember, however, that TSST-1 and SEB and SEC are made in in vitro culture (and we presume in vivo) in concentrations that may be 10,000 times higher than other staphylococcal SAgs, and this easily offsets the 100-fold difference in activity.

Do we know why this difference exists in amounts of SAgs produced by *S. aureus* strains? (Incidentally, differences also exist in production of SAgs by *S. pyogenes,* so we assume these discussions also apply to that organism.) Although incompletely studied, we have hypotheses for the differential SAg production. First, 98% of *S. aureus* strains produce one or more SAgs. This leads to the assumption that the proteins are important to the producing organisms. *S. aureus* also contains many SAg-like genes that do not yield functional proteins, most often because they lack solubility in biocompatible solutions (51). However, these genes may represent a source of recombinational precursor genes that can lead to a myriad of new SAgs, further suggesting the importance of SAgs to the microbe.

Most staphylococcal SAgs are produced in low concentration, and many if not all of these low-level SAgs are expected to be produced during the exponential phase of growth (75). For example, SEA, SEK, and SEL have been shown to be produced primarily during exponential growth of the organism, and all three of these are produced in low amounts. We hypothesize that these SAgs play important roles in early establishment of infection in the initial phase of colonization of new hosts. Both *S. aureus* and *S. pyogenes* produce many cell-associated virulence factors that are antiphagocytic through multiple mechanisms. However, these are likely to be microbial defense mechanisms of last resort because the immune system has already juxtaposed itself next to the invading microbe. It seems more advantageous for microbes to inactivate the immune system at a distance, and thus our suggested role for these SAgs as made in low concentrations and as the microbes begin their early growth in the host.

The SAgs TSST-1, SEB, and SEC are produced by *S. aureus* in high concentrations, and these SAgs cause most cases of TSS (14, 90, 98, 99). These three SAgs are not produced during the exponential phase, but instead are produced when the microbes achieve high cell densities in the postexponential phase (75). Thus, these three SAgs would be made when the organisms are most likely to be transmissible to new hosts. We hypothesize the function of these three SAgs is not to cause TSS and death of the host, but rather to ensure survival of the organisms in the first several minutes of their deposition in a new host. After that initial period of new host colonization, production of these three SAgs would be "shut off," and the low-level SAgs would become important. Thus, the organism may have been selected for having this unique strategy of SAg production. Studies should be completed to assess the validity of these hypotheses.

One final note on this aspect of our review: we have tried to induce protective antibodies in rabbits against multiple SAg injection (30-μg dose per injection), compared with immunization against a single SAg at the same dose (30 μg). None of the animals became immune to the multiple-injection regimen, possibly suggesting why so many strains make more than one SAg—that is to prevent or at least delay development of immunity. In contrast, 50% of the rabbits were immunized against the single SAg. Note that 50% of animals did not develop immunity upon immunization, even with a single SAg. This is reminiscent of menstrual TSS in which 85% of affected women do not develop immunity upon recovery and are thus susceptible to recurrences (79). This property has been attributed to high-level production of IFN-γ-inhibiting antibody production (17). However, it also seems possible that this could be the result of selective immune deficiency in such patients. This latter hypothesis is consistent with a recent study in which Parsonnet et al. demonstrated that approximately 80 to 85% of humans develop antibodies to TSST-1, but not 100% (80).

While it is clear that SAgs cause TSS, the exotoxins have been associated with many other illnesses recently (Table 4). One illness confirmed to be associated with a subset of SAgs, the SEs, is staphylococcal food poisoning (42). This illness is an intoxication caused by consuming SEs produced in food contaminated with toxin-expressing staphylococci.

The hallmark symptom is emesis following a short (1 to 6 hours) incubation period. Our understanding of the mechanism of SE-induced emesis is incomplete, in part, because the cellular target and receptor in the gastrointestinal tract have not yet been identified. However, emesis is known to depend on vagus nerve stimulation (108), and more recent evidence also suggests that SE-induced intoxication involves a variety of inflammatory mediators and neuropeptides (4, 47). SE molecular regions involved in the emetic response are likely dependent on an intact cystine loop and were discussed above. All known SEs are confirmed SAgs, and histopathology studies indicate that various types of immune cells become stimulated in the gastrointestinal tract following ingestion of the toxins (44). However, several lines of evidence suggest that SAg activity is not sufficient for induction of emesis. First, two well-characterized toxins with potent T-cell-stimulating activities, TSST-1 and SPE A, are devoid of emetic activity in the monkey feeding assay, even when large doses are administered orally (86). This experimental observation is interesting, especially considering the high degree of sequence and structural homology that SEB and SEC (emetic) share with SPE A (nonemetic). The lack of emetic activity for TSST-1 and SPE A could not be attributed to instability in the gastrointestinal tract since both toxins resist proteolysis when incubated in gastric fluid. Finally, structure–function analysis experiments with at least three different SEs have shown that T-cell stimulation and emesis induction are separable but may be determined by overlapping SE functional molecular regions (3, 33, 39).

Regarding the other illnesses listed in Table 4, their associations with SAgs have largely been made epidemiologically, and additional studies are needed to establish the role of the toxins, if any, in illness production. It is beyond the scope of this review to discuss each illness in detail, and the reader is encouraged to read the primary publications cited in Table 4. However, there are likely to be numerous other disease associations made with SAgs. Three examples are provided below.

First, *S. aureus* may cause skin infections in any individual with damaged skin, even if the damage is slight. It is an interesting subject of discussion as to whether *S. aureus* can cause the damaged skin in some cases, or whether the damaged skin always precedes the *S. aureus* infection. In either case, the offending microbes have been shown to produce SAgs in affected body sites. *S. aureus* strains have been highly associated with atopic dermatitis, and injection of the same SAgs made by the associated *S. aureus* strains has the ability to induce atopic reactions in these humans (37, 38). The question becomes: What other skin infections might *S. aureus* cause? Based on the observation that group A streptococcal SAgs have been associated with guttate psoriasis (12, 30, 59, 81), it is possible that *S. aureus* SAgs may be associated with other forms of psoriasis. In addition, at least one study has suggested the association of staphylococcal SAgs with cutaneous T-cell lymphoma (43).

As a second example, we have noted that many of the group V SAgs made by *S. aureus* skew T cells bearing Vβ5-TCR (43, 76–78). This Vβ-TCR is also skewed in patients with Crohn's disease. Prior to its association with *Clostridium difficile* infection, pseudomembranous enterocolitis (in clindamycin-treated patients) was associated with staphylococcal enterotoxins, notably SEB. Studies should be performed to evaluate the association of Crohn's disease and other forms of enterocolitis with staphylococcal SAgs.

Finally, recent studies have been exploring the possible role of group A streptococcal SAgs in obsessive compulsive and other nervous system disorders (1, 23, 24, 46, 110). In 1979, Schlievert et al. demonstrated that rheumatogenic strains of group A strepotococci produce the SAg SPE C (92). More recently, it has been shown that the M18 strains of group A streptococci associated with rheumatic fever in the Untied States produce SPEs L and M in addition to SPE C (104). In addition, a prior study suggested that SPE C has the ability to penetrate into the central nervous system of rabbits, possibly contributing to Syndenham's chorea associated with rheumatic fever (101). Studies have also demonstrated the SAg SEA has the ability to exacerbate development of experimental allergic encephalomyelitis in a mouse model of multiple sclerosis (88, 89). Finally, it has been suggested that certain individuals who become infected with M18 group A streptococci develop obsessive compulsive and other nervous system disorders (46). All these data collectively point to the association of SPEs with nervous system disorders, but the story is incomplete.

SAg CAUSATION OF HUMAN DISEASES BEGINS WITH INTERACTION AT MUCOSAL AND SKIN SURFACES

The last aspect of our presentation of new horizons for SAg research is based on the premise that human diseases caused by SAgs begin with their interaction with epithelial cells. Both group A streptococci and *S. aureus* cause infections that begin on skin and mucous membranes and, as stated above, most of these organisms make SAgs.

In this discussion, we will use *S. aureus* as the model organism. Up to 50% of humans may have *S. aureus* in the anterior nares (63), and as many as one-half of those strains may make TSST-1. As many as 20 to 30% of the strains may make SEB or SEC. During influenza season, these three SAgs may cause TSS and purpura fulminans, or contribute to necrotizing pneumonia following *S. aureus* superinfection of respiratory tissue (6, 25, 50, 64). In addition, as many as 5% of menstruating women have TSST-1 + *S. aureus* vaginally (97), and these organisms clearly cause menstrual TSS. For *S. aureus* to cause menstrual TSS the following conditions must occur:

1. *S. aureus* with the capability of making TSST-1 must colonize the human vaginal mucosa.
2. TSST-1 must be produced by those *S. aureus*.
3. TSST-1 must penetrate the vaginal mucosa; the organism remains on the mucosa.
4. TSST-1 must cross-bridge MHC II and Vβ2-TCR to cause massive cytokine release and TSS.

As stated above, studies have indicated that TSST-1 is produced by as many as 5% of vaginal *S. aureus* (80, 97). In addition, studies suggest that the environmental conditions of the human vagina may facilitate toxin production in the presence of menses and tampon use (94). After having penetrated the vaginal epithelium, TSST-1 cross-bridging MHC II and Vβ2-TCR leads to TSS. However, the aspect of TSS that has received the least amount of attention is the interaction of the toxin with the vaginal epithelium. The human vaginal mucosa is composed of stratified nonkeratinized squamous epithelium and is many layers thick, with its barrier function provided by combinations of layers of lipid vesicles (26). Recent studies suggest that small amounts of TSST-1 may penetrate through mucosal tissue, with greater amounts penetrating into the tissue, and possibly serving as a SAg reservoir (26). The understanding of the mechanism of TSST-1 penetration of mucosal tissue is incomplete. Our prior studies have shown that TSST-1 is more capable of penetrating rabbit vaginal mucosal tissue than SEC and SPE A (95). The reason for the difference is unclear. It has been shown that epithelial cells have the ability to transcytose SAgs (103), and it has been hypothesized that a dodecapeptide region (see Color Plate 1) mediates this effect. Clearly SEs cause vomiting and diarrhea when administered orally to monkeys (13). It has been suggested that this effect depends on SE penetration of mucosal tissue with subsequent stimulation of the vagus nerve (32). All of these studies suggest that mucosal tissue has the ability to bind to SAgs.

The cell type present in mucosal tissue in the highest concentration is the epithelial cell. Limited studies have been performed to study interaction of SAgs with such cell types. Our studies have investigated the ability of SAgs to bind to human vaginal epithelial cells (82). The basis for our studies was derived from the above-mentioned studies, but also prior work that suggested SAgs bind human epithelial and endothelial cells (52–54, 56, 82).

The recent study by Peterson et al. confirmed that human vaginal epithelial cells contain approximately 10^4 SAg receptors per cell (82). The ability of these cells to bind SAgs depended on a dodecapeptide of amino acids contained within all SAgs, though not of identical sequence. This dodecapeptide region was previously discussed by Arad et al. as important in T-cell superantigenicity (8–10). The dodecapeptide region is separated spatially from SAg domains required for MHC II and Vβ-TCR binding (Color Plate 1). The identity of the epithelial cell receptor for this dodecapeptide domain has not been elucidated but merits study. The consequence of the interaction has been studied, however.

TSST-1, SEB, and SPE A, as representative SAgs, interacted with the vaginal epithelial cell receptor to cause production of proinflammatory cytokines (82). It was hypothesized that this interaction leads to low-level, localized inflammation that opens the mucosal barrier to SAg penetration. Other staphylococcal exotoxins and exoenzymes may facilitate this process.

Clearly, additional studies are necessary to clarify all aspects of the interaction with mucosal and skin surfaces. These studies are likely to more fully define the extent of SAg involvement in human illnesses, and at the same time characterize the mechanism of SAg penetration of these surfaces.

Acknowledgments. This work was supported by U.S. Public Health Service research grants HL36611 and P20RR15587 from the National Heart, Lung, and Blood Institute and the National Center for Research Resources.

REFERENCES

1. **Abali, O., H. Nazik, K. Gurkan, E. Unuvar, M. Sidal, B. Ongen, F. Oguz, and U. Tuzun.** 2006. Group A beta hemolytic streptococcal infections and obsessive-compulsive symptoms in a Turkish pediatric population. *Psychiatry Clin. Neurosci.* **60:**103–105.

2. **Acharya, K. R., E. F. Passalacqua, E. Y. Jones, K. Harlos, D. I. Stuart, R. D. Brehm, and H. S. Tranter.** 1994. Structural basis of superantigen action inferred from crystal structure of toxic-shock syndrome toxin-1. *Nature* **367:**94–97.

3. **Alber, G., D. K. Hammer, and B. Fleischer.** 1990. Relationship between enterotoxic- and T lymphocyte-stimulating activity of staphylococcal enterotoxin B. *J. Immunol.* **144:**4501–4506.

4. **Alber, G., P. H. Scheuber, B. Reck, B. Sailer-Kramer, A. Hartmann, and D. K. Hammer.** 1989. Role of substance P in immediate-type skin reactions induced by staphylococcal enterotoxin B in unsensitized monkeys. *J. Allergy Clin. Immunol.* **84:**880–885.

5. **Anonymous.** 1993. CDC defines group A streptococcal toxic shock syndrome. *Am. Fam. Physician* **47:**1643–1644.

6. **Anonymous.** 1999. From the Centers for Disease Control and Prevention. Four pediatric deaths from community-acquired methicillin-resistant *Staphylococcus aureus*—Minnesota and North Dakota, 1997–1999. *JAMA* **282:**1123–1125.

7. **Anonymous.** 2003. Methicillin-resistant *Staphylococcus aureus* infections in correctional facilities—Georgia, California, and Texas, 2001–2003. *Morb. Mortal. Wkly. Rep.* **52:**992–996.

8. **Arad, G., D. Hillman, R. Levy, and R. Kaempfer.** 2004. Broad-spectrum immunity against superantigens is elicited in mice protected from lethal shock by a superantigen antagonist peptide. *Immunol. Lett.* **91:**141–145.

9. **Arad, G., D. Hillman, R. Levy, and R. Kaempfer.** 2001. Superantigen antagonist blocks Th1 cytokine gene induction and lethal shock. *J. Leukoc. Biol.* **69:**921–927.

10. **Arad, G., R. Levy, D. Hillman, and R. Kaempfer.** 2000. Superantigen antagonist protects against lethal shock and defines a new domain for T-cell activation. *Nat. Med.* **6:**414–421.

11. **Assimacopoulos, A. P., J. A. Stoehr, and P. M. Schlievert.** 1997. Mitogenic factors from group G streptococci associated with scarlet fever and streptococcal toxic shock syndrome. *Adv. Exp. Med. Biol.* **418:**109–114.

12. **Baker, B. S., S. Bokth, A. Powles, J. J. Garioch, H. Lewis, H. Valdimarsson, and L. Fry.** 1993. Group A streptococcal antigen-specific T lymphocytes in guttate psoriatic lesions. *Br. J. Dermatol.* **128:**493–499.

13. **Bergdoll, M. S.** 1988. Monkey feeding test for staphylococcal enterotoxin. *Methods Enzymol.* **165:**324–333.

14. **Bergdoll, M. S., B. A. Crass, R. F. Reiser, R. N. Robbins, and J. P. Davis.** 1981. A new staphylococcal enterotoxin, enterotoxin F, associated with toxic-shock-syndrome *Staphylococcus aureus* isolates. *Lancet* **1:**1017–1021.

15. **Bernstein, J. M., M. Ballow, P. M. Schlievert, G. Rich, C. Allen, and D. Dryja.** 2003. A superantigen hypothesis for the pathogenesis of chronic hyperplastic sinusitis with massive nasal polyposis. *Am. J. Rhinol.* **17:**321–326.

16. **Blomster-Hautamaa, D. A., B. N. Kreiswirth, J. S. Kornblum, R. P. Novick, and P. M. Schlievert.** 1986. The nucleotide and partial amino acid sequence of toxic shock syndrome toxin-1. *J. Biol. Chem.* **261:**15783–15786.

17. **Bohach, G. A., D. J. Fast, R. D. Nelson, and P. M. Schlievert.** 1990. Staphylococcal and streptococcal pyrogenic toxins involved in toxic shock syndrome and related illnesses. *Crit. Rev. Microbiol.* **17:**251–272.

18. **Choi, Y., J. A. Lafferty, J. R. Clements, J. K. Todd, E. W. Gelfand, J. Kappler, P. Marrack, and B. L. Kotzin.** 1990. Selective expansion of T cells expressing V beta 2 in toxic shock syndrome. *J. Exp. Med.* **172:**981–984.

19. **Cole, B. C.** 1991. The immunobiology of *Mycoplasma arthritidis* and its superantigen MAM. *Curr. Top. Microbiol. Immunol.* **174:**107–119.

20. **Cole, B. C., and C. L. Atkin.** 1991. The *Mycoplasma arthritidis* T-cell mitogen, MAM: a model superantigen. *Immunol. Today* **12:**271–276.

21. **Cone, L. A., D. R. Woodard, R. G. Byrd, K. Schulz, S. M. Kopp, and P. M. Schlievert.** 1992. A recalcitrant, erythematous, desquamating disorder associated with toxin-producing staphylococci in patients with AIDS. *J. Infect. Dis.* **165:**638–643.

22. **Cone, L. A., D. R. Woodard, P. M. Schlievert, and G. S. Tomory.** 1987. Clinical and bacteriologic observations of a toxic shock-like syndrome due to *Streptococcus pyogenes*. *N. Engl. J. Med.* **317:**146–149.

23. **Dale, R. C.** 2005. Post-streptococcal autoimmune disorders of the central nervous system. *Dev. Med. Child Neurol.* **47:**785–791.

24. **Dale, R. C., I. Heyman, G. Giovannoni, and A. W. Church.** 2005. Incidence of anti-brain antibodies in children with obsessive-compulsive disorder. *Br. J. Psychiatry* **187:**314–319.

25. **Daum, R. S., T. Ito, K. Hiramatsu, F. Hussain, K. Mongkolrattanothai, M. Jamklang, and S. Boyle-Vavra.** 2002. A novel methicillin-resistance cassette in community-acquired methicillin-resistant *Staphylococcus aureus* isolates of diverse genetic backgrounds. *J. Infect. Dis.* **186:**1344–1347.

26. **Davis, C. C., M. J. Kremer, P. M. Schlievert, and C. A. Squier.** 2003. Penetration of toxic shock syndrome toxin-1 across porcine vaginal mucosa ex vivo: permeability characteristics, toxin distribution, and tissue damage. *Am. J. Obstet. Gynecol.* **189:**1785–1791.

27. **Davis, J. P., P. J. Chesney, P. J. Wand, and M. LaVenture.** 1980. Toxic-shock syndrome: epidemiologic features, recurrence, risk factors, and prevention. *N. Engl. J. Med.* **303:**1429–1435.

28. **Dinges, M. M., J. Jessurun, and P. M. Schlievert.** 1998. Comparisons of mouse and rabbit models of toxic shock syndrome. *Int. Congr. Symp. Ser.* **229:**167–168.

29. **Dinges, M. M., and P. M. Schlievert.** 2001. Comparative analysis of lipopolysaccharide-induced tumor necrosis factor alpha activity in serum and lethality in mice and rabbits pretreated with the staphylococcal superantigen toxic shock syndrome toxin 1. *Infect. Immun.* **69:**7169–7172.

30. **England, R. J., D. R. Strachan, and L. C. Knight.** 1997. Streptococcal tonsillitis and its association with psoriasis: a review. *Clin. Otolaryngol. Allied Sci.* **22:**532–535.

31. **Giantonio, B. J., R. K. Alpaugh, J. Schultz, C. McAleer, D. W. Newton, B. Shannon, Y. Guedez, M. Kotb, L. Vitek, R. Persson, P. O. Gunnarsson, T. Kalland, M. Dohlsten, B. Persson, and L. M. Weiner.** 1997. Superantigen-based immunotherapy: a phase I trial of PNU-214565, a monoclonal antibody-staphylococcal enterotoxin A recombinant fusion protein, in advanced pancreatic and colorectal cancer. *J. Clin. Oncol.* **15:**1994–2007.

32. **Hamad, A. R., P. Marrack, and J. W. Kappler.** 1997. Transcytosis of staphylococcal superantigen toxins. *J. Exp. Med.* **185:**1447–1454.

33. **Harris, T. O., D. Grossman, J. W. Kappler, P. Marrack, R. R. Rich, and M. J. Betley.** 1993. Lack of complete correlation between emetic and T-cell-stimulatory activities of staphylococcal enterotoxins. *Infect. Immun.* **61:**3175–3183.

34. **Hasegawa, T., K. Torii, S. Hashikawa, Y. Iinuma, and M. Ohta.** 2002. Cloning and characterization of two novel DNases from *Streptococcus pyogenes. Arch. Microbiol.* **177:**451–456.

35. **Herz, U., R. Ruckert, K. Wollenhaupt, T. Tschernig, U. Neuhaus-Steinmetz, R. Pabst, and H. Renz.** 1999. Airway exposure to bacterial superantigen (SEB) induces lymphocyte-dependent airway inflammation associated with increased airway responsiveness—a model for non-allergic asthma. *Eur. J. Immunol.* **29:** 1021–1031.

36. **Hirooka, E. Y., E. E. Muller, J. C. Freitas, E. Vicente, Y. Yoshimoto, and M. S. Bergdoll.** 1988. Enterotoxigenicity of *Staphylococcus intermedius* of canine origin. *Int. J. Food Microbiol.* **7:**185–191.

37. **Hofer, M. F., R. J. Harbeck, P. M. Schlievert, and D. Y. Leung.** 1999. Staphylococcal toxins augment specific IgE responses by atopic patients exposed to allergen. *J. Invest. Dermatol.* **112:**171–176.

38. **Hofer, M. F., M. R. Lester, P. M. Schlievert, and D. Y. Leung.** 1995. Upregulation of IgE synthesis by staphylococcal toxic shock syndrome toxin-1 in peripheral blood mononuclear cells from patients with atopic dermatitis. *Clin. Exp. Allergy* **25:**1218–1227.

39. **Hovde, C. J., J. C. Marr, M. L. Hoffmann, S. P. Hackett, Y. I. Chi, K. K. Crum, D. L. Stevens, C. V. Stauffacher, and G. A. Bohach.** 1994. Investigation of the role of the disulphide bond in the activity and structure of staphylococcal enterotoxin C1. *Mol. Microbiol.* **13:**897–909.

40. **Igwe, E. I., P. L. Shewmaker, R. R. Facklam, M. M. Farley, C. van Beneden, and B. Beall.** 2003. Identification of superantigen genes speM, ssa, and smeZ in invasive strains of beta-hemolytic group C and G streptococci recovered from humans. *FEMS Microbiol. Lett.* **229:**259–264.

41. **Iwasaki, M., H. Igarashi, Y. Hinuma, and T. Yutsudo.** 1993. Cloning, characterization and overexpression of a *Streptococcus pyogenes* gene encoding a new type of mitogenic factor. *FEBS Lett.* **331:**187–192.

42. **Jablonski, L. M., and G.A. Bohach.** 2001. *Staphylococcus aureus*, p. 410–434. *In* M. D. L. Beuchat and T. Montville (ed.), *Fundamental of Food Microbiology.* ASM Press, Washington, D.C.

43. **Jackow, C. M., J. C. Cather, V. Hearne, A. T. Asano, J. M. Musser, and M. Duvic.** 1997. Association of erythrodermic cutaneous T-cell lymphoma, superantigen-positive *Staphylococcus aureus*, and oligoclonal T-cell receptor V beta gene expansion. *Blood* **89:**32–40. (Erratum, **89:**3496.)

44. **Kent, T. H.** 1966. Staphylococcal enterotoxin gastroenteritis in rhesus monkeys. *Am. J. Pathol.* **48:**387–407.

45. **Kim, J., R. G. Urban, J. L. Strominger, and D. C. Wiley.** 1994. Toxic shock syndrome toxin-1 complexed with a class II major histocompatibility molecule HLA-DR1. *Science* **266:**1870–1874.

46. **Kim, S. W., J. E. Grant, S. I. Kim, T. A. Swanson, G. A. Bernstein, W. B. Jaszcz, K. A. Williams, and P. M. Schlievert.** 2004. A possible association of recurrent streptococcal infections and acute onset of obsessive-compulsive disorder. *J. Neuropsychiatry Clin. Neurosci.* **16:**252–260.

47. **Komisar, J., J. Rivera, A. Vega, and J. Tseng.** 1992. Effects of staphylococcal enterotoxin B on rodent mast cells. *Infect. Immun.* **60:**2969–2975.

48. **Kotb, M., A. Norrby-Teglund, A. McGeer, H. El-Sherbini, M. T. Dorak, A. Khurshid, K. Green, J. Peeples, J. Wade, G. Thomson, B. Schwartz, and D. E. Low.** 2002. An immunogenetic and molecular basis for differences in outcomes of invasive group A streptococcal infections. *Nat. Med.* **8:**1398–1404.

49. **Kotzin, B. L., D. Y. Leung, J. Kappler, and P. Marrack.** 1993. Superantigens and their potential role in human disease. *Adv. Immunol.* **54:**99–166.

50. **Kravitz, G., D. J. Dries, M. L. Peterson, and P. M. Schlievert.** 2005. Purpura fulminans due to *Staphylococcus aureus. Clin. Infect. Dis.* **40:**941–947.

51. **Kuroda, M., T. Ohta, I. Uchiyama, T. Baba, H. Yuzawa, I. Kobayashi, L. Cui, A. Oguchi, K. Aoki, Y. Nagai, J. Lian, T. Ito, M. Kanamori, H. Matsumaru, A. Maruyama, H. Murakami, A. Hosoyama,**

Y. Mizutani-Ui, N. K. Takahashi, T. Sawano, R. Inoue, C. Kaito, K. Sekimizu, H. Hirakawa, S. Kuhara, S. Goto, J. Yabuzaki, M. Kanehisa, A. Yamashita, K. Oshima, K. Furuya, C. Yoshino, T. Shiba, M. Hattori, N. Ogasawara, H. Hayashi, and K. Hiramatsu. 2001. Whole genome sequencing of meticillin-resistant *Staphylococcus aureus. Lancet* **357:**1225–1240.

52. **Kushnaryov, V. M., M. S. Bergdoll, H. S. MacDonald, J. Vellinga, and R. Reiser.** 1984. Study of staphylococcal toxic shock syndrome toxin in human epithelial cell culture. *J. Infect. Dis.* **150:**535–545.

53. **Kushnaryov, V. M., H. S. MacDonald, R. Reiser, and M. S. Bergdoll.** 1984. Staphylococcal toxic shock toxin specifically binds to cultured human epithelial cells and is rapidly internalized. *Infect. Immun.* **45:**566–571.

54. **Kushnaryov, V. M., H. S. MacDonald, R. F. Reiser, and M. S. Bergdoll.** 1989. Reaction of toxic shock syndrome toxin 1 with endothelium of human umbilical cord vein. *Rev. Infect. Dis.* **11**(Suppl. 1)**:**S282–S287.

55. **Lee, P. K., B. N. Kreiswirth, J. R. Deringer, S. J. Projan, W. Eisner, B. L. Smith, E. Carlson, R. P. Novick, and P. M. Schlievert.** 1992. Nucleotide sequences and biologic properties of toxic shock syndrome toxin 1 from ovine- and bovine-associated *Staphylococcus aureus. J. Infect. Dis.* **165:**1056–1063.

56. **Lee, P. K., G. M. Vercellotti, J. R. Deringer, and P. M. Schlievert.** 1991. Effects of staphylococcal toxic shock syndrome toxin 1 on aortic endothelial cells. *J. Infect. Dis.* **164:**711–719.

57. **Leung, D. Y., H. C. Meissner, D. R. Fulton, D. L. Murray, B. L. Kotzin, and P. M. Schlievert.** 1993. Toxic shock syndrome toxin-secreting *Staphylococcus aureus* in Kawasaki syndrome. *Lancet* **342:**1385–1388.

58. **Leung, D. Y., H. C. Meissner, S. T. Shulman, W. H. Mason, M. A. Gerber, M. P. Glode, B. L. Myones, J. G. Wheeler, R. Ruthazer, and P. M. Schlievert.** 2002. Prevalence of superantigen-secreting bacteria in patients with Kawasaki disease. *J. Pediatr.* **140:**742–746.

59. **Leung, D. Y., J. B. Travers, R. Giorno, D. A. Norris, R. Skinner, J. Aelion, L. V. Kazemi, M. H. Kim, A. E. Trumble, M. Kotb, et al.** 1995. Evidence for a streptococcal superantigen-driven process in acute guttate psoriasis. *J. Clin. Invest.* **96:**2106–2112.

60. **Li, H., A. Llera, D. Tsuchiya, L. Leder, X. Ysern, P. M. Schlievert, K. Karjalainen, and R. A. Mariuzza.** 1998. Three-dimensional structure of the complex between a T cell receptor beta chain and the superantigen staphylococcal enterotoxin B. *Immunity* **9:**807–816.

61. **Lina, G., G. A. Bohach, S. P. Nair, K. Hiramatsu, E. Jouvin-Marche, and R. Mariuzza.** 2004. Standard nomenclature for the superantigens expressed by Staphylococcus. *J. Infect. Dis.* **189:**2334–2336.

62. **Lindsay, J.** 1996. Infectious agents and sudden infant death syndrome (SIDS): an update. *Mol. Med. Today* **2:**94–95.

63. **Lowy, F. D.** 1998. *Staphylococcus aureus* infections. *N. Engl. J. Med.* **339:**520–532.

64. **MacDonald, K. L., M. T. Osterholm, C. W. Hedberg, C. G. Schrock, G. F. Peterson, J. M. Jentzen, S. A. Leonard, and P. M. Schlievert.** 1987. Toxic shock syndrome. A newly recognized complication of influenza and influenzalike illness. *JAMA* **257:**1053–1058.

65. **Malchiodi, E. L., E. Eisenstein, B. A. Fields, D. H. Ohlendorf, P. M. Schlievert, K. Karjalainen, and R. A. Mariuzza.** 1995. Superantigen binding to a T cell receptor beta chain of known three-dimensional structure. *J. Exp. Med.* **182:**1833–1845.

66. **Manders, S. M., W. R. Heymann, E. Atillasoy, J. Kleeman, and P. M. Schlievert.** 1996. Recurrent toxin-mediated perineal erythema. *Arch. Dermatol.* **132:**57–60.

67. **Marrack, P., and J. Kappler.** 1990. The staphylococcal enterotoxins and their relatives. *Science* **248:**705–711.

68. **Marrack, P., E. Kushnir, and J. Kappler.** 1991. A maternally inherited superantigen encoded by a mammary tumour virus. *Nature* **349:**524–526.

69. **McCormick, J. K., and P. M. Schlievert.** 2006. Toxins and superantigens of group A streptococci, p. 47–58. *In* V. A. Fischetti, R. P. Novick, J. J. Ferretti, D. A. Portnoy, and J. I. Rood (ed.), *Gram-Positive Pathogens.* American Society for Microbiology, Washington, D.C.

70. **McCormick, J. K., T. J. Tripp, A. S. Llera, E. J. Sundberg, M. M. Dinges, R. A. Mariuzza, and P. M. Schlievert.** 2003. Functional analysis of the TCR binding domain of toxic shock syndrome toxin-1 predicts further diversity in MHC class II/superantigen/TCR ternary complexes. *J. Immunol.* **171:**1385–1392.

71. **McCormick, J. K., J. M. Yarwood, and P. M. Schlievert.** 2001. Toxic shock syndrome and bacterial superantigens: an update. *Annu. Rev. Microbiol.* **55:**77–104.

72. **Mitchell, D. T., D. G. Levitt, P. M. Schlievert, and D. H. Ohlendorf.** 2000. Structural evidence for the evolution of pyrogenic toxin superantigens. *J. Mol. Evol.* **51:**520–531.

73. **Newbould, M. J., J. Malam, J. M. McIllmurray, J. A. Morris, D. R. Telford, and A. J. Barson.** 1989. Immunohistological localisation of staphylococcal toxic shock syndrome toxin (TSST-1) antigen in sudden infant death syndrome. *J. Clin. Pathol.* **42:**935–939.

74. **Norrby-Teglund, A., D. Newton, M. Kotb, S. E. Holm, and M. Norgren.** 1994. Superantigenic properties of the group A streptococcal exotoxin SpeF (MF). *Infect. Immun.* **62:**5227–5233.

75. **Novick, R. P.** 2000. Pathogenicity factors and their regulation., p. 392–407. *In* R. P. Novick, V. A. Fischetti, J. J. Ferretti, D. A. Portnoy, and J. I. Rood (ed.), *Gram-Positive Pathogens.* ASM Press, Washington, D.C.

76. **Orwin, P. M., J. R. Fitzgerald, D. Y. Leung, J. A. Gutierrez, G. A. Bohach, and P. M. Schlievert.** 2003. Characterization of Staphylococcus aureus enterotoxin L. *Infect. Immun.* **71:**2916–2919.

77. **Orwin, P. M., D. Y. Leung, H. L. Donahue, R. P. Novick, and P. M. Schlievert.** 2001. Biochemical and biological properties of staphylococcal enterotoxin K. *Infect. Immun.* **69:**360–366.

78. **Orwin, P. M., D. Y. Leung, T. J. Tripp, G. A. Bohach, C. A. Earhart, D. H. Ohlendorf, and P. M. Schlievert.** 2002. Characterization of a novel staphylococcal enterotoxin-like superantigen, a member of the group V subfamily of pyrogenic toxins. *Biochemistry* **41:**14033–14040.

79. **Osterholm, M. T., J. P. Davis, R. W. Gibson, J. S. Mandel, L. A. Wintermeyer, C. M. Helms, J. C. Forfang, J. Rondeau, and J. M. Vergeront.** 1982. Tri-state toxic-state syndrome study. I. Epidemiologic findings. *J. Infect. Dis.* **145:**431–440.

80. **Parsonnet, J., M. A. Hansmann, M. L. Delaney, P. A. Modern, A. M. Dubois, W. Wieland-Alter, K. W. Wissemann, J. E. Wild, M. B. Jones, J. L. Seymour, and A. B. Onderdonk.** 2005. Prevalence of toxic shock syndrome toxin 1-producing *Staphylococcus aureus* and the presence of antibodies to this superantigen in menstruating women. *J. Clin. Microbiol.* **43:**4628–4634.

81. **Patrizi, A., A. M. Costa, L. Fiorillo, and I. Neri.** 1994. Perianal streptococcal dermatitis associated with guttate psoriasis and/or balanoposthitis: a study of five cases. *Pediatr. Dermatol.* **11:**168–171.

82. **Peterson, M., K. Ault, M. J. Kremer, A. J. Klingelhutz, C. C. Davis, C. A. Squier, and Schlievert, P. M.** 2005. Innate immune system is activated by stimulation of vaginal epithelial cells with *Staphylococcus aureus* and toxic shock syndrome toxin-1. *Infect. Immun.* **73:**2164–2174.

83. **Prasad, G. S., C. A. Earhart, D. L. Murray, R. P. Novick, P. M. Schlievert, and D. H. Ohlendorf.** 1993. Structure of toxic shock syndrome toxin 1. *Biochemistry* **32:**13761–13766.

84. **Proft, T., P. D. Webb, V. Handley, and J. D. Fraser.** 2003. Two novel superantigens found in both group A and group C Streptococcus. *Infect. Immun.* **71:**1361–1369.

85. **Reingold, A. L., N. T. Hargrett, B. B. Dan, K. N. Shands, B. Y. Strickland, and C. V. Broome.** 1982. Nonmenstrual toxic shock syndrome: a review of 130 cases. *Ann. Intern. Med.* **96:**871–874.

86. **Sachse, S., P. Seidel, D. Gerlach, E. Gunther, J. Rodel, E. Straube, and K. H. Schmidt.** 2002. Superantigen-like gene(s) in human pathogenic *Streptococcus dysgalactiae,* subsp. *equisimilis*: genomic localisation of the gene encoding streptococcal pyrogenic exotoxin G (*speG(dys)*). *FEMS Immunol. Med. Microbiol.* **34:** 159–167.

87. **Scherer, M. T., L. Ignatowicz, G. M. Winslow, J. W. Kappler, and P. Marrack.** 1993. Superantigens: bacterial and viral proteins that manipulate the immune system. *Annu. Rev. Cell Biol.* **9:**101–128.

88. **Schiffenbauer, J., H. M. Johnson, E. J. Butfiloski, L. Wegrzyn, and J. M. Soos.** 1993. Staphylococcal enterotoxins can reactivate experimental allergic encephalomyelitis. *Proc. Natl. Acad. Sci. USA* **90:**8543–8546.

89. **Schiffenbauer, J., J. Soos, and H. Johnson.** 1998. The possible role of bacterial superantigens in the pathogenesis of autoimmune disorders. *Immunol. Today* **19:**117–120.

90. **Schlievert, P. M.** 1986. Staphylococcal enterotoxin B and toxic-shock syndrome toxin-1 are significantly associated with non-menstrual TSS. *Lancet* **1:**1149–1150.

91. **Schlievert, P. M., K. M. Bettin, and D. W. Watson.** 1978. Effect of antipyretics on group A streptococcal pyrogenic exotoxin fever production and ability to enhance lethal endotoxin shock. *Proc. Soc. Exp. Biol. Med.* **157:**472–475.

92. **Schlievert, P. M., K. M. Bettin, and D. W. Watson.** 1979. Production of pyrogenic exotoxin by groups of streptococci: association with group A. *J. Infect. Dis.* **140:**676–681.

93. **Schlievert, P. M., K. M. Bettin, and D. W. Watson.** 1979. Reinterpretation of the Dick test: role of group A streptococcal pyrogenic exotoxin. *Infect. Immun.* **26:**467–472.

94. **Schlievert, P. M., and D. A. Blomster.** 1983. Production of staphylococcal pyrogenic exotoxin type C: influence of physical and chemical factors. *J. Infect. Dis.* **147:**236–242.

95. **Schlievert, P. M., L. M. Jablonski, M. Roggiani, I. Sadler, S. Callantine, D. T. Mitchell, D. H. Ohlendorf, and G. A. Bohach.** 2000. Pyrogenic toxin superantigen site specificity in toxic shock syndrome and food poisoning in animals. *Infect. Immun.* **68:**3630–3634.

96. **Schlievert, P. M., M. Y. Kotb, and D. L. Stevens.** 2000. Streptococcal superantigens: streptococcal toxic shock syndrome. *In* M. W. Cunningham and R. S. Fujinami (ed.), *Effects of Microbes on the Immune System.* Lippincott Williams & Wilkins, Philadelphia, Pa.

97. **Schlievert, P. M., M. T. Osterholm, J. A. Kelly, and R. D. Nishimura.** 1982. Toxin and enzyme characterization of Staphylococcus aureus isolates from patients with and without toxic shock syndrome. *Ann. Intern. Med.* **96:**937–940.

98. **Schlievert, P. M., K. N. Shands, B. B. Dan, G. P. Schmid, and R. D. Nishimura.** 1981. Identification and characterization of an exotoxin from *Staphylococcus aureus* associated with toxic-shock syndrome. *J. Infect. Dis.* **143:**509–516.

99. **Schlievert, P. M., T. J. Tripp, and M. L. Peterson.** 2004. Reemergence of staphylococcal toxic shock syndrome in Minneapolis-St. Paul, Minnesota, during the 2000–2003 surveillance period. *J. Clin. Microbiol.* **42:**2875–2876.

100. **Schlievert, P. M., and D. W. Watson.** 1979. Biogenic amine involvement in pyrogenicity and enhancement of lethal endotoxin shock by group A streptococcal pyrogenic exotoxin. *Proc. Soc. Exp. Biol. Med.* **162:**269–274.

101. **Schlievert, P. M., and D. W. Watson.** 1978. Group A streptococcal pyrogenic exotoxin: pyrogenicity, alteration of blood-brain barrier, and separation of sites for pyrogenicity and enhancement of lethal endotoxin shock. *Infect. Immun.* **21:**753–763.

102. **Shands, K. N., G. P. Schmid, B. B. Dan, D. Blum, R. J. Guidotti, N. T. Hargrett, R. L. Anderson, D. L. Hill, C. V. Broome, J. D. Band, and D. W. Fraser.** 1980. Toxic-shock syndrome in menstruating women: association with tampon use and *Staphylococcus aureus* and clinical features in 52 cases. *N. Engl. J. Med.* **303:**1436–1442.

103. **Shupp, J. W., M. Jett, and C. H. Pontzer.** 2002. Identification of a transcytosis epitope on staphylococcal enterotoxins. *Infect. Immun.* **70:**2178–2186.

104. **Smoot, L. M., J. K. McCormick, J. C. Smoot, N. P. Hoe, I. Strickland, R. L. Cole, K. D. Barbian, C. A. Earhart, D. H. Ohlendorf, L. G. Veasy, H. R. Hill, D. Y. Leung, P. M. Schlievert, and J. M. Musser.** 2002. Characterization of two novel pyrogenic toxin superantigens made by an acute rheumatic fever clone of *Streptococcus pyogenes* associated with multiple disease outbreaks. *Infect. Immun.* **70:**7095–7104.

105. **Sriskandan, S., M. Unnikrishnan, T. Krausz, and J. Cohen.** 2000. Mitogenic factor (MF) is the major DNase of serotype M89 *Streptococcus pyogenes*. *Microbiology* **146**(Pt 11)**:**2785–2792.

106. **Stevens, D. L., M. H. Tanner, J. Winship, R. Swarts, K. M. Ries, P. M. Schlievert, and E. Kaplan.** 1989. Severe group A streptococcal infections associated with a toxic shock-like syndrome and scarlet fever toxin A. *N. Engl. J. Med.* **321:**1–7.

107. **Stuart, P. M., R. K. Munn, E. DeMoll, and J. G. Woodward.** 1995. Characterization of human T-cell responses to Yersinia enterocolitica superantigen. *Hum. Immunol.* **43:**269–275.

108. **Sugiyama, H., and T. Hayama.** 1965. Abdominal viscera as site of emetic action from staphylococcal enterotoxin in the monkey. *J. Infect. Dis.* **115:**330–336.

109. **Sundberg, E. J., H. Li, A. S. Llera, J. K. McCormick, J. Tormo, P. M. Schlievert, K. Karjalainen, and R. A. Mariuzza.** 2002. Structures of two streptococcal superantigens bound to TCR beta chains reveal diversity in the architecture of T cell signaling complexes. *Structure* **10:**687–699.

110. **Swedo, S. E., and P. J. Grant.** 2005. Annotation: PANDAS: a model for human autoimmune disease. *J. Child Psychol. Psychiatry* **46:**227–234.

111. **Todd, J. K., F. A. Kapral, M. Fishaut, and T. R. Welch.** 1978. Toxic shock syndrome associated with phage group 1 staphylococci. *Lancet* **2:**1116–1118.

112. **Tomai, M. A., P. M. Schlievert, and M. Kotb.** 1992. Distinct T-cell receptor V beta gene usage by human T lymphocytes stimulated with the streptococcal pyrogenic exotoxins and pep M5 protein. *Infect. Immun.* **60:**701–705.

113. **Toyosaki, T., T. Yoshioka, Y. Tsuruta, T. Yutsudo, M. Iwasaki, and R. Suzuki.** 1996. Definition of the mitogenic factor (MF) as a novel streptococcal superantigen that is different from streptococcal pyrogenic exotoxins A, B, and C. *Eur. J. Immunol.* **26:**2693–2701.

114. **Uchiyama, T., T. Miyoshi-Akiyama, H. Kato, W. Fujimaki, K. Imanishi, and X. J. Yan.** 1993. Super-antigenic properties of a novel mitogenic substance produced by *Yersinia pseudotuberculosis* isolated from patients manifesting acute and systemic symptoms. *J. Immunol.* **151:**4407–4413.

115. **Vath, G. M., C. A. Earhart, J. V. Rago, M. H. Kim, G. A. Bohach, P. M. Schlievert, and D. H. Ohlen-dorf.** 1997. The structure of the superantigen exfoliative toxin A suggests a novel regulation as a serine pro-tease. *Biochemistry* **36:**1559–1566.

116. **Yutsudo, T., H. Murai, J. Gonzalez, T. Takao, Y. Shimonishi, Y. Takeda, H. Igarashi, and Y. Hinuma.** 1992. A new type of mitogenic factor produced by *Streptococcus pyogenes*. *FEBS Lett.* **308:**30–34.

Superantigens: Molecular Basis for Their Role in Human Diseases
Edited by Malak Kotb and John D. Fraser
© 2007 ASM Press, Washington, D.C.

Chapter 3

Mycoplasma arthritidis-Derived Superantigen (MAM), a Unique Class of Superantigen That Bridges Innate and Adaptive Immunity

Barry C. Cole and Hong-Hua Mu

INTRODUCTION

This review begins with an outline of the original observations that led to the discovery of *Mycoplasma arthritidis*-derived superantigen (MAM) and discusses the structural basis of its interaction with class II major histocompatibility complex (MHC) molecules and T-cell receptors (TCRs). Next, we review recent work from our laboratory on the interaction of MAM with Toll-like receptors and their importance in control of innate and adaptive immunity and in disease expression. Finally, we will revisit the issue of the potential role of MAM-like superantigens (SAgs) in autoimmune disease and how this might relate to recent findings on Toll-like receptor (TLR) control of adaptive immunity.

THE ORGANISM, *MYCOPLASMA ARTHRITIDIS*

The genus *Mycoplasma* is included in the family *Mycoplasmataceae*, a member of the *Mollicutes,* which is characterized by organisms that possess a limited genome resulting from successive deletions in the genome of their bacterial ancestors. The species of the genus *Mycoplasma* therefore depend on the cells of their animal hosts to provide essential nutrients, and growth in vitro requires complex media including animal serum that supplies cholesterol lipoproteins and other growth factors. The mycoplasmas are ubiquitous parasites or commensals of mammalian and other vertebrate hosts, in which they cause acute to chronic, often fatal diseases that can be difficult to treat. Many species exhibit a triad of syndromes ranging from musculoskeletal arthritides, pulmonary disease, and genitourinary syndromes (56). There are at least three established pathogens in humans: *Mycoplasma pneumoniae* is the cause of often chronic, primary atypical pneumonia. *Ureaplasma* (a related genus) *urealyticum* and *Mycoplasma hominis* are agents of postpartum

Barry C. Cole and Hong-Hua Mu • Division of Rheumatology, University of Utah School of Medicine, Salt Lake City, UT 84132.

fever, premature or low-weight births, urethritis, and prostatitis (48). Although my-coplasma species often occur as commensals, they are common secondary invaders espe-cially in the immunocompromised host causing an acute to chronic arthritis. *Mycoplasma arthritidis* is a pathogen of rodents causing acute to chronic arthritis, toxic shock, and a necrotizing fasciitis-like syndrome in specific genetically defined mouse and rat strains. These disease manifestations are strongly influenced by the interaction of the *M. arthri-tidis* SAg MAM with specific MHC alleles (TCR) (12).

EARLY WORK ON THE MAM SAg

The initial discovery of a unique mitogenic moiety in *M. arthritidis* was first made in 1977 (reviewed in reference 15) when it was shown that the organism could induce a lympho-cyte-mediated, cytotoxic reaction in murine cells that differed from the traditionial MHC-restricted specificity for expressed MHC alleles on fibroblasts. This observation was closely related to another observation in which the mitogenic potential of the organism and *M. arthritidis* culture supernatants (MAS) derived from them was dependent on specific MHC alleles (18). In both cases, cytotoxicity and mitogenicity were mediated by lympho-cytes that expressed $H-2^d$ or $H-2^k$ but not those expressing $H-2^b$. Inasmuch as the MHC re-striction seen was different from classical MHC restriction patterns for antigens and the lack of restriction seen for lectin mitogens, the observations indicated that MAS activated lymphocytes through a novel pathway. Subsequent studies using congenic and recombi-nant mice demonstrated that the active moiety in *M. arthritidis* was strongly dependent on the Ia 7 serological specificity, now known to be borne on the class II H-2Ea chain that is present in mice expressing $H-2^d$ (BALB/c) and $H-2^k$ (CBA) alleles but is absent in mice expressing $H-2^b$ (C57BL6). Shortly thereafter it was shown that the biologic activity could be removed from *M. arthritidis* supernatants by absorption with lymphocytes from mice expressing $H-2^k$ and $H-2^d$ but not from $H-2^b$ cells, thus providing the first evidence that MAM binds to H-2E molecules (17). Subsequent studies demonstrated that the moiety from *M. arthritidis* activated T cells and that activation by MAS, although dependent on accessory cells, did not require metabolic processing as for traditional antigens since for-malin-treated cells (14), L cells transfected with H-2E, and liposomes bearing H-2 E coated onto glass beads could present MAS to T cells (8), again indicating a physical asso-ciation of the active component with class II MHC molecules. Early studies also estab-lished that MAS could activate human T cells (30) and that the human HLA-DR molecule, the equivalent of murine H-2E, also presented MAM to human T cells almost as well as to murine T cells (70, 73). MAM was recognized by T cells through the Vβ-chain segments of the TCR (20) as for bacterial SAgs (86). Partial purification of the *M. arthritidis* mito-gen, now called MAM, was achieved in 1994 (5) and the molecule was sequenced in 1996 (21). *M. arthritidis* and MAM were also shown to be potent activators of macrophages (1, 31, 71), NK cells (32), and B cells (29, 82).

STRUCTURAL PROPERTIES AND INTERACTION
WITH CLASS II MHC MOLECULES

The MAM SAg, like other SAgs, forms an association with MHC molecules on antigen-presenting cells (APCs) and with T cells via their TCR Vβ-chains which leads to T-cell ac-tivation and production of inflammatory cytokines. However this trimolecular complex also impacts B-cell function by virtue of expressed MHC receptors on their cell surfaces. The derivation of the MAM sequence was an important first step in understanding the molecular basis of its interaction with both MHC and TCR molecules (21). It immediately became apparent that MAM was phylogenetically unrelated to any of the other known SAg classes, possibly explaining properties that make this molecule distinct from the pyrogenic staphylococcal and streptococcal SAgs. By using a series of overlapping synthetic peptides it was shown that MAM_{11-38} and MAM_{71-95} could interfere with the ability of the intact molecule to stimulate lymphocytes. The MAM_{11-38} peptide shared some short epitopes from other bacterial and endogenous viral SAgs (21), which were known to be associated with binding to class II HLA-DR or HLA-DQ molecules (44, 45). The MAM_{71-95} sequence contained the legume lectin motif that is thought to be responsible for T-cell activation stimulated by phytohemagglutinin (PHA) and concanavalin A (ConA) (21). Work by Bernatchez et al. (9) had suggested that MAM binding to class II MHC might be Zn^{2+} dependent and that the binding sites for MAM and SEA might be similar. It was confirmed that the N-terminal region of MAM played a role in binding to human HLA-DR but that a C-terminal region was responsible for TCR recognition. Further studies on MAM again showed that residues within the active N-terminal peptides (21) were responsible for MHC binding and that Zn^{2+} binding sites on MAM were involved and promoted dimer formation (34, 50, 51).

Although MAM preferentially utilizes the murine H-2Eα chain, which is highly conserved between different H-2E alleles, and is almost identical with the human HLA-DRα chain, both α- and β-chains of the murine H-2A molecules and the human HLA-DQ molecules are polymorphic. Through use of congenic, recombinant, and transgenic mice expressing different murine H-2A and human HLA-DQ alleles, but which lacked the H-2Eα or HLD-DRα chains, it was shown that the response to MAM was highly specific in that it activated cells from mice expressing H-2A[d, r, p or b] and HLA-DQw6 but not from H-2A[f, k, s or q] mice, and only weakly activated cells from HLA-DQw8 (24). Although SEA and SEB activated cells expressing all murine H-2A and human HLA-DQ alleles, the responses of cells from mice bearing only H-2A were very low and required 10^3-fold or higher concentrations of SAg as compared with MAM. In contrast, cells from mice expressing both human HLA-DQ alleles responded very highly to SEA and SEB.

An important advance in understanding the structure of MAM was made possible following analysis of the X-ray crystallographic structure of MAM complexed with class II HLA-DR molecules. MAM was found to possess a unique structure unlike other bacterial superantigens consisting of two α-helical domains that formed a novel fold. Also, two MAM molecules could cross-link two MHC molecules producing a dimerized MAM/MHC complex, confirming that MAM represented a new class of SAg (87).

INTERACTION WITH TCR MOLECULES

Early work established that MAM could activate both murine and human T cells and that the specific Vβ-chains of the TCR were responsible. As for other SAgs, MAM exhibited a characteristic pattern of T-cell receptor usage. Not unexpectedly, those human Vβ TCR chains that bore the most homology with the murine Vβ chains that were used by MAM were also used by their human counterparts (6, 36, 70). There was a clear hierarchical usage of these receptors (16). Thus, in Vβ[b] mice that express most of the known murine Vβ TCR chains, except those eliminated by somatic deletions due to endogenous MMTV

SAgs, MAM preferentially activated cells bearing Vβ 8.2, 8.1, and 8.3 chains, followed by Vβ 6 and Vβ 5.1. In mice of the Vβ^a haplotype that have genomic deletions of the Vβ 8 family and the Vβ 5.1 TCR, the percentage of T cells responding to Vβ 6 was markedly increased and evidence of usage of Vβ 1, Vβ 7, and Vβ 16 was now apparent. Finally, using Vβ^c mice that have genomic deletions of Vβ 5, 6, and the 8 family, MAM now preferentially utilized cells bearing the Vβ 7 chain followed by Vβ 1, and to a lesser degree by Vβ 4. These observations suggest that the MAM is a versatile molecule with an ability to adapt to the Vβ specificities displayed by its host. Subsequent studies indicated that the CDR3 region of the TCR also played a role in MAM-induced activation of T cells (40), and that Vα-chains and the Jβ region in combination with some Vβ-chains might also influence T-cell activation (70). These findings were found to be consistent with the recently proposed model for the MHC/MAM/TCR complex, resulting from crystallographic analysis of MAM-complexed HLA-DR (87). In addition, follow-up studies on the crystal structures of MAM-reactive versus MAM-non-reactive Vβ-chains suggested that the CDR2 and framework region 3 may also be involved in MAM/TCR binding (55). It was also found that there were significant differences in the structure of the Vβ domains, i.e., CDR1, CDR2, and framework region 3, in TCRs that recognized MAM versus those that did not.

MAM INTERACTIONS WITH INNATE AND ADAPTIVE IMMUNITY

Mouse Strain Specificity in the Adaptive Immune Response to MAM in Vivo

Very early work had established that the BALB/c mouse was relatively resistant to arthritis induced by *M. arthritidis* whereas the C3H mouse (substrain unknown) was susceptible (26). After recently confirming this using the C3H/HeJ and BALB/c strains (Fig. 1), studies were conducted to determine whether differences in susceptibility to *M. arthritidis* involved in vitro or in vivo cytokine profile responses to MAM. Splenocytes from naïve mice of both strains produced identical levels of both type 1 inflammatory cytokines (interleukin-2 [IL-2], gamma interferon [IFN-γ], tumor necrosis factor alpha [TNF-α]) and type 2 "protective" cytokines (IL-4, IL-6, IL-10) in response to MAM in vitro. However, the in vivo adaptive cytokine response to MAM was markedly different in BALB/c mice than in C3H/HeJ mice. Thus splenocytes from BALB/c mice injected intravenously (i.v.) with MAM, and challenged with MAM in vitro, after one to three days, exhibited a typical type 2 cytokine profile, whereas C3H/HeJ mouse splenocytes secreted an inflammatory type 1 cytokine profile (62). The change to a type 1 cytokine profile in C3H/HeJ mice was also associated with a marked increase in serum levels of IgG2a which is known to be enhanced by IFN-γ and which promotes antibody-dependent cytotoxicity. Since the BALB/c mouse (*lps^n*) is sometimes considered to be a type 2 mouse, i.e., it preferentially produces type 2 immune responses to various microbial agents by a mechanism involving high levels of endogenous glucocorticoids, or more recently a defect in the IL-12p40 receptor β2-chain (38), we considered that the high response in C3H/HeJ mice might be due to another mechanism, possibly the fact that this mouse has a mutation in the *lps^n* gene (*lps^d*) that confers hyporeactivity to lipopolysaccharide (LPS) (68). Thus, the experiments were repeated by comparing the adaptive immune response of splenocytes from MAM-injected wild-type C3H/HeSnJ mice (*lps^n*) with those from mutant C3H/HeJ (*lps^d*) mice rechallenged with MAM in vitro. This time, the cells from the C3H/HeSnJ wild-type *lps^n* mouse gave a type 2 cytokine adaptive response whereas again, those from the mutant *lps^d* mouse exhib-

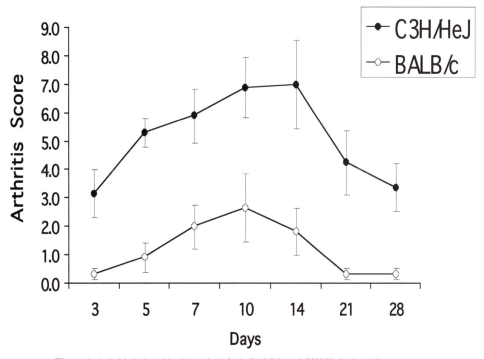

Figure 1. Arthritis induced by *M. arthritidis* in BALB/c and C3H/HeJ mice. Mice were injected i.v. with 1×10^8 CFU *M. arthritidis* and scored for arthritis as described for 28 days. Mean scores for BALB/c ($\circ$) and C3H/HeJ ($\bullet$) mice $\pm$SEM are shown. C3H/HeJ mice were significantly more susceptible at all time periods ($P < 0.002$). Reprinted from *Infection and Immunity* (62) with permission of the publisher.

ited a type 1 cytokine profile (Fig. 2). It was also demonstrated that the early innate response to MAM, as evidenced by induction of serum cytokines 90 minutes after i.v. injection, was also markedly different in lps^n versus lps^d mice in that C3H/HeSnJ sera again exhibited predominantly type 2 cytokines, whereas C3H/HeJ sera showed higher levels of type 1 cytokines (Fig. 3).

So, what is the relationship between the response of these mice to LPS and to MAM? It was shown in 1998 (68) that the lps^d mutation in the C3H/HeJ mouse is due to a single mutation that renders the lps^d mouse (C3H/HeJ) hyporesponsive to LPS-induced toxicity and to production of inflammatory cytokines. At first, it seemed paradoxical that cells from these same LPS-hyporesponsive mice could produce elevated inflammatory cytokines in response to MAM as compared with wild-type lps^n mice that respond normally to LPS. In contrast, lps^n mice were more resistant to disease induced by *M. arthritidis* and produced type 2 cytokines in response to MAM. We thus hypothesized that MAM could interact with TLR4 resulting in a differential outcome in immune responses in lps^n versus lps^d mice (63).

The cells of the innate immune system play an instrumental role not only in recognizing pathogen-associated molecular patterns on invading organisms sometimes resulting in a potent inflammatory response (58), but also in directing the subsequent adaptive immune

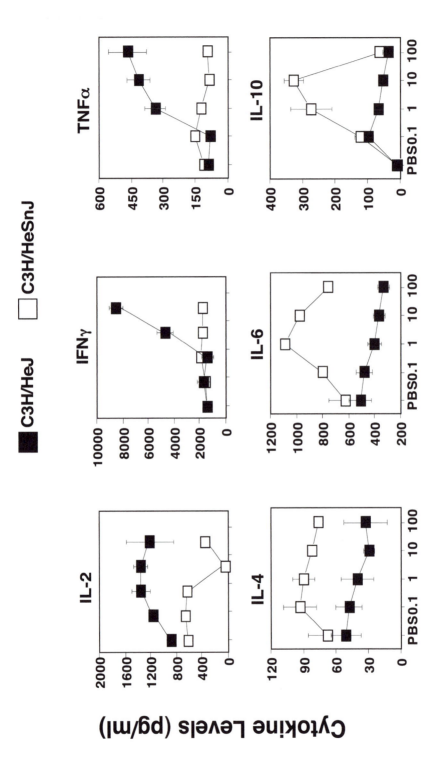

Figure 2. Inducible cytokines in cells from MAM-injected mice 3 days postinjection. Splenocytes (10^7 cells/ml) from C3H/HeJ and C3H/HeSnJ mice injected 72 hours previously with MAM (0.1 to 100 ng/mouse) were rechallenged in vitro with a second dose of MAM (1 ng/ml) for an additional 24 h. Inducible cytokines (IL-2, IFN-γ, TNF-α, IL-4, -6 and -10) were analyzed by ELISA. Splenocytes from three to five mice were included in each experiment for each specific dose point; the data shown are representative of three different experiments. Reprinted from *Infection and Immunity* (63) with permission of the publisher.

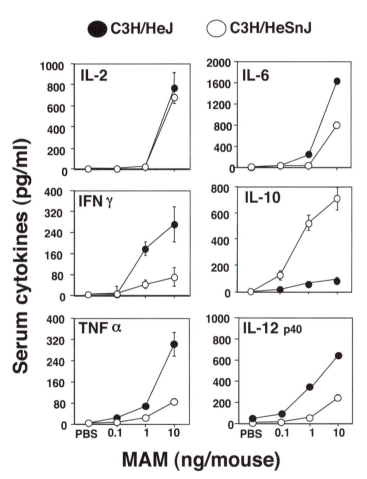

Figure 3. Early serum cytokines induced by MAM in C3H/HeSnJ and C3H/HeJ mice. Mice were injected i.v. with diluent PBS and MAM at doses of 0.1, 1, or 10 ng/mouse. After 90 minutes, mice were exsanguinated under anesthesia and the sera were collected for cytokine assays for IL-2, IL-6, IFN-γ, IL-10, TNF-α, and IL-12p40. Sera from three to five mice were assayed in each experiment for each specific dose point. Similar results were seen in three repeat experiments. Reprinted from *Infection and Immunity* (63) with permission of the publisher.

response, thus selecting the signaling pathways that ultimately determine disease outcome (59). The Toll-like receptors (TLRs) on cells of the innate immune system are mammalian homologues of Toll (68), a type 1 transmembrane receptor that was first described in *Drosophila* (3). The specificity of different TLRs in mediating responses to diverse microbial and endogenous ligands activates signaling pathways that trigger the release of cytokines and up-regulation of costimulatory molecules that influence the nature of the adaptive immune response. Many microbial lipoproteins can activate macrophages and dendritic cells (DCs) via TLR2 in collaboration with TLR1 or TLR6 thus resulting in an inflammatory response (80); other ligands such as some LPS species can utilize TLR4 (10), which can lead to severe endotoxemia.

Our findings described above on the differential adaptive immune responses of cells from MAM-injected C3H/HeSnJ (lps^n) and C3H/HeJ (lps^d) mice provided indirect evidence that MAM might interact with TLRs. Several earlier and recent studies had established that *M. arthritidis* and MAM were capable of activating both human and murine macrophages and monocytes (31, 63, 71). More direct evidence for a MAM/TLR interaction was recently documented (61) by showing that treatment of RAW 264.7 monocytic cells (TLR2+/4+) with MAM resulted in up-regulation of both TLR2 and TLR4. Similar results were obtained by using macrophages from C3H/HeSnJ mice (TLR2+4+), whereas macrophages from TLR4-defective C3H/HeJ mice expressed a much greater increase in TLR2 and, as expected, no increase in TLR4 (Fig. 4). The marked increase in TLR2 ex-

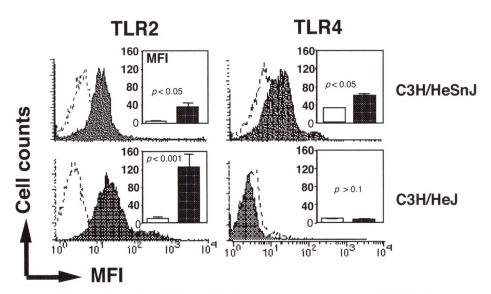

Figure 4. Expression of TLR2 and TLR4 by macrophages in response to MAM. Peritoneal macrophages from C3H/HeSnJ (TLR2$^{+/+}$/TLR4$^{+/+}$) and C3H/HeJ (TLR2$^{+/+}$/TLR4$^{-/-}$) were treated with MAM (100 ng/ml) or NS for 18 h and then stained and analyzed for expression of TLR2 and TLR4. Flow cytometry was conducted, as before, for the expression of both TLR2 and TLR4. Insertions are the mean results of mean fluorescence intensity (MFI) ± SEM of three experiments. Reprinted from *Cellular Microbiology* (61) with permission of the publisher.

pression was also associated with elevated levels of IL-12p40 release from MAM-treated cells. In addition, antibody to both TLR2 and TLR4 partially inhibited the response of RAW 264.7 cells to MAM, but a combination of antibodies completely inhibited all responses. By testing the ability of MAM to activate peritoneal macrophages from mutant C3H/HeJ (TLR2+/4−), C3H/HeJ, TLR2 KO (TLR2−/4−), C3H/HeN (TLR2+4+) and C3H/HeN, TLR2 KO (TLR2−/4+) mice, we demonstrated that MAM-induced macrophage activation occurred in the absence of TLR2 and in the absence of TLR4, but not when both were absent. The results confirmed that unlike most microbial TLR agonists, MAM could utilize both TLR2 and TLR4 (61).

The finding that, in the absence of TLR4, macrophages treated with MAM expressed more TLR2 and had elevated inflammatory cytokine levels suggested that TLR4 might cross-regulate TLR2. This was, in fact, found to be the case since blockade of TLR4 on C3H/HeN mice (TLR2+/4+) with anti-TLR4 antibody resulted in a marked increase both in expression of TLR2 and in production of IL-12p40, a molecule that promotes type 1 inflammatory adaptive immune responses (Fig. 5). Also, macrophages from C3H/HeN TLR2 KO mice failed to produce IL-12p40 in response to MAM. The results of all of these studies indicate that the presence of TLR4 down-regulates TLR2 expression and function in innate cells treated with MAM. In contrast, TLR4 alone, or together with TLR2, leads to production of IL-10, a promoter of type 2 adaptive responses. Thus, TLR4 appears to play a major role in maintaining homeostasis by reducing the induction of proinflammatory cytokines and possibly also in alleviating inflammatory disease by down-regulation of TLR2 expression and function as proposed previously (63).

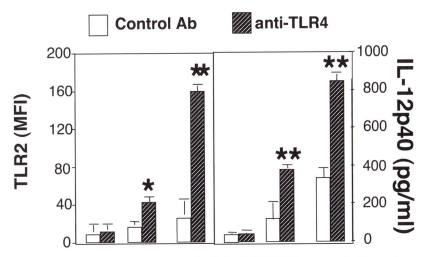

Figure 5. Regulation of TLR2 and IL-12p40 by MAM/TLR4 interaction. Resident peritoneal macrophages from C3H/HeN mice were pretreated with anti-mouse TLR4 (20 µg/ml) for 2 h. MAM (1 and 10 ng/ml, final concentration) was then added, followed by incubation for a further 18 h. Surface expression of TLR2 by macrophages was analyzed by flow cytometric analysis and the culture supernatants were assessed for IL-12p40. The data are the mean ±SEM for three experiments (*$P < 0.05$; **$P < 0.01$). Each experiment contained cells pooled from three to five mice. Reprinted from *Cellular Microbiology* (61) with permission of the publisher.

MAM-Induced Regulation of B7-1 and B7-2 Is Mediated through TLRs

Antigen-induced activation of T cells leading to cytokine production and proliferation requires signals delivered by APC, i.e., macrophages or DCs, through costimulatory molecules such as B7-1 (CD80) and B7-2 (CD86) that are related membrane-bound molecules. Both act as ligands for CD28 on T-cell surfaces and deliver the signals required for activation of resting T cells (53). Studies have suggested that both B7-1 and B7-2 appear to deliver equivalent functional costimulatory signals in vitro since they are similar in their ability to induce T-cell proliferation as well as IL-2 production (52, 54). However, other evidence indicates that the functional outcome of B7-1- and B7-2-mediated signaling appears to be distinct (27, 35, 49, 67). Inasmuch as MAM can differentially interact with TLR2 and TLR4, resulting in either type 1 or type 2 immune responses, the question arises whether MAM/TLR interactions can influence B7-1 or B7-2 expression and/or function. Injections of MAM into mice expressing only TLR2 (C3H/HeJ) up-regulated expression of B7-1 but not B7-2 on peritoneal adherent cells and resulted in elevated secretion of IFN-γ. In contrast, B7-1 expression was lower on cells from C3H/HeSnJ mice, and a marked increase in the type 2 cytokine, IL-10, was observed. Thus these findings suggest an important role for TLR expression in cytokine selection via B7-1 versus B7-2. The downstream importance of B7-1 and B7-2 on innate cells in directing adaptive immune responses to MAM was also clearly demonstrated. Thus, treatment of C3H/HeJ (TLR2+/4−) mice with antibody to B7-1 prior to injection of MAM changed the type 1 cytokine response to in vitro challenge of splenocytes to MAM to a type 2 cytokine profile, whereas antibody to B7-2, or control antibody, was without effect (Fig. 6). Furthermore, the controlling role of MAM/TLR interactions in this process was again demonstrated in that cells from mice expressing TLR2+/4+ similarly injected with anti-B7-1 and MAM exhibited a shift from a weak neutral cytokine profile to a predominantly type 1 cytokine profile (Fig. 6).

Is Class II MHC a Coreceptor for MAM Signaling through TLR?

Numerous studies have clearly established that MAM, in its role as a typical SAg, binds to select MHC molecules which then present it to T cells, thus initiating a chain of events that leads to an acute inflammatory response, enhanced humoral immunity, and precipitation of autoimmune disease (see below). However, MAM has other unique attributes in that it is the only SAg that has been shown, to date, to interact directly with Toll-like receptors. A key question therefore is whether the diverse interactions between MAM and specific class II MHC alleles can modify the MAM, TLR, and TCR interactions. TLR4 agonists such as LPS are known to require CD14 as a coreceptor, whereas microbial lipoproteins that typically use TLR2 require instead an association with either TLR6 or diacylated lipopeptides such as MALP-2 derived from *Mycoplasma fermentans* (81). However, triacylated lipopeptides such as Pam3-Cys-Ser-(Lys)4, the synthetic bacterial lipopeptide analogue from *Escherichia coli*, require TLR1 as well as TLR2 and also need CD-14. MAM which utilizes both TLR2 and TLR4 does not require CD14 as a coreceptor (61). MAM cannot activate CHO cells transfected with either TLR2 or TLR4 in combination with CD14 as evidenced by failure to up-regulate CD25, an indicator molecule for TLR activation through NFκB; this is in contrast with MALP-2, which activates CHO cells bearing only TLR2 with CD14, and with lipid A (the active LPS moiety), which activates CHO cells

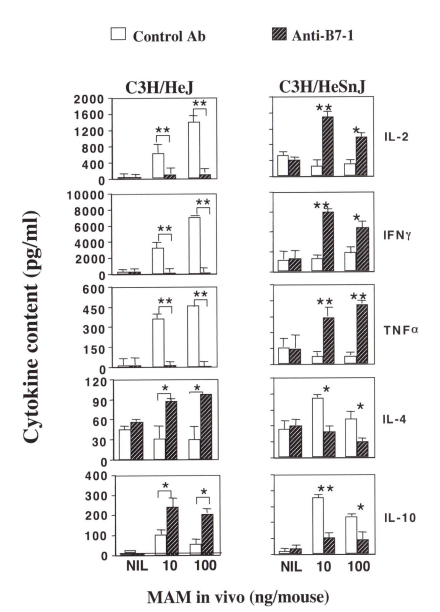

Figure 6. Effect of in vivo treatment with anti-B7-1 antibody on inducible cytokine pro-files induced in cells from MAM-injected mice. Mice were injected with varying doses of MAM after treatment with anti-B7-1 or isotype-matched anti-mouse antibody (250 μg of each mAb per mouse, respectively) on two separate occasions. Twenty-four hours after MAM injection, splenocytes (10^7 cells/ml) were isolated and rechallenged in vitro with MAM (2.5 ng/ml) and culture supernatants were assayed for cytokines IL-2, IFN-γ, TNF-α, IL-4, and IL-10. The data shown are pooled from three different experiments (*$P <$ 0.05; **$P <$ 0.01). Reprinted from *Cellular Microbiology* (60) with permission of the pub-lisher.

bearing only TLR4 and CD14. Furthermore MAM is unable to activate either splenic cells (using IL-2 induction) or macrophages (using TNF-α induction) in cells from SJL mice (TLR2+/TLR4+) which lack H-2E and possess a MAM nonresponsive H-2A allele (24, 61). As depicted in Fig. 7, we propose therefore, that MAM can cross-link MHC with either TLR2 or TLR4 leading to an MyD88-dependent type 1 inflammatory cytokine response with TLR2 or an MyD88-independent type 2 cytokine response with TLR4; the latter differs from the inflammatory MyD88-dependent pathway mediated by LPS through TLR4 and may reflect different coreceptor usage. The mechanism(s) involved in MAM/TLR4 suppression of MAM/TLR-2-mediated inflammatory responses remain(s) to be determined.

In view of the demonstrated allelic specificity of MAM for MHC molecules it is also tempting to project that these polymorphisms may influence the outcome of the MAM/TLR interactions. Our recent findings on differential cytokine profiles to MAM in mice carrying different human MHC alleles provide support for this idea (see section on MAM and autoimmunity). In this event, MHC participation in agonist/TLR interactions may introduce a whole new level of complexity into the specificity and selectivity of innate immune responses.

INTERACTION OF OTHER SUPERANTIGENS WITH TLRs

In preliminary studies, we failed to find evidence that SEA or SEB could differentially influence cytokine profiles in lps^n versus lps^d mice, but evidence was obtained for up-regulation of macrophage and DC cell surface markers (H.-H. Mu and B. C. Cole, unpublished observations, 2000 and 2005). Many different TLR agonists including MAM can cause up-regulation of TLRs on macrophage and DC cell surfaces prior to activation and release of inflammatory and regulatory cytokines. Muraille et al. (65) reported that bacterial SAgs could cause maturation of DC in vivo by a T-cell-dependent mechanism. It is also known that SAgs can synergize with LPS resulting in often fatal toxic effects (11). Rossi et al. (72) also reported that preinjecting mice with SEA or SEB primed DCs to produce higher levels of TNF-α and IL-12p40 when exposed to LPS, a TLR4 agonist. This effect was also T cell dependent and was probably mediated by production of IFN-γ or other cytokines that are known to up-regulate cell surface markers on DC. Other investigators have shown that LPS stimulation of antigen-specific T cells through TLR4 promotes T-cell survival, clonal expansion, and differentiation into memory cells (57). In another study, it was recently reported that streptococcal and staphylococcal SAgs could up-regulate TLR4 expression on human monocytes by ligation of class II MHC and in so doing enhanced the proinflammatory cytokine responses to LPS (42). These synergistic effects occurred at low toxin levels that would be expected during a natural infection. In addition, unlike the murine model of toxic shock induced by bacterial SAgs, neither IFN-γ nor T cells were required for synergy (42). Thus, the ability of SAgs to augment the responses of innate immune cells to their TLR agonists is only one of the mechanisms by which SAgs contribute to disease.

ROLE OF MAM IN DISEASE INDUCED BY *M. ARTHRITIDIS*

MAM by itself does not induce overt clinical disease except when injected locally into rodent joints resulting in a transient inflammatory response, indicating that disease induced by *M. arthritidis* requires additional pathogenetic moieties. Other factors known

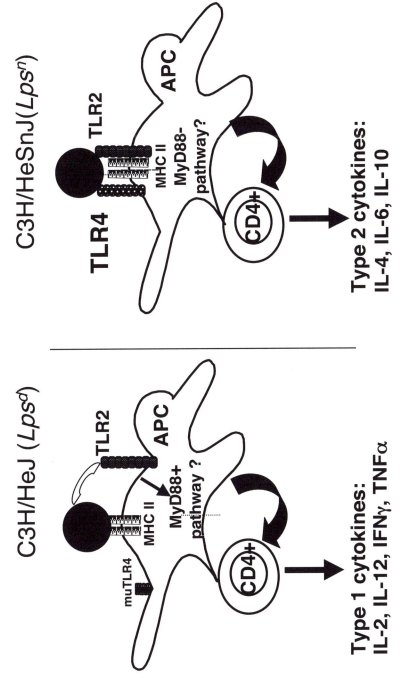

Figure 7. Proposed models for MAM selection of cytokine profiles triggered through different TLRs.

to contribute to *M. arthritidis* disease include the Maa1 and Maa2 phase-variable adhesins, the MAV-1 virus (83–85) and recently a TLR2-utilizing, macrophage- and DC-activating lipoprotein present on the cell membrane that induces proinflammatory cytokines both in vitro and in vivo (22). MAM, however, can influence disease outcome mediated by live *M. arthritidis*, and by itself can profoundly change the immune status of the host as described above, even triggering autoimmune disease (see section below). The role of MAM in susceptibility to toxic shock and necrotizing fasciitis induced by *M. arthritidis* in mice was first established by using various inbred and congenic mice that differentially expressed the highly conserved α-chain of the murine H-2E molecule that is preferentially utilized by MAM. Thus, mice that fail to express H-2E exhibited significantly less severe disease (23, 25).

The first indication that TLRs might be involved in disease susceptibility, as well as in MAM activation of innate cells, was in our finding that C3H/HeJ mice, which have a defective TLR4 molecule, were much more susceptible to toxic shock and arthritis induced by *M. arthritidis* than were wild-type C3H/HeSnJ or C3H/HeN mice (TLR2+/4+) (63). These results correlated closely with the ability of MAM to induce a type 1 adaptive cytokine response in the TLR2+/4− mice, but a type 2 response in TLR2+/4+ mice. Also, the ability of TLR4 to down-regulate the proinflammatory MAM/TLR2 function in vivo suggests that the presence of TLR4 may protect against disease. The second observation was that antibody to B7-1 suppressed disease caused by *M. arthritidis* and changed in vivo responses both to MAM and to live *M. arthritidis* from a type 1 to a type 2 cytokine profile. There was also evidence that antibody to B7-2 increased disease severity induced by *M. arthritidis* (60). Furthermore, as summarized in Table 1, the use of inbred mice and mouse strains with various deletions of TLR2 and TLR4 has established that mice lacking TLR2 are less susceptible to disease than those possessing TLR2 and TLR4 and that no disease is seen when both TLRs are absent. Thus, a strong correlation exists between MAM-induced innate and adaptive immune response in vivo and the ability of *M. arthritidis* to cause disease in mice differentially expressing TLR2 and TLR4.

MAM AND AUTOIMMUNITY

The ability of SAgs to activate a high proportion of specific SAg-reactive T-cell clones and also to act as polyclonal B-cell activators led to the suggestion that they might be candidates for the triggering of autoimmune disease (37, 46, 47, 69, 74, 76). Friedman and col-

Table 1. Disease caused by *M. arthritidis*

Mouse strain	TLR2	TLR4	Toxicity	Arthritis	Adaptive cytokine profile	
					MAM	LPS
C3H/HeJ	+[a]	−	+++	+++	type 1	type 2
C3H/HeSnJ	+	+	+	+	type 2	type 1
C3H/HeN	+	+	+	+	type 2	type 1
C3H/HeJ.TLR2−/−	−	−	−	−	none	none
C3H/HeN.TLR2−/−	−	+	−	−	type 2	NT

[a]For TLR2 and TLR4, +, present; −, absent. For toxicity and arthritis, +, mild; +++, severe; −, absent.

leagues found that MAM was able to effectively cross-link B cells with T cells, resulting in a polyclonal B-cell activation of human peripheral lymphocytes with secretion of large amounts of immunoglobulin G (IgG) and IgM (29). It was postulated that this interaction between T-helper cells and B cells could ultimately lead to an increase in antibodies to multiple antigens and, in particular, to multivalent self-antigens such as DNA as is seen in lupus erythematosus (37). Subsequent findings described below in mice and humans continue to support the notion that SAgs might indeed play a role autoimmune disease.

Triggering and Exacerbation of Murine Collagen-Induced Arthritis (CIA)

Work by David and colleagues on CIA, which is induced in susceptible mouse strains (i.e., the B10RIII mouse, H-2^r) by two immunizations with type II collagen, had established that joint inflammation was associated with the presence of T cells in arthritic joints that bore the TCR Vβ 6, 7, and 8 chains (7, 39). In addition, it was shown that MAM could clonally expand T-cell subsets bearing these same Vβ-chains in vitro and/or as in vivo in the CIA-susceptible B10.RIIIS (H-2^r) mouse. To determine whether MAM could influence CIA by expanding collagen-reactive T cells, mice that had largely recovered from CIA 4 to 6 months after previous immunization with collagen developed a flare in disease just 3 days after i.v. injection with MAM (19). Mice that had initially failed to develop CIA now developed arthritis. In addition, mice suboptimally immunized against collagen, and which also did not develop arthritis, exhibited disease when challenged with MAM. Mice injected with SEB, albeit in high doses, which also utilizes the Vβ 8 gene family, developed enhanced arthritis, whereas SEA, which utilizes neither Vβ 8 nor Vβ 6 chains, failed to influence disease. The results suggest that the enhanced arthritis in collagen-immunized mice mediated by MAM or SEB was due to activation of collagen-specific, Vβ-bearing T cells rather than by a nonspecific effect as would have occurred with the SEA SAg. In addition, the increase in antibody to collagen in MAM-activated CIA also suggested a role for B cells in arthritis development as has been proposed for the CIA model of autoimmunity (78). This would be consistent with other observations that clearly indicate the ability of MAM to initiate a T-cell-dependent polyclonal activation of B cells (82).

Role of SAgs in Human Autoimmune Disease

As reviewed previously (47, 69, 74, 76) many investigators have found evidence that T cells expressing certain Vβ-chains are enriched in synovial tissues from patients with rheumatoid arthritis (RA). Of particular interest was the finding of Paliard et al. (66), who reported that human Vβ 14 was decreased in the peripheral circulation but was increased in synovial fluid. Also Howell et al. (43) reported that activated T cells from synovial tissues exhibited an increase in those expressing Vβ 14 as well as Vβ 3 and Vβ 17. The human Vβ 3 and Vβ 14 are the equivalent of murine Vβ 7 and Vβ 8, and human Vβ 17 is related to murine Vβ 6. Thus, similar Vβ polymorphisms may be involved in both murine CIA and human RA. Of relevance is that MAM activates both human and murine T cells bearing all of these Vβ-chains (6, 16, 36, 70). In view of these observations, a search for antibodies against SAgs in the sera from humans suffering from a variety of rheumatic autoimmune diseases was undertaken. Antibodies to MAM were significantly elevated in patients with RA as compared with healthy individuals or patients exhibiting systemic lupus erythematosus, ankylosing spondylitis, psoriatic arthritis, or Reiter's syndrome. However, there was no difference between anti-MAM antibodies in the sera of RF+ versus RF-RA patients. Antibodies to SEB which also utilizes human Vβ 14 were also elevated in sera from both RA and lupus patients whereas antibodies to SEA, which activates T cells expressing different Vβ-chains, were not significantly elevated over those seen in the control individuals.

The significance of these observations is hard to assess because other reports fail to implicate the same Vβ-chains in RA. Also, different sources of tissues and methodologies have been used confounding a reliable analysis. Despite the ability of MAM to activate those T cells that bear CIA-reactive and RA-associated Vβ-chains and the ability of MAM to activate CIA, it is not clear why human RA patients should specifically express antibodies to a SAg of murine origin. One possibility is that there might be a MAM-like SAg present in an as-yet unidentified human mycoplasma species that is capable of invading the joint. However, in view of the ability of numerous mycoplasma species to cause acute to chronic joint disease in many animals, the idea has persisted that these organisms might play a role in the human arthritides, especially in RA. Although human mycoplasma species are one of the most common agents of serious joint infections in immunocompromised individuals (79), evidence linking these organisms to human RA has been conflicting (13, 41, 75).

A recent observation that has relevance to the potential role of MAM-like SAgs in human RA is that in preliminary studies transgenic mice bearing the HLA-DR and HLA-DQ alleles that predispose to RA develop a type 1 adaptive cytokine profile in response to MAM, whereas cells from MAM-injected mice bearing those alleles that protect against RA develop a type 2 cytokine profile (B. C. Cole, H.-H. Mu, and C. S. David, manuscript in preparation). These observations, if confirmed, clearly imply that allelic differences in human MHC class II genes also influence cytokine profiles in response to MAM representing yet another potential link between MAM and human autoimmune disease and possibly confirming a role for MHC molecules in influencing MAM control of innate and adaptive immunity through an interaction with TLRs.

What is the relevance for human disease of our finding that mice expressing a TLR4 mutation develop an increased inflammatory response to *M. arthritidis*? There is increasing evidence that TLRs might also influence the susceptibility of humans to infectious and inflammatory disease (2, 77) since polymorphisms in human TLR4 have been shown to be associated with endotoxin hyporesponsiveness (4) and susceptibility to septic shock induced by gram-negative organisms (28). The involvement of TLRs in artherosclerosis is also being reported (33, 64). In addition, the protective role of a functional TLR4 receptor on TLR2-mediated inflammation as seen in the mouse model with MAM may also have relevance to understanding the processes that protect the normal human host from inflammatory disease.

CONCLUDING REMARKS

The sequence data on the MAM SAg clearly indicate that it is phylogenetically unrelated to any of the other SAgs and recent crystallograhic studies on the structure showing a MAM dimer complexed with two class II MHC HLA-DR molecules confirm its novel structure and its being representative of a new class of SAg. MAM, to date, is the only known SAg to interact with TLRs (2 and 4) and with MHC molecules; these interactions through costimulatory molecules may profoundly influence the subsequent direction of the adaptive immune response and resulting disease expression in hosts infected with *M. arthritidis*. Future elucidation of the role of cross-talk between MAM/TLR2 and MAM/TLR4 interactions with the other virulence factors of this organism is likely to greatly enhance our understanding of microbial-mediated inflammatory disease.

Since *M. arthritidis* is a natural pathogen of rodents, the experimental model is particularly valuable to study these issues. The marked selectivity of MAM for specific MHC alleles, T-cell receptor chains, TLRs, and costimulatory molecules, as well as the availability of mice differentially expressing these molecules, will allow study of the signal transduction pathways which determine the outcome of these interactions. On a final note, we believe that due to the less effective interaction of the SAgs derived from bacteria of human origin with murine cells, caution should be expressed in the applicability of the latter findings to the human situation.

Acknowledgments. The work cited in this chapter was supported by grants AI 12103 and AR 02255 from the National Institutes of Health, Bethesda, MD, and by grants from the Nora Eccles Treadwell Foundation. B.C.C. is the Nora Eccles Harrison Professor in Rheumatology.

REFERENCES

1. **al-Daccak, R., K. Mehindate, J. Hebert, L. Rink, S. Mecheri, and W. Mourad.** 1994. *Mycoplasma arthritidis*-derived superantigen induces proinflammatory monokine gene expression in the THP-1 human monocytic cell line. *Infect. Immun.* **62:**2409–2416.

2. **Anders, H. J., D. Zecher, R. D. Pawar, and P. S. Patole.** 2005. Molecular mechanisms of autoimmunity triggered by microbial infection. *Arthritis Res. Ther.* **7:**215–224.

3. **Anderson, K. V., L. Bokla, and C. Nusslein-Volhard.** 1985. Establishment of dorsal-ventral polarity in the Drosophila embryo: the induction of polarity by the Toll gene product. *Cell* **42:**791–798.

4. **Arbour, N. C., E. Lorenz, B. C. Schutte, J. Zabner, J. N. Kline, M. Jones, K. Frees, J. L. Watt, and D. A. Schwartz.** 2000. TLR4 mutations are associated with endotoxin hyporesponsiveness in humans. *Nat. Genet.* **25:**187–191.

5. **Atkin, C. L., S. Wei, and B. C. Cole.** 1994. The Mycoplasma arthritidis superantigen MAM: purification and identification of an active peptide. *Infect. Immun.* **62:**5367–5375.

6. **Baccala, R., L. R. Smith, M. Vestberg, P. A. Peterson, B. C. Cole, and A. N. Theofilopoulos.** 1992. *Mycoplasma arthritidis* mitogen. Vβ engaged in mice, rats, and humans, and requirement of HLA-DRα for presentation. *Arthritis Rheum.* **35:**434–442.

7. **Banerjee, S., T. M. Haqqi, H. S. Luthra, J. M. Stuart, and C. S. David.** 1988. Possible role of Vβ T cell receptor genes in susceptibility to collagen-induced arthritis in mice. *J. Exp. Med.* **167:**832–839.

8. **Bekoff, M. C., B. C. Cole, and H. M. Grey.** 1987. Studies on the mechanism of stimulation of T cells by the *Mycoplasma arthritidis*-derived mitogen. Role of class II IE molecules. *J. Immunol.* **139:**3189–3194.

9. **Bernatchez, C., R. Al-Daccak, P. E. Mayer, K. Mehindate, L. Rink, S. Mecheri, and W. Mourad.** 1997. Functional analysis of Mycoplasma arthritidis-derived mitogen interactions with class II molecules. *Infect. Immun.* **65:**2000–2005.

10. **Beutler, B.** 2000. Tlr4: central component of the sole mammalian LPS sensor. *Curr. Opin. Immunol.* **12:**20–26.

11. **Blank, C., A. Luz, S. Bendigs, A. Erdmann, H. Wagner, and K. Heeg.** 1997. Superantigen and endotoxin synergize in the induction of lethal shock. *Eur. J. Immunol.* **27:**825–833.

12. **Cole, B. C.** 1991. The immunobiology of *Mycoplasma arthritidis* and its superantigen MAM. *Curr. Top. Microbiol. Immunol.* **174:**107–119.

13. **Cole, B. C.** 1999. Mycoplasma-induced arthritis in animals: relevance to understanding the etiologies of the human rheumatic diseases. *Rev. Rhum. Engl. Ed.* **66:**45S–49S.

14. **Cole, B. C., B. A. Araneo, and G. J. Sullivan.** 1986. Stimulation of mouse lymphocytes by a mitogen derived from *Mycoplasma arthritidis*. IV. Murine T hybridoma cells exhibit differential accessory cell requirements for activation by *M. arthritidis* T cell mitogen, concanavalin A, or egg-white lysozyme. *J. Immunol.* **136:**3572–3578.

15. **Cole, B. C., and C. L. Atkin.** 1991. The Mycoplasma arthritidis T-cell mitogen, MAM: a model superantigen. *Immunol. Today* **12:**271–276.

16. **Cole, B. C., R. A. Balderas, E. A. Ahmed, D. Kono, and A. N. Theofilopoulos.** 1993. Genomic composition and allelic polymorphisms influence V beta usage by the Mycoplasma arthritidis superantigen. *J. Immunol.* **150:**3291–3299.

17. **Cole, B. C., R. A. Daynes, and J. R. Ward.** 1982. Stimulation of mouse lymphocytes by a mitogen derived from *Mycoplasma arthritidis* III. Ir gene control of lymphocyte transformation correlates with binding of the mitogen to specific IA bearing cells. *J. Immunol.* **129:**1352–1359.

18. **Cole, B. C., R. A. Daynes, and J. R. Ward.** 1981. Stimulation of mouse lymphocytes by a mitogen derived from Mycoplasma arthritidis. I. Transformation is associated with an H-2-linked gene that maps to the I-E/I-C subregion. *J. Immunol.* **127:**1931–1936.

19. **Cole, B. C., and M. M. Griffiths.** 1993. Triggering and exacerbation of autoimmune arthritis by the *Mycoplasma arthritidis* superantigen MAM. *Arthritis Rheum.* **36:**994–1002.

20. **Cole, B. C., D. R. Kartchner, and D. J. Wells.** 1989. Stimulation of mouse lymphocytes by a mitogen derived from Mycoplasma arthritidis. VII. Responsiveness is associated with expression of a product(s) of the V beta 8 gene family present on the T cell receptor alpha/beta for antigen. *J. Immunol.* **142:**4131–4137.

21. **Cole, B. C., K. L. Knudtson, A. Oliphant, A. D. Sawitzke, A. Pole, M. Manohar, L. S. Benson, E. Ahmed, and C. L. Atkin.** 1996. The sequence of the Mycoplasma arthritidis superantigen, MAM: Identification of functional domains and comparison with microbial superantigens and plant lectin mitogens. *J. Exp. Med.* **183:**1105–1110.

22. **Cole, B. C., H. H. Mu, N. D. Pennock, A. Hasebe, F. V. Chan, L. R. Washburn, and M. R. Peltier.** 2005. Isolation and partial purification of macrophage- and dendritic cell-activating components from Mycoplasma arthritidis: association with organism virulence and involvement with Toll-like receptor 2. *Infect. Immun.* **73:**6039–6047.

23. **Cole, B. C., M. W. Piepkorn, and E. C. Wright.** 1985. Influence of genes of the major histocompatibility complex on ulcerative dermal necrosis induced in mice by *Mycoplasma arthritidis*. *J. Invest. Dermatol.* **85:**357–361.

24. **Cole, B. C., A. D. Sawitzke, E. A. Ahmed, C. L. Atkin, and C. S. David.** 1997. Allelic polymorphisms at the H-2A and HLA-DQ loci influence the response of murine lymphocytes to the Mycoplasma arthritidis superantigen MAM. *Infect. Immun.* **65:**4190–4198.

25. **Cole, B. C., R. N. Thorpe, L. A. Hassell, and J. R. Ward.** 1983. Toxicity but not arthritogenicity of *Mycoplasma arthritidis* for mice associates with the haplotype expressed at the major histocompatibility complex. *Infect. Immun.* **41:**1010–1015.

26. **Cole, B. C., J. R. Ward, and L. Golightly-Rowland.** 1973. Factors influencing the susceptibility of mice to Mycoplasma arthritidis. *Infect. Immun.* **7:**218–225.

27. **Collins, A. V., D. W. Brodie, R. J. Gilbert, A. Iaboni, R. Manso-Sancho, B. Walse, D. I. Stuart, P. A. van der Merwe, and S. J. Davis.** 2002. The interaction properties of costimulatory molecules revisited. *Immunity* **17:**201–210.

28. **Cook, D. N., D. S. Pisetsky, and D. A. Schwartz.** 2004. Toll-like receptors in the pathogenesis of human disease. *Nat. Immunol.* **5:**975–979.

29. **Crow, M. K., G. Zagon, Z. Chu, B. Ravina, J. R. Tumang, B. C. Cole, and S. M. Friedman.** 1992. Human B cell differentiation induced by microbial superantigens: unselected peripheral blood lymphocytes secrete polyclonal immunoglobulin in response to Mycoplasma arthritidis mitogen. *Autoimmunity* **14:**23–32.

30. **Daynes, R. A., J. M. Novak, and B. C. Cole.** 1982. Comparison of the cellular requirements for human T cell transformation by a soluble mitogen derived from Mycoplasma arthritidis and concanavalin A. *J. Immunol.* **129:**936–938.

31. **Dietz, J. N., and B. C. Cole.** 1982. Direct activation of the J774.1 murine macrophage cell line by *Mycoplasma arthritidis*. *Infect. Immun.* **37:**811–819.

32. **D'Orazio, J. A., B. C. Cole, and J. Stein-Streilein.** 1996. Mycoplasma arthritidis mitogen Up-regulates human NK cell activity. *Infect. Immun.* **64:**441–447.

33. **Edfeldt, K., J. Swedenborg, G. K. Hansson, and Z. Q. Yan.** 2002. Expression of toll-like receptors in human atherosclerotic lesions: a possible pathway for plaque activation. *Circulation* **105:**1158–1161.

34. **Etongue-Mayer, P., M. A. Langlois, M. Ouellette, H. Li, S. Younes, R. Al-Daccak, and W. Mourad.** 2002. Involvement of zinc in the binding of Mycoplasma arthritidis-derived mitogen to the proximity of the HLA-DR binding groove regardless of histidine 81 of the beta chain. *Eur. J. Immunol.* **32:**50–58.

35. **Freeman, G. J., V. A. Boussiotis, A. Anumanthan, G. M. Bernstein, X. Y. Ke, P. D. Rennert, G. S. Gray, J. G. Gribben, and L. M. Nadler.** 1995. B7-1 and B7-2 do not deliver identical costimulatory signals, since B7-2 but not B7-1 preferentially costimulates the initial production of IL-4. *Immunity* **2:**523–532.

36. **Friedman, S. M., M. K. Crow, J. R. Tumang, M. Tumang, Y. Q. Xu, A. S. Hodtsev, B. C. Cole, and D. N. Posnett.** 1991. Characterization of human T cells reactive with the *Mycoplasma arthritidis*-derived superantigen (MAM): generation of a monoclonal antibody against Vβ7, the T cell receptor gene product expressed by a large fraction of MAM-reactive human T cells. *J. Exp. Med.* **174:**891–900.

37. **Friedman, S. M., D. N. Posnett, J. R. Tumang, B. C. Cole, and M. K. Crow.** 1991. A potential role for microbial superantigens in the pathogenesis of systemic autoimmune disease. *Arthritis Rheum.* **34:**468–480.

38. **Guler, M. L., N. G. Jacobson, U. Gubler, and K. M. Murphy.** 1997. T cell genetic background determines maintenance of IL-12 signaling: effects on BALB/c and B10.D2 T helper cell type 1 phenotype development. *J. Immunol.* **159:**1767–1774.

39. **Haqqi, T. M., G. D. Anderson, S. Banerjee, and C. S. David.** 1992. Restricted heterogeneity in T-cell antigen receptor Vβ gene useage in the lymph nodes and arthritic joints of mice. *Proc. Natl. Acad. Sci. USA* **89:**1253–1255.

40. **Hodtsev, A. S., Y. Choi, E. Spanopoulou, and D. Posnett.** 1998. Mycoplasma superantigen is a CDR3-dependent ligand for the T cell antigen receptor. *J. Exp. Med.* **187:**319–327.

41. **Hoffman, R. W., F. X. O'Sullivan, K. R. Schafermeyer, T. L. Moore, D. Roussell, R. Watson-McKown, M. F. Kim, and K. S. Wise.** 1997. Mycoplasma infection and rheumatoid arthritis: analysis of their relationship using immunoblotting and an ultrasensitive polymerase chain reaction detection method. *Arthritis Rheum.* **40:**1219–1228.

42. **Hopkins, P. A., J. D. Fraser, A. C. Pridmore, H. H. Russell, R. C. Read, and S. Sriskandan.** 2005. Superantigen recognition by HLA class II on monocytes up-regulates toll-like receptor 4 and enhances proinflammatory responses to endotoxin. *Blood* **105:**3655–3662.

43. **Howell, M. D., J. P. Diveley, K. A. Lundeen, A. Esty, S. T. Winters, D. J. Carlo, and S. W. Brostoff.** 1991. Limited T-cell receptor β-chain heterogeneity among interleukin 2 receptor-positive synovial T cells suggests a role for superantigen in rheumatoid arthritis. *Proc. Natl. Acad. Sci. USA* **88:**10921–10925.

44. **Kappler, J. W., A. Herman, J. Clements, and P. Marrack.** 1992. Mutations defining functional regions of the superantigen staphylococcal enterotoxin B. *J. Exp. Med.* **175:**387–396.

45. **Kline, J. B., and C. M. Collins.** 1996. Analysis of the superantigenic activity of mutant and allelic forms of streptococcal pyrogenic exotoxin A. *Infect. Immun.* **64:**861–869.

46. **Kotzin, B.** 1993. Presented at the Keystone Conference.

47. **Kotzin, B. L., D. Y. Leung, J. Kappler, and P. Marrack.** 1993. Superantigens and their potential role in human disease. *Adv. Immunol.* **54:**99–166.

48. **Krause, D., and D. Taylo-Robinson.** 1992. Mycoplasma which infect humans, p. 417–444. *In* J. Maniloff (ed.), *Mycoplasma: Molecular Biology and Pathogenesis.* American Society for Microbiology, Washington, D.C.

49. **Kuchroo, V., M. Das, J. Brown, A. Ranger, S. Zamvil, R. Sobel, H. Weiner, N. Nabavi, and L. Glimcher.** 1995. B7-1 and B7-2 costimulatory molecules activate differentially the Th1/Th2 developmental pathways: application to autoimmune disease therapy. *Cell* **80:**707–718.

50. **Langlois, M. A., Y. El Fakhry, and W. Mourad.** 2003. Zinc-binding sites in the N terminus of Mycoplasma arthritidis-derived mitogen permit the dimer formation required for high affinity binding to HLA-DR and for T cell activation. *J. Biol. Chem.* **278:**22309–22315.

51. **Langlois, M. A., P. Etongue-Mayer, M. Ouellette, and W. Mourad.** 2000. Binding of Mycoplasma arthritidis-derived mitogen to human MHC class II molecules via its N terminus is modulated by invariant chain expression and its C terminus is required for T cell activation. *Eur. J. Immunol.* **30:**1748–1756.

52. **Lanier, L. L., S. O'Fallon, C. Somoza, J. H. Phillips, P. S. Linsley, K. Okumura, D. Ito, and M. Azuma.** 1995. CD80 (B7) and CD86 (B70) provide similar costimulatory signals for T cell proliferation, cytokine production, and generation of CTL. *J. Immunol.* **154:**97–105.

53. **Lenschow, D. J., T. L. Walunas, and J. A. Bluestone.** 1996. CD28/B7 system of T cell costimulation. *Annu. Rev. Immunol.* **14:**233–258.

54. **Levine, B. L., Y. Ueda, N. Craighead, M. L. Huang, and C. H. June.** 1995. CD28 ligands CD80 (B7-1) and CD86 (B7-2) induce long-term autocrine growth of CD4+ T cells and induce similar patterns of cytokine secretion in vitro. *Int. Immunol.* **7:**891–904.

55. **Li, H., S. Van Vranken, Y. Zhao, Z. Li, Y. Guo, L. Eisele, and Y. Li.** 2005. Crystal structures of T cell receptor (beta) chains related to rheumatoid arthritis. *Protein Sci.* **14:**3025–3038.

56. **Maniloff, J., R. McElhaney, R. Lloyd, and J. Baseman (ed.).** 1992. *Mycoplasmas: Molecular Biology and Pathogenesis,* 1st ed. American Society for Microbiology, Washington, D.C.

57. **Maxwell, J. R., R. J. Rossi, S. J. McSorley, and A. T. Vella.** 2004. T cell clonal conditioning: a phase occurring early after antigen presentation but before clonal expansion is impacted by Toll-like receptor stimulation. *J. Immunol.* **172:**248–259.

58. **Medzhitov, R., and C. Janeway, Jr.** 2000. Innate immune recognition: mechanisms and pathways. *Immunol. Rev.* **173:**89–97.

59. **Medzhitov, R., and C. A. Janeway, Jr.** 1998. Innate immune recognition and control of adaptive immune responses. *Semin. Immunol.* **10:**351–353.

60. **Mu, H. H., J. Humphreys, F. V. Chan, and B. C. Cole.** 2006. TLR2 and TLR4 differentially regulate B7-1 resulting in distinct cytokine responses to the mycoplasma superantigen MAM as well as to disease induced by Mycoplasma arthritidis. *Cell. Microbiol.* **8:**414–426.

61. **Mu, H. H., N. D. Pennock, J. Humphreys, C. J. Kirschning, and B. C. Cole.** 2005. Engagement of Toll-like receptors by mycoplasmal superantigen: downregulation of TLR2 by MAM/TLR4 interaction. *Cell. Microbiol.* **7:**789–797.

62. **Mu, H. H., A. D. Sawitzke, and B. C. Cole.** 2000. Modulation of cytokine profiles by the Mycoplasma superantigen Mycoplasma arthritidis mitogen parallels susceptibility to arthritis induced by M. arthritidis. *Infect. Immun.* **68:**1142–1149.

63. **Mu, H. H., A. D. Sawitzke, and B. C. Cole.** 2001. Presence of Lps(d) mutation influences cytokine regulation in vivo by the Mycoplasma arthritidis mitogen superantigen and lethal toxicity in mice infected with M. arthritidis. *Infect. Immun.* **69:**3837–3844.

64. **Mullick, A. E., P. S. Tobias, and L. K. Curtiss.** 2005. Modulation of atherosclerosis in mice by Toll-like receptor 2. *J. Clin. Invest.* **115:**3149–3156.

65. **Muraille, E., C. De Trez, B. Pajak, M. Brait, J. Urbain, and O. Leo.** 2002. T cell-dependent maturation of dendritic cells in response to bacterial superantigens. *J. Immunol.* **168:**4352–4360.

66. **Paliard, X., S. G. West, J. A. Lafferty, J. R. Clements, J. W. Kappler, P. Marrack, and B. L. Kotzin.** 1991. Evidence for the effects of a superantigen in rheumatoid arthritis. *Science* **253:**325–329.

67. **Pentcheva-Hoang, T., J. G. Egen, K. Wojnoonski, and J. P. Allison.** 2004. B7-1 and B7-2 selectively recruit CTLA-4 and CD28 to the immunological synapse. *Immunity* **21:**401–413.

68. **Poltorak, A., X. He, I. Smirnova, M. Y. Liu, C. V. Huffel, X. Du, D. Birdwell, E. Alejos, M. Silva, C. Galanos, M. Freudenberg, P. Ricciardi-Castagnoli, B. Layton, and B. Beutler.** 1998. Defective LPS signaling in C3H/HeJ and C57BL/10ScCr mice: mutations in Tlr4 gene. *Science* **282:**2085–2088.

69. **Posnett, D. N.** 1993. Do superantigens play a role in autoimmunity? *Semin. Immunol.* **5:**65–72.

70. **Posnett, D. N., A. S. Hodtsev, S. Kabak, S. M. Friedman, B. C. Cole, and N. Bhardwaj.** 1993. Interaction of Mycoplasma arthritidis superantigen with human T cells. *Clin. Infect. Dis.* **17**(Suppl .1)**:**S170–S175.

71. **Rink, L., J. Luhm, M. Koester, and H. Kirchner.** 1996. Induction of a cytokine network by superantigens with parallel TH1 and TH2 stimulation. *J. Interferon. Cytokine Res.* **16:**41–47.

72. **Rossi, R. J., G. Muralimohan, J. R. Maxwell, and A. T. Vella.** 2004. Staphylococcal enterotoxins condition cells of the innate immune system for Toll-like receptor 4 stimulation. *Int. Immunol.* **16:**1751–1760.

73. **Sawada, T., R. Pergolizzi, K. Ito, J. Silver, C. Atkin, B. C. Cole, and M. D. Chang.** 1995. Replacement of the DR alpha chain with the E alpha chain enhances presentation of Mycoplasma arthritidis superantigen by the human class II DR molecule. *Infect. Immun.* **63:**3367–3372.

74. **Sawitzke, A. D., H. Mu, and B. Cole.** 1999. Superantigens and autoimmune disease: are they involved? *Curr. Opin. Infect. Dis.* **12:**213–219.

75. **Schaeverbeke, T., M. Clerc, L. Lequen, A. Charron, C. Bebear, B. de Barbeyrac, B. Bannwarth, and J. Dehais.** 1998. Genotypic characterization of seven strains of Mycoplasma fermentans isolated from synovial fluids of patients with arthritis. *J. Clin. Microbiol.* **36:**1226–1231.

76. **Schiffenbauer, J., H. Johnson, and J. Soos.** 1997. Superantigens in autoimmunity: their role as etiologic agents, p. 525–549. *In* Y. Leung, B. Huber, and P. Schlievert (ed.), *Superantigens: Molecular Biology, Immunology, and Relevance to Human Disease*. Marcel Dekker, Inc, New York, N.Y.

77. **Schroder, N. W., and R. R. Schumann.** 2005. Single nucleotide polymorphisms of Toll-like receptors and susceptibility to infectious disease. *Lancet Infect. Dis.* **5:**156–164.

78. **Seki, N., Y. Sudo, T. Yoshioka, S. Sugihara, T. Fujitsu, S. Sakuma, T. Ogawa, T. Hamaoka, H. Senoh, and H. Fijiwara.** 1988. Type II collagen-induced murine arthritis. I. Induction and perpetuation of arthritis require synergy between humoral and cell-mediated immunity. *J. Immunol.* **140:**1477–1484.

79. **Sordet, C., A. Cantagrel, T. Schaeverbeke, and J. Sibilia.** 2005. Bone and joint disease associated with primary immune deficiencies. *Joint Bone Spine* **72:**503–514.

80. **Takeda, K., T. Kaisho, and S. Akira.** 2003. Toll-like receptors. *Annu. Rev. Immunol.* **21:**335–376.

81. **Takeuchi, O., A. Kaufmann, K. Grote, T. Kawai, K. Hoshino, M. Morr, P. F. Muhlradt, and S. Akira.** 2000. Cutting edge: preferentially the R-stereoisomer of the mycoplasmal lipopeptide macrophage-activating lipopeptide-2 activates immune cells through a toll-like receptor 2- and MyD88-dependent signaling pathway. *J. Immunol.* **164:**554–557.

82. **Tumang, J. R., E. P. Cherniack, D. M. Gietl, B. C. Cole, C. Russo, M. K. Crow, and S. M. Friedman.** 1991. T helper cell-dependent, microbial superantigen-induced murine B cell activation: polyclonal and antigen-specific antibody responses. *J. Immunol.* **147:**432–438.

83. **Voelker, L., K. Weaver, L. Ehle, and L. Washburn.** 1995. Association of lysogenic bacteriophage MAV1 with virulence of Mycoplasma arthritidis. *Infect. Immun.* **63:**4016–4023.

84. **Washburn, L. R., E. J. Miller, and K. E. Weaver.** 2000. Molecular characterization of Mycoplasma arthritidis membrane lipoprotein MAA1. *Infect. Immun.* **68:**437–442.

85. **Washburn, L. R., K. E. Weaver, E. J. Weaver, W. Donelan, and S. Al-Sheboul.** 1998. Molecular characterization of Mycoplasma arthritidis variable surface protein MAA2. *Infect. Immun.* **66:**2576–2586.

86. **White, J., A. Herman, A. M. Pullen, R. Kubo, J. W. Kappler, and P. Marrack.** 1989. The Vβ-specific superantigen staphylococcal enterotoxin B: stimulation of mature T cells and clonal deletion in neonatal mice. *Cell* **56:**27–35.

87. **Zhao, Y., Z. Li, S. J. Drozd, Y. Guo, W. Mourad, and H. Li.** 2004. Crystal structure of Mycoplasma arthritidis mitogen complexed with HLA-DR1 reveals a novel superantigen fold and a dimerized superantigen-MHC complex. *Structure (Camb.)* **12:**277–288.

Chapter 4

Viral Superantigens in Mice and Humans

Albert K. Tai and Brigitte T. Huber

Adaptive immunity relies on the antigen-specific B cell (BCR) and T cell (TCR) receptors to survey for pathogenic events. Upon recognition of a microbe by these receptors, an immune response is initiated, resulting in the differentiation of the antigen-specific lymphocytes into effector cells, which eliminate the pathogen. The antigen-specific memory cells that are generated ensure that a more rigorous and effective immune response is mounted should the same pathogen be encountered again. Since the immune receptors play such a critical role in the host defense against pathogens, it is not surprising that various microbes have evolved means to interfere with the proper function of these receptors. One of these mechanisms is the production and/or use of superantigens (SAgs), a class of immune deregulating antigens that interact with the TCR in an unusual manner. The most prominent feature of this interaction is the TCR Vβ specificity. Compared with the recognition of a conventional antigen, which is mediated through the antigen-binding site, consisting of both α- and β-chains of the TCR, the recognition of a SAg appears to rely solely on the Vβ-region of the TCR. Furthermore, T cells expressing TCRs sharing the same or closely related Vβ-chains can all be stimulated by a particular SAg. According to the IMGT database, there are 23 and 18 functional TCR Vβ-families in humans and mice, respectively. Thus, a given SAg can stimulate up to 5 to 25% of the total peripheral T cells, compared with less than 0.01% that are reactive to a conventional antigen. In addition to the Vβ specificity, several other features distinguish a SAg-induced response from a conventional immune reaction. While presentation by major histocompatibility complex (MHC) proteins is required for proper recognition of both SAgs and conventional peptide antigens by T cells, presentation of SAgs is not MHC restricted. Moreover, conventional antigen processing is not required for SAg presentation by MHC II; instead, SAgs bind to the TCR and MHC II outside of the antigen-binding site.

SAgs that stimulate B cells have also been defined. Similar to their T-cell counterparts, these B-cell SAgs exhibit distinctive features, such as stimulation of a significantly higher

Albert K. Tai and Brigitte T. Huber • Department of Pathology, Tufts University School of Medicine, Boston, MA 02111.

frequency of B cells in a VH-chain-restricted manner, and they bind to the BCR outside the conventional antigen-binding site (115).

ORGANISMS THAT ENCODE SAgs

The majority of known SAgs are of either bacterial or viral origin, the prototypes being the bacterial pathogens *Staphylococcus aureus* and *Streptococcus pyogenes* and the murine mammary tumor virus (MMTV). SAgs have also been isolated from other bacterial pathogens, such as *Mycoplasma arthritidis* (109), *Yersinia enterocolitica* and *pseudotuberculosis* (72, 97, 120, 127), *Plasmodium falciparum* (17), *Clostridium perfringens* (19, 134), and *Toxoplasma gondii* (36), as well as from other viral pathogens, such as rabies virus (*Rhabdoviridae*). Recently, a plant SAg, *Urtica dioica* agglutinin (UDA), has been isolated from the rhizomes of the stinging nettle (*Urtica dioica*) (48, 49, 112), suggesting that SAg production is not restricted to microscopic pathogens, but may be more widespread in nature than currently known. One critical difference between bacterial and viral SAgs is their origin of production. While bacterial SAgs are secreted by the pathogens and bind to MHC II extracellularly for presentation (28, 77, 89, 93, 137), the viral SAgs are produced intracellularly, presumably associating with MHC II during biosynthesis (11, 12, 27, 68, 138). Nevertheless, although these molecules are evolutionarily distinct, they share very similar mechanisms of action and have comparable effects on the host immune system. The viral SAgs in humans and mice are the subject of discussion of this chapter, and a list of the known viral pathogens encoding SAgs and their corresponding Vβ or VH specificities is shown in Table 1.

VIRAL PATHOGENS ASSOCIATED WITH, BUT NOT ENCODING, A SAg

The organisms discussed above encode their own SAgs; however, there are others that are associated with a SAg-like activity, but do not encode a SAg. These include several members of the herpesvirus (*Herpesviridae*) family, such as Epstein-Barr Virus (EBV), cytomegalovirus (CMV), and murine herpesvirus (MHV)-68 (39, 58, 125).

Our laboratory has reported an EBV-associated SAg activity with human Vβ13 specificity (125). The SAg responsible for this activity was subsequently cloned, not from the EBV genome, but from the *env* gene of a human endogenous retrovirus (HERV), demonstrating the possible exploitation of endogenous SAgs by exogenous viral pathogens (123). SAg activity with a specificity of human Vβ12 has also been associated with CMV in vitro (39); nevertheless, the viral gene product responsible for this observed SAg activity has not been identified, leading to the postulate that CMV infection may result in the induction of a human endogenous SAg. In addition, MHV-68, an infectious mononucleosis (IM)-inducing murine γ-herpesvirus closely related to EBV, seems to be associated with a SAg-like activity (58, 90, 132). The IM induced upon latent MHV-68 infection is characterized by a polyclonal expansion of CD8$^+$ Vβ4$^+$ T cells in most mouse strains, with the exception of DBA/2. The Vβ-specific expansion points to the involvement of a SAg, although this activity does not seem to be encoded by the viral genome, nor does it depend on MHC I or MHC II for presentation to T cells (30). Nevertheless, the authors have not ruled out the possibility that this putative SAg may be

Table 1. Vβ specificity of exogenous and endogenous viral SAgs

Virus	SAg	Vβ / VH specificity[a]	References
MMTV			Reviewed in references 1 and 63; reported in 53, 100, 114, and 129
Endogenous			
Mtv-1		mVβ 3	
Mtv-2		mVβ 14	
Mtv-3		mVβ 3, 17	
Mtv-6		mVβ 3, 17	
Mtv-7		mVβ 6, 7, 8.1, 9	
Mtv-8		mVβ 11, 12	
Mtv-9		mVβ 5, 11, 12	
Mtv-11		mVβ 11, 12	
Mtv-13		mVβ 3	
Mtv-29		mVβ 16	
Mtv-43		mVβ 6, 7, 8.1, 9	
Mtv-44		mVβ 6	
Mtv-48		mVβ 2	
Mtv-51		mVβ 2	
Exogenous			
MMTV-C3H		mVβ 14, 15	
MMTV-SW		mVβ 6, 7, 8.1, 9	
MMTV-BALB2		mVβ 2	
MMTV-BALB14		mVβ 14	
MMTV-LA		mVβ 6, 7, 8.1, 9	
Rabies virus	Nucleocapsid/N protein	hVβ8 mVβ6	84, 85
HIV	gp120	hVH3	9
	gp160	hVβ 3, 12, 14, 15	3
HERV-K18	Envelope	hVβ 13, 7, 9 mVβ 3, 7	119, 123, 126
HERV-W	Envelope	hVβ16	103

[a]hVβ, human Vβ; mVβ, murine Vβ.

able to be presented by either MHC I or II, similar to what has been observed with UDA (110). More recently, the loci controlling the activation of CD8$^+$ Vβ4$^+$ T cells upon MHV-68 infection were mapped to the murine chromosomes 6 and 17, suggesting that a host-derived gene product may be responsible for this activity (57).

The use of host-derived SAgs is not restricted to herpesviruses. It has been reported that the murine leukemia virus (MuLV, *Retroviridae*), the causative agent of murine acquired immune deficiency syndrome (AIDS), is also associated with a SAg activity upon infection (70). It has been subsequently demonstrated that this SAg activity is not encoded within the virus itself (41), but is contributed by an endogenous MMTV SAg (50). However, the implication of the SAg expression in murine AIDS pathogenesis remains unclear (95). In addition, SAg activity has been observed during acute measles virus (*Paramyxoviridae*) infection (29), although no additional data supporting this notion are available at the time of writing.

MMTV SAg

MMTV is a nonacute transforming milk-borne retroviral pathogen, transmitted horizontally from the infected mother to its suckling offspring. The pathogen first enters its host through the gut and is transported to the mammary glands, where it infects the epithelium. The retrovirus undergoes lytic amplification in the infected epithelial cells in response to the hormones produced by the host during pregnancy and lactation. As a result, retroviral particles are released from the infected epithelial cells into the milk and surrounding tissue. A high retroviral titer is generated that increases the frequency of (re)infection of the surrounding mammary epithelium and random proviral integrations, eventually disrupting the proper function of a unique set of cellular proto-oncogenes, such as *int-1,* that leads to the development of mammary tumors in the host. Both B and T cells are required for the pathogen to reach the mammary gland epithelium from the initial site of infection, as demonstrated by resistance to MMTV infection in mice lacking either B or T cells. The initial infection of B cells allows transcription of the retroviral proteins, including the SAg, and the expression and presentation of the SAg by the infected B cells activates the SAg-reactive T cells in the vicinity. The activated T cells express stimulatory membrane-bound proteins, such as CD40 ligand, and produce cytokines, such as interleukin-4 (IL-4), which, in turn, provide the signals required for the activation of the infected B cells. B- and T-cell stimulation allows retroviral amplification, which is essential for the transportation of MMTV to the mammary gland. In this model, through the direct and indirect activation of B and T cells, respectively, the SAg provides the essential environment for pathogen amplification and translocation to the target tissue, thus playing an indispensable role in the MMTV life cycle, as MMTV lacking a functional SAg is incapable of productive infection. While the exogenous virus encoded SAg is critical for the viral infection, the expression of endogenous MMTV SAgs leads to thymic deletion of T cells with the corresponding Vβ-chains, hence rendering the mice resistant to infection by exogenous MMTV encoding SAgs with the same Vβ specificity (1, 33, 69).

Recently, the cloning of MMTV-like sequences from human breast cancer tissue has been reported (91, 135, 136), but no indication of SAg encoding sequences has been found, and the potential implication of the presence of these viral sequences remains to be elucidated.

RABIES VIRUS SAgs

The rabies virus N protein, encoded within the viral structural protein nucleocapsid (NC), has SAg activity, stimulating human Vβ8$^+$ and murine Vβ6$^+$ T cells (84, 85, 94). To investigate whether the SAg contributes to the susceptibility for viral infection, Vβ6$^+$ and Vβ8$^+$ T cells were adoptively transferred into mice lacking these T-cell populations, followed by exposure to rabies virus. While the nonreconstituted and Vβ8$^+$ T-cell-reconstituted mice survived, all the mice reconstituted with Vβ6$^+$ T cells were dead by day 18 (85). In another experimental setting it was shown that mice with (CBA/H) or without (CBA/J) Vβ6$^+$ T cells differed in their susceptibility to rabies virus infection, in that the latter, but not the former, were resistant (83). These results clearly demonstrate that susceptibility to rabies virus infection and/or its pathogenesis, as measured by paralytic attack, depend on the presence of Vβ6$^+$ T cells, and thus the N protein SAg. However, whether these findings can apply to rabies infection in other species, including humans, remains to be elucidated.

HUMAN IMMUNODEFICIENCY VIRUS TYPE 1 (HIV-1) SAgs

An HIV-associated SAg was first suspected when the Vβ repertoire from the peripheral blood mononuclear cells of AIDS patients showed marked reduction of several Vβ subsets, as compared with healthy controls (71). Subsequently, the HIV glycoprotein, gp160, was identified as a SAg that is specific for human Vβ3, 12, 14, 15 and, to a lesser extent, Vβ17 and 20 (3). Since then, experimental evidence for and against these data has been reported (3, 15, 16, 20, 31, 32, 34, 38, 55, 80, 105–107, 118, 131). Later, HIV gp120 was shown to have B-cell SAg activity with specificity for the VH3 family (9, 10, 54, 78, 98, 99, 130). HIV gp160 and gp120 have both been implicated in the pathogenesis of AIDS. It has also been reported that HIV-1 preferentially replicates in the gp160 SAg-activated T cells (87, 105), while gp120 expression has been associated with the gradual reduction of VH3$^+$ B cells (10, 40) and VH3 antibody production (76), as well as the development of VH3$^+$ AIDS-related Burkitt's lymphoma (4).

HERV SAgs

Transposable elements constitute approximately 42% of the human genome, the majority of them being retroelements. HERV and HERV-derived sequences, such as solitary long terminal repeats (LTRs), are a subclass of retroelements that make up approximately 8% of the human genome (86, 133). HERV shares structural similarity with the modern-day retrovirus and in general is regarded as footprint of ancient retroviral infection that gained access to the germ line. Because of their primeval origin, most of their sequences have accumulated numerous mutations, and most of the viral open reading frames (ORFs) are nonfunctional; thus, no HERV-derived infectious retrovirus has ever been reported. Nevertheless, HERVs are still biologically active, and small numbers of intact ORFs, derived from different HERV families, have been documented. Within these intact ORFs, two SAgs, the envelope protein (Env) of HERV-K18 (123) and HERV-W (103), were identified.

HERV-W ENV SAg

HERV-W was first characterized because of its sequence homology to the multiple sclerosis-associated retrovirus-like (MSRV) particle, originally isolated from the plasma of MS patients (14). The HERV-W Env SAg stimulates human Vβ16$^+$ T cells in vitro, regardless of the HLA-DR haplotype of the antigen-presenting cells (APCs). These observations coincide with the properties of a classical T-cell SAg, suggesting that the HERV-W Env may be a SAg (103).

The HERV-W Env protein has been proposed to play an etiological role in MS, and the expression of HERV-W Env and Gag can be demonstrated in the MS lesions in situ (104). It has been observed that the capsid (Gag) protein is expressed at a baseline level in normal human brain tissue, while a significant accumulation of Gag protein was seen in MS lesions. The Env protein was found to be restricted to the microglia in normal brain tissue, but is expressed transiently in macrophage within the MS lesions. Furthermore, the HERV-W *env* and *gag* genes are transactivated in neuronal and brain endothelial cell lines upon herpes simplex virus-1 (HSV-1) infection in vitro (111), suggesting that the expression of HERV-W-derived proteins can be regulated by environmental factors, such as viral infection. When humanized serve-combined immunodeficient (SCID) mice were injected with recombined MSRV protein intraperitoneally, they succumbed to brain hemorrhage, but the symptoms were alleviated upon T-cell depletion, suggesting a role of T cells in the development of the hemorrhage (45). Taken together, these results indicate that the expression of HERV-W-derived proteins is associated with MS, and MSRV is capable of inducing brain pathology in a T-cell-dependent manner, albeit different from the lesions observed in MS patients. Nevertheless, it remains to be directly demonstrated whether the HERV-W Env is a SAg that is responsible for the pathogenesis, as it also possesses fusogenic activity, which is important for the formation of the placenta (96).

HERV-K18 Env SAg

The HERV-K18 Env SAg stimulates human T cells and T-cell hybridomas bearing $hV\beta13^+$ and $hV\beta7^+$ and, to a lesser extent, $hV\beta9^+$ TCRs, as demonstrated by in vitro experimental systems (119, 123). More recently, the superantigenicity of HERV-K18 Env has been confirmed in the murine system, stimulating $mV\beta3^+$ T-cell hybridomas in vitro in the context of both human and murine APCs. In addition, transgenic mice expressing HERV-K18 Env partially delete $V\beta3^+$ and $V\beta7^+$ T cells, a hallmark of endogenous SAg expression (126).

HERV-K18, a type I HERV-K provirus, maps to chromosome 1q23.1-24.1, within the first intron of the EBV-inducible cellular gene, *cd48*. The HERV-K18 provirus is in the opposite transcriptional orientation of *cd48* (Fig. 1) (59). Possibly because of its proximity to the location of an EBV-specific enhancer within the regulatory region of *cd48*, HERV-K18 *env* is transactivated upon EBV infection. The transcription of HERV-K *env* can also be induced in human B cells upon alpha interferon (IFN-α) treatment (119) and immunoglobulin M (IgM) or IgM/CD40 cross-linking (126). Through the work of our laboratory, we now have a better understanding of the regulation of HERV-K18 *env* by EBV. Our data indicate that the EBV latent membrane protein, LMP-2A, can transactivate the transcription of HERV-K18 *env* (122). Furthermore, we have shown that HERV-K18 *env* transcription can also be induced via the signal given by the B-cell membrane protein CD21, the cellular receptor for EBV (44, 47). Hence, HERV-K18 *env* transcription is probably induced very early on during viral entry through the interaction of the EBV Env glycoprotein, gp350, and CD21 (67). In addition, we have shown that LMP-2A transactivates HERV-K18 *env* through the EBV-specific enhancer within the *cd48* promoter, but not the proviral LTR (F. C. Hsiao, A. K. Tai, and B. T. Huber, submitted for publication). Although EBV leads to the activation of HERV-K18 *env* at multiple stages of the viral infection, the benefits gained by EBV through the transactivation of this SAg remain to be investigated. Nevertheless, the fact that EBV induces an ancient functional endogenous SAg is very likely to have an impact on the host immune system as a result of infection.

There are three known allelic forms of HERV-K *env*, K18.1, K18.2, and K18.3, that are unevenly distributed within the Caucasian population, with frequencies of 46.6%, 42.5%, and 10.8%, respectively (119). Both alleles K18.2 and K18.3 are predicted to encode Env proteins of 560 amino acids, containing a surface unit (SU) and a transmembrane (TM) domain of a typical retroviral Env protein. The allele K18.1, on the other hand, is predicted to encode a truncated Env protein of 153 amino acids as a result of mutations that converted the codon for tryptophan at position 154 into a stop codon. Thus, it contains approximately half of the SU domain, but lacks the entire TM section (see Fig. 1). Because of this truncation, the allele K18.1 is predicted to have biochemical properties different from the other

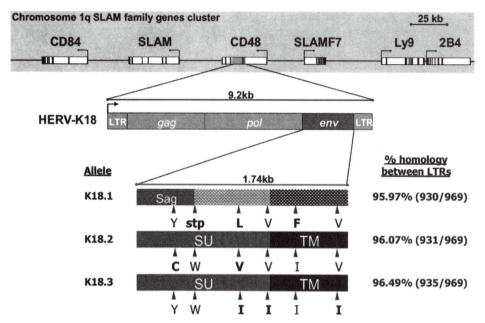

Figure 1. The HERV-K18 provirus. The HERV-K18 provirus is mapped to the chromosomal region 1q23.1-24.1, within the SLAM family gene cluster. Specifically, it is located within the first intron of the cellular gene, *cd48*, but is in opposite transcriptional orientation. It is 9.2 kb and contains a functional ORF for the *env* gene only. There are three alleles of HERV-K18 *env*: K18.1, K18.2, and K18.3. Both K18.2 and K18.3 are predicted to encode a full-length Env protein of 560 amino acids. On the other hand, K18.1 is predicted to encode a truncated Env protein of 153 amino acids, as a result of a mutation converting the codon for tryptophan at position 154 into a stop codon. The three alleles are highly homologous to each other. The degree of homology between the two proviral LTRs encoding each allele is shown.

two alleles. First, K18.1 is expected to be soluble due to the lack of the TM domain. Second, it has been demonstrated that the retroviral Env proteins homotrimerize to form a functional unit. From the Env crystal structures of several retroviruses, including HERV-FRD (108), it has been surmised that the formation of this homotrimer relies heavily on the interactions between the TM domains (79). Since surface expression and fusogenic activity have been demonstrated for the Env proteins of several members of the HERV-K family (37), it is likely that alleles K18.2 and K18.3, but not K18.1, have a similar potential to form homotrimers. A schematic diagram comparing the three alleles of HERV-K18 *env* is shown in Fig. 1. The SAg activity of HERV-K18 Env is encoded within the 153 amino acids of the SU domain, as all three alleles of HERV-K 18 Env possess SAg activity.

Since three alleles of HERV-K18 Env have predicted differences in biochemical and probably superantigenic properties, and their distribution is uneven within the healthy Caucasian population, a potential selective pressure on these alleles during evolution is speculated. Because of its unique properties, HERV-K18 Env may be involved in the development of certain diseases, fulfilling several criteria. First, HERV alleles are inherited in a Mendelian fashion; thus, diseases with documented genetic influences were considered. SAg- and HERV-implicated diseases were also reasonable candidates. Last, but not least, EBV association was considered. Several autoimmune diseases fulfill these criteria, such as MS and systemic lupus erythematosus (SLE). We have recently completed a prospective case-controlled study, comparing the allelic and genotypic distribution of HERV-K18 *env* in healthy Caucasians and MS patients (A. K. Tai, E. O'Reilly, K. A. Alroy, K. L. Munger, B. T. Huber, and A. Ascherio, submitted for publication). In this study we observed that the genotypic distribution of the HERV-K18 Env violates the Hardy–Weinberg equilibrium; furthermore, we discovered a significant difference in the HERV-K18 Env allelic and genotypic distribution between control and patient cohorts. We observed a similar deviation of the allelic and genotypic distribution of HERV-K18 Env in SLE patients as in MS patients (our unpublished observations).

What is the potential mechanism by which HERV-K18 Env SAg may be involved in the pathogenesis of these diseases? We can get a glimpse of how the HERV-K18 Env SAg alleles may influence the host immune response by extending our knowledge of the function of other SAgs. First, SAgs have been reported to alter the proper function of CD4 T cells, such as the induction of proliferation and anergy (46), differentiation of T cells into regulatory T cells (Treg) (101), as well as the ability to bias Th1/Th2 differentiation in a dose-dependent or APC-dependent manner in vitro (21, 51). Furthermore, it has been reported that SAgs promote germinal center formation when expressed by B cells (116). In addition, SAgs can induce T cells and APCs to produce various cytokines, including proinflammatory cytokines, such as TNF-α (2, 5, 56, 62), interleukin-1 (IL-1) (7, 8, 24, 64), chemokines, such as MIP-1 (82), MCP-1 (75, 82) and RANTES (75), and other homeostatic cytokines, such as IL-4 (25), IL-5 (60), IL-6 (117), IL-8 (81, 117), IL-10 (66), IL-12 (42), IL-18 (5), IFN-γ (66), and G-CSF (117). The expression of surface molecules with regulatory functions, such as CD40L on T cells (74) and GITR-like ligand on Treg cells (26), has also been reported to be regulated by SAgs. Furthermore, nitric oxide (NO), a mediator of activation-induced cell death, can be induced in macrophages upon SAg treatment (22, 43, 139). These are possible means through which HERV-K18 Env may alter the host immune response.

The potential role of HERV-K18 Env SAg in EBV-associated lymphoproliferative disorders and malignancies has been reviewed previously (124). We would, however, like to propose a model of how HERV-K18 Env may contribute to the development of autoimmunity.

AN AFFINITY MODEL FOR A WEAK ENDOGENOUS VIRAL SAg

Although classified as a SAg, the specific T-cell stimulation by the HERV-K18 Env is relatively weak. We have reproducibly demonstrated its human and murine Vβ specificities in vitro by T-cell hybridoma assays and measurement of an early activation event in primary T cells and in vivo by the partial deletion observed in the HERV-K18 transgenic mice (126). Nevertheless, a SAg-induced Vβ-specific T-cell proliferation has yet to be demonstrated. Keeping this in mind, we would like to address a potentially operative model of HERV-K18 Env by proposing that HERV-K18 Env binding to an existing TCR:peptide MHC (pMHC) complex alters the affinity between the TCR and its ligand and, therefore, the TCR signal strength, thus altering the outcome of this interaction.

It has been well documented that the strength of the TCR signal influences the T-cell development in the thymus, Th1 and Th2 cell differentiation in the periphery, as well as the development of autoimmunity (52, 65, 73, 128). As the TCR signal strength is a function of the affinity between the pMHC complex and the TCR, we hypothesize that the HERV-K18 Env SAg alters the signal strength of the TCR by binding to and stabilizing the TCR:pMHC complex, thus resulting in an improper immune response and contributing to the development of autoimmune diseases.

During thymic maturation, only T cells that receive signals above a certain threshold survive by undergoing positive selection. The signal strength then becomes important for lineage commitment: those with a lower/shorter signal are thought to become CD8$^+$ T cells, while those with a higher/longer signal commit to the CD4 lineage (reviewed in reference 52). At this point, the developing T cells are subjected to negative selection, and those that receive very strong signals through their TCRs are considered autoreactive and are eliminated, while the thymocytes receiving a moderate signal survive, migrate to the periphery, and become naïve T cells. Expression of a strong endogenous SAg during the negative selection process often results in thymic deletion of the entire population of T-cell expression TCR Vβ-chains that are reactive to the SAg, while a weak SAg activity leads to partial deletion or anergy of the reactive T cells. Once the naïve T cells encounter a specific antigen, the high-affinity interaction between the TCR and a pMHC complex results in T-cell activation. For the naïve CD4 T cells, it has been demonstrated that a weak signal above the activation threshold, with CD28 costimulation, leads to development of Th2 cells, while a strong signal above threshold leads to Th1 development, regardless of CD28 involvement (18, 128).

A classical SAg, such as SEB, gives a strong signal through the TCR and is able to induce T-cell activation, as well as anergy. Self-antigens and epitopes have low affinity and are thus incapable of giving an activation signal to naïve T cells. Foreign antigens/epitopes, on the other hand, represent a heterogenic population with a large range of affinities, from too low to induce naïve T-cell activation to high enough for the induction of a Th1 response. Foreign antigens/epitopes with an affinity similar to those of self-antigens/epitopes may include those that are structurally similar to self-antigens (molecular mimicry).

Assuming that the signal strength of the TCR is the only variable in this model, it dictates the outcome of a T-cell response to a conventional antigen. In the absence of SAg, the T cell would respond appropriately as a direct consequence of the affinity between TCR and pMHC. However, when a weak SAg, e.g., HERV-K18 Env, comes into the picture, the binding of the SAg to the TCR:pMHC complex further stabilizes the interaction, thereby forming a SAg:TCR:pMHC supercomplex that shifts the affinity toward the higher end, which is interpreted by the T cell as a higher TCR signal. This shift in affinity and, hence, signal strength transmitted via the TCR to the T cell can result in various outcomes, depending on the combined affinity of the TCR:pMHC complex and the TCR:SAg. For antigens with far lower affinity than the activation threshold, no T cell activation is induced, even in the presence of additional affinity contributed by the binding of the SAg. For those with affinity only slightly lower than the activation threshold, the additional affinity given by the SAg may be sufficient to induce activation of the T cell. This may lead to the breakdown of self-tolerance, if the response is against a self-antigen, or the process of molecular mimicry, if the response is against a foreign antigen that is structurally similar to a self-antigen. Antigens with affinity inducing a Th2 response may now be capable of inducing a Th1 response with the additional affinity given by the SAg. These events may all result in an inappropriate immune response, leading to pathogenic events in the host.

After the initiation of a primary immune response, memory T cells with the same specificity, but a lower activation threshold, are generated. Whether or not SAg is still required to activate these memory T cells depends on the affinity contributed by the SAg during the primary response. If the affinity is low, then the SAg may not be needed for subsequent memory T-cell activation, and a continued state of activation may result. If the contribution is high, then it is likely that stabilization by the SAg is still required to stimulate memory T cells; thus, relapses or flares of the symptoms may correlate with the expression of the SAg.

The affinity contributed by a SAg, for instance HERV-K18 Env, is the function of several parameters. These include the differential affinity for various TCR Vβ-chains and MHC II haplotypes (61, 88, 92, 102, 113, 121), as well as the TCR Vα-chain (6, 13, 23, 35), which have all been documented to affect the stability of the interaction of a SAg with the TCR.

Additionally, the three alleles of HERV-K18 differ in their capacity to form homotrimers and, thus, oligomerization of TCR:pMHC, which, in turn, influences the TCR strength by varying the avidity. Finally, the induction of HERV-K18 Env by exogenous and endogenous signals, such as other EBV viral infections (via IFN-α) and hormones, may provide a mechanism for how external stimuli trigger or influence the course of human autoimmune diseases. The model discussed above provides a means to explain how HERV-K18 Env may contribute to the development of human autoimmunity and offers an explanation for the heterogeneity observed in these patients and the contribution of both environmental and genetic factors.

REFERENCES

1. **Acha-Orbea, H., and H. R. MacDonald.** 1995. Superantigens of mouse mammary tumor virus. *Annu. Rev. Immunol.* **13:**459–486.
2. **Akatsuka, H., K. Imanishi, K. Inada, H. Yamashita, M. Yoshida, and T. Uchiyama.** 1994. Production of tumour necrosis factors by human T cells stimulated by a superantigen, toxic shock syndrome toxin-1. *Clin. Exp. Immunol.* **96:**422–426.
3. **Akolkar, P. N., N. Chirmule, B. Gulwani-Akolkar, S. Pahwa, V. S. Kalyanaraman, R. Pergolizzi, S. Macphail, and J. Silver.** 1995. V beta-specific activation of T cells by the HIV glycoprotein gp 160. *Scand. J. Immunol.* **41:**487–498.
4. **Amariglio, N., A. Vonsover, I. Hakim, Y. Neumann, Z. Mark, F. Brok-Simoni, I. Ben-Bassat, and G. Rechavi.** 1994. Immunoglobulin VH3-positive AIDS-related Burkitt's lymphoma: a possible role for the HIV gp120 superantigen. *Acta Haematol.* **91:**103–105.
5. **Aubert, V., D. Schneeberger, A. Sauty, J. Winter, P. Sperisen, J. D. Aubert, and F. Spertini.** 2000. Induction of tumor necrosis factor alpha and interleukin-8 gene expression in bronchial epithelial cells by toxic shock syndrome toxin 1. *Infect. Immun.* **68:**120–124.
6. **Aude-Garcia, C., A. Attinger, D. Housset, H. R. MacDonald, H. Acha-Orbea, P. N. Marche, and E. Jouvin-Marche.** 2000. Pairing of Vbeta6 with certain Valpha2 family members prevents T cell deletion by Mtv-7 superantigen. *Mol. Immunol.* **37:**1005–1012.
7. **Beezhold, D. H., G. K. Best, P. F. Bonventre, and M. Thompson.** 1987. Synergistic induction of interleukin-1 by endotoxin and toxic shock syndrome toxin-1 using rat macrophages. *Infect. Immun.* **55:**2865–2869.
8. **Beezhold, D. H., G. K. Best, P. F. Bonventre, and M. Thompson.** 1989. Endotoxin enhancement of toxic shock syndrome toxin 1-induced secretion of interleukin 1 by murine macrophages. *Rev. Infect. Dis.* **11**(Suppl. 1):S289–S293.
9. **Berberian, L., L. Goodglick, T. J. Kipps, and J. Braun.** 1993. Immunoglobulin VH3 gene products: natural ligands for HIV gp120. *Science* **261:**1588–1591.
10. **Berberian, L., J. Shukla, R. Jefferis, and J. Braun.** 1994. Effects of HIV infection on VH3 (D12 idiotope) B cells in vivo. *J Acquir. Immune Defic. Syndr.* **7:**641–646.

11. **Beutner, U., B. McLellan, E. Kraus, and B. T. Huber.** 1996. Lack of MMTV superantigen presentation in MHC class II-deficient mice. *Cell. Immunol.* **168:**141–147.

12. **Beutner, U., C. Rudy, and B. T. Huber.** 1992. Molecular characterization of Mls-1. *Int. Rev. Immunol.* **8:**279–288.

13. **Blackman, M. A., and D. L. Woodland.** 1996. Role of the T cell receptor alpha-chain in superantigen recognition. *Immunol. Res.* **15:**98–113.

14. **Blond, J. L., F. Beseme, L. Duret, O. Bouton, F. Bedin, H. Perron, B. Mandrand, and F. Mallet.** 1999. Molecular characterization and placental expression of HERV-W, a new human endogenous retrovirus family. *J. Virol.* **73:**1175–1185.

15. **Boldt-Houle, D. M., B. D. Jamieson, G. M. Aldrovandi, C. R. Rinaldo, Jr., G. D. Ehrlich, and J. A. Zack.** 1997. Loss of T cell receptor Vbeta repertoires in HIV type 1-infected SCID-hu mice. *AIDS Res. Hum. Retroviruses* **13:**125–134.

16. **Boldt-Houle, D. M., C. R. Rinaldo, Jr., and G. D. Ehrlich.** 1993. Random depletion of T cells that bear specific T cell receptor V beta sequences in AIDS patients. *J. Leukoc. Biol.* **54:**486–491.

17. **Boubou, M. I., A. Collette, D. Voegtle, D. Mazier, P. A. Cazenave, and S. Pied.** 1999. T cell response in malaria pathogenesis: selective increase in T cells carrying the TCR V(beta)8 during experimental cerebral malaria. *Int. Immunol.* **11:**1553–1562.

18. **Boutin, Y., D. Leitenberg, X. Tao, and K. Bottomly.** 1997. Distinct biochemical signals characterize agonist- and altered peptide ligand-induced differentiation of naive CD4+ T cells into Th1 and Th2 subsets. *J. Immunol.* **159:**5802–5809.

19. **Bowness, P., P. A. Moss, H. Tranter, J. I. Bell, and A. J. McMichael.** 1992. Clostridium perfringens enterotoxin is a superantigen reactive with human T cell receptors V beta 6.9 and V beta 22. *J. Exp. Med.* **176:**893–896.

20. **Boyer, V., L. R. Smith, F. Ferre, P. Pezzoli, R. J. Trauger, F. C. Jensen, and D. J. Carlo.** 1993. T cell receptor V beta repertoire in HIV-infection individuals: lack of evidence for selective V beta deletion. *Clin. Exp. Immunol.* **92:**437–441.

21. **Brandt, K., J. van der Bosch, R. Fliegert, and S. Gehring.** 2002. TSST-1 induces Th1 or Th2 differentiation in naive CD4+ T cells in a dose- and APC-dependent manner. *Scand. J. Immunol.* **56:**572–579.

22. **Bras, A., L. Rodriguez-Borlado, A. Gonzalez-Garcia, and A. C. Martinez.** 1997. Nitric oxide regulates clonal expansion and activation-induced cell death triggered by staphylococcal enterotoxin B. *Infect. Immun.* **65:**4030–4037.

23. **Bravo de Alba, Y., P. N. Marche, P. A. Cazenave, I. Cloutier, R. P. Sekaly, and J. Thibodeau.** 1997. V alpha domain modulates the multiple topologies of mouse T cell receptor V beta20/staphylococcal enterotoxins A and E complexes. *Eur. J. Immunol.* **27:**92–99.

24. **Buyalos, R. P., E. M. Rutanen, E. Tsui, and J. Halme.** 1991. Release of tumor necrosis factor alpha by human peritoneal macrophages in response to toxic shock syndrome toxin-1. *Obstet. Gynecol.* **78:**182–186.

25. **Campbell, D. E., and A. S. Kemp.** 1997. Proliferation and production of interferon-gamma (IFN-gamma) and IL-4 in response to Staphylococcus aureus and staphylococcal superantigen in childhood atopic dermatitis. *Clin. Exp. Immunol.* **107:**392–397.

26. **Cardona, I. D., E. Goleva, L. S. Ou, and D. Y. Leung.** 2006. Staphylococcal enterotoxin B inhibits regulatory T cells by inducing glucocorticoid-induced TNF receptor-related protein ligand on monocytes. *J. Allergy Clin. Immunol.* **117:**688–695.

27. **Choi, Y., P. Marrack, and J. W. Kappler.** 1992. Structural analysis of a mouse mammary tumor virus superantigen. *J. Exp. Med.* **175:**847–852.

28. **Choi, Y. W., B. Kotzin, L. Herron, J. Callahan, P. Marrack, and J. Kappler.** 1989. Interaction of Staphylococcus aureus toxin "superantigens" with human T cells. *Proc. Natl. Acad. Sci. USA* **86:**8941–8945.

29. **Chwae, Y. J., I. H. Choi, D. S. Kim, E. C. Shin, D. H. Kwon, S. J. Kim, and J. D. Kim.** 1998. Clonal expansion of T-cells in measles. *Immunol. Lett.* **63:**147–152.

30. **Coppola, M. A., E. Flano, P. Nguyen, C. L. Hardy, R. D. Cardin, N. Shastri, D. L. Woodland, and M. A. Blackman.** 1999. Apparent MHC-independent stimulation of CD8+ T cells in vivo during latent murine gammaherpesvirus infection. *J. Immunol.* **163:**1481–1489.

31. **Cossarizza, A., C. Ortolani, C. Mussini, G. Guaraldi, N. Mongiardo, V. Borghi, D. Barbieri, E. Bellesia, M. G. Franceschini, B. De Rienzo, et al.** 1995. Lack of selective V beta deletion in CD4+ or CD8+ lymphocytes and functional integrity of T-cell repertoire during acute HIV syndrome. *AIDS* **9:**547–553.

32. **Cottrez, F., A. Capron, and H. Groux.** 1996. Selective CD4+ T cell deletion after specific activation in HIV-infected individuals; protection by anti-CD28 monoclonal antibodies. *Clin. Exp. Immunol.* **105:**31–38.

33. **Czarneski, J., J. C. Rassa, and S. R. Ross.** 2003. Mouse mammary tumor virus and the immune system. *Immunol. Res.* **27:**469–480.

34. **Dadaglio, G., S. Garcia, L. Montagnier, and M. L. Gougeon.** 1994. Selective anergy of V beta 8+ T cells in human immunodeficiency virus-infected individuals. *J. Exp. Med.* **179:**413–424.

35. **Daly, K., P. Nguyen, D. Hankley, W. J. Zhang, D. L. Woodland, and M. A. Blackman.** 1995. Contribution of the TCR alpha-chain to the differential recognition of bacterial and retroviral superantigens. *J. Immunol.* **155:**27–34.

36. **Denkers, E. Y., P. Caspar, and A. Sher.** 1994. Toxoplasma gondii possesses a superantigen activity that selectively expands murine T cell receptor V beta 5-bearing CD8+ lymphocytes. *J. Exp. Med.* **180:**985–994.

37. **Dewannieux, M., S. Blaise, and T. Heidmann.** 2005. Identification of a functional envelope protein from the HERV-K family of human endogenous retroviruses. *J. Virol.* **79:**15573–15577.

38. **Dobrescu, D., S. Kabak, K. Mehta, C. H. Suh, A. Asch, P. U. Cameron, A. S. Hodtsev, and D. N. Posnett.** 1995. Human immunodeficiency virus 1 reservoir in CD4+ T cells is restricted to certain V beta subsets. *Proc. Natl. Acad. Sci. USA* **92:**5563–5567.

39. **Dobrescu, D., B. Ursea, M. Pope, A. S. Asch, and D. N. Posnett.** 1995. Enhanced HIV1 replication in V beta 12 T cells due to human cytomegalovirus in monocytes: evidence for a putative herpesvirus superantigen. *Cell* **82:**753–763.

40. **Domiati-Saad, R., and P. E. Lipsky.** 1997. B cell superantigens: potential modifiers of the normal human B cell repertoire. *Int. Rev. Immunol.* **14:**309–324.

41. **Doyon, L., C. Simard, R. P. Sekaly, and P. Jolicoeur.** 1996. Evidence that the murine AIDS defective virus does not encode a superantigen. *J. Virol.* **70:**1–9.

42. **Du, C., and S. Sriram.** 2000. Induction of interleukin-12/p40 by superantigens in macrophages is mediated by activation of nuclear factor-kappaB. *Cell. Immunol.* **199:**50–57.

43. **Fast, D. J., B. J. Shannon, M. J. Herriott, M. J. Kennedy, J. A. Rummage, and R. W. Leu.** 1991. Staphylococcal exotoxins stimulate nitric oxide-dependent murine macrophage tumoricidal activity. *Infect. Immun.* **59:**2987–2993.

44. **Fingeroth, J. D., J. J. Weis, T. F. Tedder, J. L. Strominger, P. A. Biro, and D. T. Fearon.** 1984. Epstein-Barr virus receptor of human B lymphocytes is the C3d receptor CR2. *Proc. Natl. Acad. Sci. USA* **81:**4510–4514.

45. **Firouzi, R., A. Rolland, M. Michel, E. Jouvin-Marche, J. J. Hauw, C. Malcus-Vocanson, F. Lazarini, L. Gebuhrer, J. M. Seigneurin, J. L. Touraine, K. Sanhadji, P. N. Marche, and H. Perron.** 2003. Multiple sclerosis-associated retrovirus particles cause T lymphocyte-dependent death with brain hemorrhage in humanized SCID mice model. *J. Neurovirol.* **9:**79–93.

46. **Foster, T. J.** 2005. Immune evasion by staphylococci. *Nat. Rev. Microbiol.* **3:**948–958.

47. **Frade, R., M. Barel, B. Ehlin-Henriksson, and G. Klein.** 1985. gp140, the C3d receptor of human B lymphocytes, is also the Epstein-Barr virus receptor. *Proc. Natl. Acad. Sci. USA* **82:**1490–1493.

48. **Galelli, A., M. Delcourt, M. C. Wagner, W. Peumans, and P. Truffa-Bachi.** 1995. Selective expansion followed by profound deletion of mature V beta 8.3+ T cells in vivo after exposure to the superantigenic lectin Urtica dioica agglutinin. *J. Immunol.* **154:**2600–2611.

49. **Galelli, A., and P. Truffa-Bachi.** 1993. Urtica dioica agglutinin. A superantigenic lectin from stinging nettle rhizome. *J. Immunol.* **151:**1821–1831.

50. **Gayama, S., L. Doyon, B. Vaupel, R. P. Sekaly, and O. Kanagawa.** 1998. Induction of endogenous mammary tumor virus in lymphocytes infected with murine acquired immunodeficiency syndrome virus. *Cell. Immunol.* **187:**124–130.

51. **Gehring, S., M. Schlaak, and J. van der Bosch.** 1998. A new in vitro model for studying human T cell differentiation: T(H1)/T(H2) induction following activation by superantigens. *J. Immunol. Methods* **219:**85–98.

52. **Germain, R. N.** 2002. T-cell development and the CD4-CD8 lineage decision. *Nat. Rev. Immunol.* **2:**309–322.

53. **Golovkina, T. V., I. Piazzon, I. Nepomnaschy, V. Buggiano, M. de Olano Vela, and S. R. Ross.** 1997. Generation of a tumorigenic milk-borne mouse mammary tumor virus by recombination between endogenous and exogenous viruses. *J. Virol.* **71:**3895–3903.

54. **Goodglick, L., N. Zevit, M. S. Neshat, and J. Braun.** 1995. Mapping the Ig superantigen-binding site of HIV-1 gp120. *J. Immunol.* **155:**5151–5159.

55. **Gougeon, M. L.** 1995. Chronic activation of the immune system in HIV infection: contribution to T cell apoptosis and V beta selective T cell anergy. *Curr. Top. Microbiol. Immunol.* **200:**177–193.

56. **Hackett, S. P., and D. L. Stevens.** 1993. Superantigens associated with staphylococcal and streptococcal toxic shock syndrome are potent inducers of tumor necrosis factor-beta synthesis. *J. Infect. Dis.* **168:**232–235.

57. **Hardy, C. L., L. Lu, P. Nguyen, D. L. Woodland, R. W. Williams, and M. A. Blackman.** 2001. Identification of quantitative trait loci controlling activation of TRBV4 CD8+ T cells during murine gamma-herpesvirus-induced infectious mononucleosis. *Immunogenetics* **53:**395–400.

58. **Hardy, C. L., S. L. Silins, D. L. Woodland, and M. A. Blackman.** 2000. Murine gamma-herpesvirus infection causes V(beta)4-specific CDR3-restricted clonal expansions within CD8(+) peripheral blood T lymphocytes. *Int. Immunol.* **12:**1193–1204.

59. **Hasuike, S., K. Miura, O. Miyoshi, T. Miyamoto, N. Niikawa, Y. Jinno, and M. Ishikawa.** 1999. Isolation and localization of an IDDMK1,2-22-related human endogenous retroviral gene, and identification of a CA repeat marker at its locus. *J. Hum. Genet.* **44:**343–347.

60. **Heaton, T., D. Mallon, T. Venaille, and P. Holt.** 2003. Staphylococcal enterotoxin induced IL-5 stimulation as a cofactor in the pathogenesis of atopic disease: the hygiene hypothesis in reverse? *Allergy* **58:**252–256.

61. **Held, W., G. A. Waanders, H. R. MacDonald, and H. Acha-Orbea.** 1994. MHC class II hierarchy of superantigen presentation predicts efficiency of infection with mouse mammary tumor virus. *Int. Immunol.* **6:**1403–1407.

62. **Henne, E., W. H. Campbell, and E. Carlson.** 1991. Toxic shock syndrome toxin 1 enhances synthesis of endotoxin-induced tumor necrosis factor in mice. *Infect. Immun.* **59:**2929–2933.

63. **Herman, A., J. W. Kappler, P. Marrack, and A. M. Pullen.** 1991. Superantigens: mechanism of T-cell stimulation and role in immune responses. *Annu. Rev. Immunol.* **9:**745–972.

64. **Hirose, A., T. Ikejima, and D. M. Gill.** 1985. Established macrophagelike cell lines synthesize interleukin-1 in response to toxic shock syndrome toxin. *Infect. Immun.* **50:**765–770.

65. **Hogquist, K. A.** 2001. Signal strength in thymic selection and lineage commitment. *Curr. Opin. Immunol.* **13:**225–231.

66. **Hoiden, I., and G. Moller.** 1996. CD8+ cells are the main producers of IL10 and IFN gamma after superantigen stimulation. *Scand. J. Immunol.* **44:**501–505.

67. **Hsiao, F. C., M. Lin, A. Tai, G. Chen, and B. T. Huber.** 2006. Cutting edge: Epstein-Barr Virus transactivates the HERV-K18 superantigen by docking to the human complement receptor 2 (CD21) on primary B cells. *J. Immunol.* **177:**2056–2060.

68. **Hsu, P. N., P. Wolf Bryant, N. Sutkowski, B. McLellan, H. L. Ploegh, and B. T. Huber.** 2001. Association of mouse mammary tumor virus superantigen with MHC class II during biosynthesis. *J. Immunol.* **166:**3309–3314.

69. **Huber, B. T.** 1995. The role of superantigens in virus infection. *J. Clin. Immunol.* **15:**22S–25S.

70. **Hugin, A. W., M. S. Vacchio, and H. C. Morse III.** 1991. A virus-encoded "superantigen" in a retrovirus-induced immunodeficiency syndrome of mice. *Science* **252:**424–427.

71. **Imberti, L., A. Sottini, A. Bettinardi, M. Puoti, and D. Primi.** 1991. Selective depletion in HIV infection of T cells that bear specific T cell receptor V beta sequences. *Science* **254:**860–862.

72. **Ito, Y., J. Abe, K. Yoshino, T. Takeda, and T. Kohsaka.** 1995. Sequence analysis of the gene for a novel superantigen produced by Yersinia pseudotuberculosis and expression of the recombinant protein. *J. Immunol.* **154:**5896–5906.

73. **Iwashima, M.** 2003. Kinetic perspectives of T cell antigen receptor signaling. A two-tier model for T cell full activation. *Immunol. Rev.* **191:**196–210.

74. **Jabara, H. H., and R. S. Geha.** 1996. The superantigen toxic shock syndrome toxin-1 induces CD40 ligand expression and modulates IgE isotype switching. *Int. Immunol.* **8:**1503–1510.

75. **Jedrzkiewicz, S., G. Kataeva, C. M. Hogaboam, S. L. Kunkel, R. M. Strieter, and D. M. McKay.** 1999. Superantigen immune stimulation evokes epithelial monocyte chemoattractant protein 1 and RANTES production. *Infect. Immun.* **67:**6198–6202.

76. **Juompan, L., P. Lambin, and M. Zouali.** 1998. Selective deficit in antibodies specific for the superantigen binding site of gp120 in HIV infection. *FASEB J.* **12:**1473–1480.

77. **Kappler, J., B. Kotzin, L. Herron, E. W. Gelfand, R. D. Bigler, A. Boylston, S. Carrel, D. N. Posnett, Y. Choi, and P. Marrack.** 1989. V beta-specific stimulation of human T cells by staphylococcal toxins. *Science* **244:**811–813.

78. **Karray, S., and M. Zouali.** 1997. Identification of the B cell superantigen-binding site of HIV-1 gp120. *Proc. Natl. Acad. Sci. USA* **94:**1356–1360.

79. **Kobe, B., R. J. Center, B. E. Kemp, and P. Poumbourios.** 1999. Crystal structure of human T cell leukemia virus type 1 gp21 ectodomain crystallized as a maltose-binding protein chimera reveals structural evolution of retroviral transmembrane proteins. *Proc. Natl. Acad. Sci. USA* **96:**4319–4324.

80. **Komanduri, K. V., M. D. Salha, R. P. Sekaly, and J. M. McCune.** 1997. Superantigen-mediated deletion of specific T cell receptor V beta subsets in the SCID-hu Thy/Liv mouse is induced by staphylococcal enterotoxin B, but not HIV-1. *J. Immunol.* **158:**544–549.

81. **Krakauer, T.** 1998. Interleukin-8 production by human monocytic cells in response to staphylococcal exotoxins is direct and independent of interleukin-1 and tumor necrosis factor-alpha. *J. Infect. Dis.* **178:**573–577.

82. **Krakauer, T.** 1999. Induction of CC chemokines in human peripheral blood mononuclear cells by staphylococcal exotoxins and its prevention by pentoxifylline. *J. Leukoc. Biol.* **66:**158–164.

83. **Lafon, M.** 1997. Superantigen in rabies virus and its involvement in paralysis, p. 85–102. *In* D. Y. M. Leung, B. T. Huber, and P. M. Schlievert (ed.), *Superantigens: Molecular Biology, Immunology, and Relevance to Human Disease.* Marcel Dekker, New York, N.Y.

84. **Lafon, M., M. Lafage, A. Martinez-Arends, R. Ramirez, F. Vuillier, D. Charron, V. Lotteau, and D. Scott-Algara.** 1992. Evidence for a viral superantigen in humans. *Nature* **358:**507–510.

85. **Lafon, M., D. Scott-Algara, P. N. Marche, P. A. Cazenave, and E. Jouvin-Marche.** 1994. Neonatal deletion and selective expansion of mouse T cells by exposure to rabies virus nucleocapsid superantigen. *J. Exp. Med.* **180:**1207–1215.

86. **Lander, E. S., L. M. Linton, B. Birren, C. Nusbaum, M. C. Zody, J. Baldwin, K. Devon, K. Dewar, M. Doyle, W. FitzHugh, R. Funke, D. Gage, K. Harris, A. Heaford, J. Howland, L. Kann, J. Lehoczky, R. LeVine, P. McEwan, K. McKernan, J. Meldrim, J. P. Mesirov, C. Miranda, W. Morris, J. Naylor, C. Raymond, M. Rosetti, R. Santos, A. Sheridan, C. Sougnez, N. Stange-Thomann, N. Stojanovic, A. Subramanian, D. Wyman, J. Rogers, J. Sulston, R. Ainscough, S. Beck, D. Bentley, J. Burton, C. Clee, N. Carter, A. Coulson, R. Deadman, P. Deloukas, A. Dunham, I. Dunham, R. Durbin, L. French, D. Grafham, S. Gregory, T. Hubbard, S. Humphray, A. Hunt, M. Jones, C. Lloyd, A. McMurray, L. Matthews, S. Mercer, S. Milne, J. C. Mullikin, A. Mungall, R. Plumb, M. Ross, R. Shownkeen, S. Sims, R. H. Waterston, R. K. Wilson, L. W. Hillier, J. D. McPherson, M. A. Marra, E. R. Mardis, L. A. Fulton, A. T. Chinwalla, K. H. Pepin, W. R. Gish, S. L. Chissoe, M. C. Wendl, K. D. Delehaunty, T. L. Miner, A. Delehaunty, J. B. Kramer, L. L. Cook, R. S. Fulton, D. L. Johnson, P. J. Minx, S. W. Clifton, T. Hawkins, E. Branscomb, P. Predki, P. Richardson, S. Wenning, T. Slezak, N. Doggett, J. F. Cheng, A. Olsen, S. Lucas, C. Elkin, E. Uberbacher, M. Frazier, et al.** 2001. Initial sequencing and analysis of the human genome. *Nature* **409:**860–921.

87. **Laurence, J., A. S. Hodtsev, and D. N. Posnett.** 1992. Superantigen implicated in dependence of HIV-1 replication in T cells on TCR V beta expression. *Nature* **358:**255–259.

88. **Lavoie, P. M., H. McGrath, N. H. Shoukry, P. A. Cazenave, R. P. Sekaly, and J. Thibodeau.** 2001. Quantitative relationship between MHC class II-superantigen complexes and the balance of T cell activation versus death. *J. Immunol.* **166:**7229–7237.

89. **Lavoie, P. M., J. Thibodeau, F. Erard, and R. P. Sekaly.** 1999. Understanding the mechanism of action of bacterial superantigens from a decade of research. *Immunol. Rev.* **168:**257–269.

90. **Lennon, G. P., J. E. Sillibourne, E. Furrie, M. J. Doherty, and R. A. Kay.** 2000. Antigen triggering selectively increases TCRBV gene transcription. *J. Immunol.* **165:**2020–2027.

91. **Liu, B., Y. Wang, S. M. Melana, I. Pelisson, V. Najfeld, J. F. Holland, and B. G. Pogo.** 2001. Identification of a proviral structure in human breast cancer. *Cancer Res.* **61:**1754–1759.

92. **Llewelyn, M., S. Sriskandan, M. Peakman, D. R. Ambrozak, D. C. Douek, W. W. Kwok, J. Cohen, and D. M. Altmann.** 2004. HLA class II polymorphisms determine responses to bacterial superantigens. *J. Immunol.* **172:**1719–1726.

93. **Marrack, P., M. Blackman, E. Kushnir, and J. Kappler.** 1990. The toxicity of staphylococcal enterotoxin B in mice is mediated by T cells. *J. Exp. Med.* **171:**455–464.

94. **Martinez-Arends, A., E. Astoul, M. Lafage, and M. Lafon.** 1995. Activation of human tonsil lymphocytes by rabies virus nucleocapsid superantigen. *Clin. Immunol. Immunopathol.* **77:**177–184.

95. **McCarty, T. C., S. K. Chattopadhyay, M. T. Scherer, T. N. Fredrickson, J. W. Hartley, and H. C. Morse III.** 1996. Endogenous Mtv-encoded superantigens are not required for development of murine AIDS. *J. Virol.* **70:**8148–8150.

96. **Mi, S., X. Lee, X. Li, G. M. Veldman, H. Finnerty, L. Racie, E. LaVallie, X. Y. Tang, P. Edouard, S. Howes, J. C. Keith, Jr., and J. M. McCoy.** 2000. Syncytin is a captive retroviral envelope protein involved in human placental morphogenesis. *Nature* **403:**785–789.

97. **Miyoshi-Akiyama, T., A. Abe, H. Kato, K. Kawahara, H. Narimatsu, and T. Uchiyama.** 1995. DNA sequencing of the gene encoding a bacterial superantigen, Yersinia pseudotuberculosis-derived mitogen (YPM), and characterization of the gene product, cloned YPM. *J. Immunol.* **154:**5228–5234.

98. **Muller, S., and H. Kohler.** 1997. B cell superantigens in HIV-1 infection. *Int. Rev. Immunol.* **14:**339–349.

99. **Neshat, M. N., L. Goodglick, K. Lim, and J. Braun.** 2000. Mapping the B cell superantigen binding site for HIV-1 gp120 on a V(H)3 Ig. *Int. Immunol.* **12:**305–312.

100. **Niimi, N., W. Wajjwalku, Y. Ando, N. Nakamura, M. Ueda, and Y. Yoshikai.** 1995. A novel V beta 2-specific endogenous mouse mammary tumor virus which is capable of producing a milk-borne exogenous virus. *J. Virol.* **69:**7269–7273.

101. **Noel, C., S. Florquin, M. Goldman, and M. Y. Braun.** 2001. Chronic exposure to superantigen induces regulatory CD4(+) T cells with IL-10-mediated suppressive activity. *Int. Immunol.* **13:**431–439.

102. **Norrby-Teglund, A., G. T. Nepom, and M. Kotb.** 2002. Differential presentation of group A streptococcal superantigens by HLA class II DQ and DR alleles. *Eur. J. Immunol.* **32:**2570–2577.

103. **Perron, H., E. Jouvin-Marche, M. Michel, A. Ounanian-Paraz, S. Camelo, A. Dumon, C. Jolivet-Reynaud, F. Marcel, Y. Souillet, E. Borel, L. Gebuhrer, L. Santoro, S. Marcel, J. M. Seigneurin, P. N. Marche, and M. Lafon.** 2001. Multiple sclerosis retrovirus particles and recombinant envelope trigger an abnormal immune response in vitro, by inducing polyclonal Vbeta16 T-lymphocyte activation. *Virology* **287:**321–332.

104. **Perron, H., F. Lazarini, K. Ruprecht, C. Pechoux-Longin, D. Seilhean, V. Sazdovitch, A. Creange, N. Battail-Poirot, G. Sibai, L. Santoro, M. Jolivet, J. L. Darlix, P. Rieckmann, T. Arzberger, J. J. Hauw, and H. Lassmann.** 2005. Human endogenous retrovirus (HERV)-W ENV and GAG proteins: physiological expression in human brain and pathophysiological modulation in multiple sclerosis lesions. *J. Neurovirol.* **11:**23–33.

105. **Posnett, D. N., S. Kabak, D. Dobrescu, and A. S. Hodtsev.** 1995. The HIV-1 reservoir in distinct V beta subsets of CD4 T cells: evidence for a putative superantigen. *J. Clin. Immunol.* **15:**18S–21S.

106. **Posnett, D. N., S. Kabak, A. S. Hodtsev, E. A. Goldberg, and A. Asch.** 1993. T-cell antigen receptor V beta subsets are not preferentially deleted in AIDS. *AIDS* **7:**625–631.

107. **Rebai, N., G. Pantaleo, J. F. Demarest, C. Ciurli, H. Soudeyns, J. W. Adelsberger, M. Vaccarezza, R. E. Walker, R. P. Sekaly, and A. S. Fauci.** 1994. Analysis of the T-cell receptor beta-chain variable-region (V beta) repertoire in monozygotic twins discordant for human immunodeficiency virus: evidence for perturbations of specific V beta segments in CD4+ T cells of the virus-positive twins. *Proc. Natl. Acad. Sci. USA* **91:**1529–1533.

108. **Renard, M., P. F. Varela, C. Letzelter, S. Duquerroy, F. A. Rey, and T. Heidmann.** 2005. Crystal structure of a pivotal domain of human syncytin-2, a 40 million years old endogenous retrovirus fusogenic envelope gene captured by primates. *J. Mol. Biol.* **352:**1029–1034.

109. **Rink, L., and H. Kirchner.** 1992. Mycoplasma arthritidis-derived superantigen. *Chem. Immunol.* **55:**137–145.

110. **Rovira, P., M. Buckle, J. P. Abastado, W. J. Peumans, and P. Truffa-Bachi.** 1999. Major histocompatibility class I molecules present Urtica dioica agglutinin, a superantigen of vegetal origin, to T lymphocytes. *Eur. J. Immunol.* **29:**1571–1580.

111. **Ruprecht, K., K. Obojes, V. Wengel, F. Gronen, K. S. Kim, H. Perron, J. Schneider-Schaulies, and P. Rieckmann.** 2006. Regulation of human endogenous retrovirus W protein expression by herpes simplex virus type 1: implications for multiple sclerosis. *J. Neurovirol.* **12:**65–71.

112. **Saul, F. A., P. Rovira, G. Boulot, E. J. Damme, W. J. Peumans, P. Truffa-Bachi, and G. A. Bentley.** 2000. Crystal structure of Urtica dioica agglutinin, a superantigen presented by MHC molecules of class I and class II. *Structure* **8:**593–603.

113. **Sawada, T., R. Pergolizzi, K. Ito, J. Silver, C. Atkin, B. C. Cole, and M. D. Chang.** 1995. Replacement of the DR alpha chain with the E alpha chain enhances presentation of Mycoplasma arthritidis superantigen by the human class II DR molecule. *Infect. Immun.* **63:**3367–3372.

114. **Sen, N., W. J. Simmons, R. M. Thomas, G. Erianne, D. J. Zhang, N. S. Jaeggli, C. Huang, X. Xiong, V. K. Tsiagbe, N. M. Ponzio, and G. J. Thorbecke.** 2001. META-controlled env-initiated transcripts

encoding superantigens of murine Mtv29 and Mtv7 and their possible role in B cell lymphomagenesis. *J. Immunol.* **166:**5422–5429.

115. **Silverman, G. J., J. V. Nayak, and A. La Cava.** 1997. B-cell superantigens: molecular and cellular implications. *Int. Rev. Immunol.* **14:**259–290.

116. **Simmons, W. J., M. Simms, R. Chiarle, F. Mackay, V. K. Tsiagbe, J. Browning, G. Inghirami, and G. J. Thorbecke.** 2001. Induction of germinal centers by MMTV encoded superantigen on B cells. *Dev. Immunol.* **8:**201–211.

117. **Soderquist, B., J. Kallman, H. Holmberg, T. Vikerfors, and E. Kihlstrom.** 1998. Secretion of IL-6, IL-8 and G-CSF by human endothelial cells in vitro in response to Staphylococcus aureus and staphylococcal exotoxins. *APMIS* **106:**1157–1164.

118. **Soudeyns, H., J. P. Routy, and R. P. Sekaly.** 1994. Comparative analysis of the T cell receptor V beta repertoire in various lymphoid tissues from HIV-infected patients: evidence for an HIV-associated superantigen. *Leukemia* **8**(Suppl. 1)**:**S95–S97.

119. **Stauffer, Y., S. Marguerat, F. Meylan, C. Ucla, N. Sutkowski, B. Huber, T. Pelet, and B. Conrad.** 2001. Interferon-alpha-induced endogenous superantigen. A model linking environment and autoimmunity. *Immunity* **15:**591–601.

120. **Stuart, P. M., R. K. Munn, E. DeMoll, and J. G. Woodward.** 1995. Characterization of human T-cell responses to Yersinia enterocolitica superantigen. *Hum. Immunol.* **43:**269–275.

121. **Surman, S., A. M. Deckhut, M. A. Blackman, and D. L. Woodland.** 1994. MHC-specific recognition of a bacterial superantigen by weakly reactive T cells. *J. Immunol.* **152:**4893–4902.

122. **Sutkowski, N., G. Chen, G. Calderon, and B. T. Huber.** 2004. Epstein-Barr virus latent membrane protein LMP-2A is sufficient for transactivation of the human endogenous retrovirus HERV-K18 superantigen. *J. Virol.* **78:**7852–7860.

123. **Sutkowski, N., B. Conrad, D. A. Thorley-Lawson, and B. T. Huber.** 2001. Epstein-Barr virus transactivates the human endogenous retrovirus HERV-K18 that encodes a superantigen. *Immunity* **15:**579–589.

124. **Sutkowski, N., and B. T. Huber.** 2005. EBV induces an endogenous superantigen: implications for pathogenesis, p. 233–262. *In* E. S. Robertson (ed.), *Epstein-Barr Virus*, 1st ed. Caister Academic Press, Norwich, United Kingdom.

125. **Sutkowski, N., T. Palkama, C. Ciurli, R. P. Sekaly, D. A. Thorley-Lawson, and B. T. Huber.** 1996. An Epstein-Barr virus-associated superantigen. *J. Exp. Med.* **184:**971–980.

126. **Tai, A. K., M. Lin, F. Chang, G. Chen, F. Hsiao, N. Sutkowski, and B. T. Huber.** 2006. Murine V3+ and V7+ T cell subsets are specific targets for the HERV-K18 Env superantigen. *J. Immunol.* **177:**3178–3184.

127. **Takeda, T., K. Yoshino, Y. Itoh, J. Abe, Y. Shimonishi, and T. Kohsaka.** 1995. Purification and gene cloning of a superantigen (YPM) produced by a patient strain of Yersinia pseudotuberculosis. *Contrib. Microbiol. Immunol.* **13:**331–333.

128. **Tao, X., S. Constant, P. Jorritsma, and K. Bottomly.** 1997. Strength of TCR signal determines the costimulatory requirements for Th1 and Th2 CD4+ T cell differentiation. *J. Immunol.* **159:**5956–5963.

129. **Tomonari, K., and S. Fairchild.** 1992. Positive and negative selection of Tcrb-V6+ T cells. *Immunogenetics* **36:**230–237.

130. **Townsley-Fuchs, J., M. S. Neshat, D. H. Margolin, J. Braun, and L. Goodglick.** 1997. HIV-1 gp120: a novel viral B cell superantigen. *Int. Rev. Immunol.* **14:**325–338.

131. **Trentin, L., R. Zambello, M. Facco, R. Sancetta, A. Cerutti, A. Milani, C. Tassinari, C. Crivellaro, A. Cipriani, C. Agostini, and G. Semenzato.** 1996. Skewing of the T-cell receptor repertoire in the lung of patients with HIV-1 infection. *AIDS* **10:**729–737.

132. **Tripp, R. A., A. M. Hamilton-Easton, R. D. Cardin, P. Nguyen, F. G. Behm, D. L. Woodland, P. C. Doherty, and M. A. Blackman.** 1997. Pathogenesis of an infectious mononucleosis-like disease induced by a murine gamma-herpesvirus: role for a viral superantigen? *J. Exp. Med.* **185:**1641–1650.

133. **Venter, J. C., M. D. Adams, E. W. Myers, P. W. Li, R. J. Mural, G. G. Sutton, H. O. Smith, M. Yandell, C. A. Evans, R. A. Holt, J. D. Gocayne, P. Amanatides, R. M. Ballew, D. H. Huson, J. R. Wortman, Q. Zhang, C. D. Kodira, X. H. Zheng, L. Chen, M. Skupski, G. Subramanian, P. D. Thomas, J. Zhang, G. L. Gabor Miklos, C. Nelson, S. Broder, A. G. Clark, J. Nadeau, V. A. McKusick, N. Zinder, A. J. Levine, R. J. Roberts, M. Simon, C. Slayman, M. Hunkapiller, R. Bolanos, A. Delcher, I. Dew, D. Fasulo, M. Flanigan, L. Florea, A. Halpern, S. Hannenhalli, S. Kravitz, S. Levy, C. Mobarry, K. Reinert, K. Remington, J. Abu-Threideh, E. Beasley, K. Biddick, V. Bonazzi, R. Brandon, M. Cargill, I. Chandramouliswaran, R. Charlab, K. Chaturvedi, Z. Deng, V. Di Francesco, P. Dunn, K. Eilbeck,

C. Evangelista, A. E. Gabrielian, W. Gan, W. Ge, F. Gong, Z. Gu, P. Guan, T. J. Heiman, M. E. Higgins, R. R. Ji, Z. Ke, K. A. Ketchum, Z. Lai, Y. Lei, Z. Li, J. Li, Y. Liang, X. Lin, F. Lu, G. V. Merkulov, N. Milshina, H. M. Moore, A. K. Naik, V. A. Narayan, B. Neelam, D. Nusskern, D. B. Rusch, S. Salzberg, W. Shao, B. Shue, J. Sun, Z. Wang, A. Wang, X. Wang, J. Wang, M. Wei, R. Wides, C. Xiao, C. Yan, et al. 2001. The sequence of the human genome. *Science* **291:**1304–1351.

134. **Wallace, F. M., A. S. Mach, A. M. Keller, and J. A. Lindsay.** 1999. Evidence for Clostridium perfringens enterotoxin (CPE) inducing a mitogenic and cytokine response in vitro and a cytokine response in vivo. *Curr. Microbiol.* **38:**96–100.

135. **Wang, Y., J. D. Jiang, D. Xu, Y. Li, C. Qu, J. F. Holland, and B. G. Pogo.** 2004. A mouse mammary tumor virus-like long terminal repeat superantigen in human breast cancer. *Cancer Res.* **64:**4105–4111.

136. **Wang, Y., I. Pelisson, S. M. Melana, J. F. Holland, and B. G. Pogo.** 2001. Detection of MMTV-like LTR and LTR-env gene sequences in human breast cancer. *Int. J. Oncol.* **18:**1041–1044.

137. **White, J., A. Herman, A. M. Pullen, R. Kubo, J. W. Kappler, and P. Marrack.** 1989. The V beta-specific superantigen staphylococcal enterotoxin B: stimulation of mature T cells and clonal deletion in neonatal mice. *Cell* **56:**27–35.

138. **Winslow, G. M., M. T. Scherer, J. W. Kappler, and P. Marrack.** 1992. Detection and biochemical characterization of the mouse mammary tumor virus 7 superantigen (Mls-1a). *Cell* **71:**719–730.

139. **Zembowicz, A., and J. R. Vane.** 1992. Induction of nitric oxide synthase activity by toxic shock syndrome toxin 1 in a macrophage-monocyte cell line. *Proc. Natl. Acad. Sci. USA* **89:**2051–2055.

Superantigens: Molecular Basis for Their Role in Human Diseases
Edited by Malak Kotb and John D. Fraser
© 2007 ASM Press, Washington, D.C.

Chapter 5

Superantigens from Gram-Negative Bacteria and the Diseases That They Cause

Takehiko Uchiyama, Tohru Miyoshi-Akiyama, and Hidehiro Ueshiba

INTRODUCTION

The superantigen (SAg) concept was proposed in 1989 (14, 15) for several bacterial protein toxins from *Staphylococcus aureus*, including toxic shock syndrome (TSS) toxin-1 (TSST-1), the major causative toxin of TSS (33). Many bacterial SAgs have been identified subsequently, and most of them are products of gram-positive cocci (24, 33). *Yersinia pseudotuberculosis*-derived mitogens (YPMs) a, b, and c, however, have been identified as SAgs from gram-negative bacteria (1). At very low doses (1 pg/ml or more) most SAgs activate a vast number of human T cells in a T-cell receptor (TCR) β-chain Vβ-element-selective manner in direct association with major histocompatibility complex (MHC) class II molecules expressed on the surface of antigen-presenting cells (APCs) (33). The T-cell activation by SAgs triggers the pathological changes that are based on multiple organ failure, seen in several infectious diseases, such as acute and systemic *Y. pseudotuberculosis* infection (1, 35), TSS in children and adults (33, 34), and TSS in neonates, neonatal TSS-like exanthematous disease (NTED) (30). In this chapter we review progress in research on YPMs and the diseases caused by them. We also discuss research findings in TSS and NTED, because these findings provide clues to the pathogenic mechanism of systemic *Y. pseudotuberculosis* infection.

YPMs AND THE TERTIARY STRUCTURE OF YPMa
Discovery of YPMs and YPM Genes

The initial step in the discovery of YPMa was closely related with the pathogenic mechanism of systemic *Y. pseudotuberculosis* infection. A hypothesis that overactivation of T cells by TSST-1 is a primary cause of the abnormal changes in TSS (34) strongly suggested

Takehiko Uchiyama • Department of Human Science, Tokiwa University, Mito, 310-8585, Japan. *Tohru Miyoshi-Akiyama* • Department of Infectious Disease, International Medical Center of Japan, Tokyo, 162-8655, Japan. *Hidehiro Ueshiba* • Institute of Laboratory Animals, Tokyo Women's Medical University, Tokyo, 162-8666, Japan.

that a toxin with SAg activity is involved in the pathogenic mechanism of the disease. In 1993, two research groups in Japan succeeded in identifying a novel SAg, YPMa, from clinical strains (3, 23, 35), and the YPMa gene and the amino acid sequence of YPMa were identified in 1995 (13, 21). Sequencing of the YPM gene revealed that it encodes a protein composed of 131 amino acid residues with a molecular weight 14.5 kDa (Fig. 1). Homology analyses revealed that homology between the amino acid sequences of YPMa and other well-known SAgs is quite low. Subsequently, two variants of YPMa, YPMb (25) and YPMc (5), were identified (Fig. 1). YPMb is one amino acid shorter than YPMa, and alignment of the amino acid sequences of the mature YPMa and YPMb proteins revealed 83% homology between them (25). YPMc has the same amino acid sequence as YPMa except for one amino acid substitution (5). It was reported in the 1990s that some strains of *Yersinia enterocolitica*, which cause gastroenteritis, produce a SAg, as cited in reference 5. To date the product has not been characterized at either the protein level or the gene level.

Genes encoding SAgs are frequently carried within mobile genetic elements, especially bacteriophages (1), and several features of YPMs strongly suggest involvement of mobile genetic elements in carrying the SAg genes. First, YPM genes have not been present in all *Y. pseudotuberculosis* strains examined (11, 36, 38). Second, their guanine and cytosine

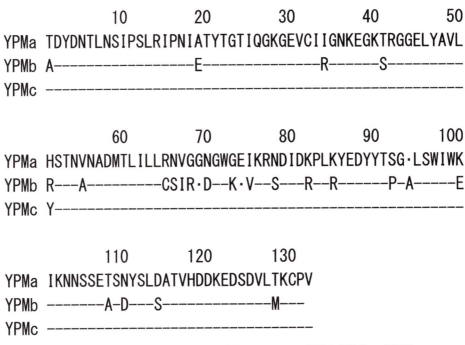

Figure 1. Deduced amino acid sequences of the mature types of YPMa, YPMb, and YPMc. Amino acids are represented by the single-letter code. Numbering of the amino acids starts at the amino terminus of the mature types of YPMa, YPMb, and YPMc. Identical amino acids compared with YPMa are indicated with dashes (–). Dots (·) indicate deletions. YPMa, from references 13 and 21; YPMb, from reference 25; YPMc, from reference 5.

(GC) content is significantly lower (34.6 to 35.3%) than in the genomic core (46.5%) (5). Third, an analysis of a 17.1-kb DNA segment encompassing the YPM genes strongly suggested active involvement of genetic elements in insertion of the YPM genes into the *Y. pseudotuberculosis* chromosome (4).

Tertiary Structure of YPMa

Most SAgs from gram-positive bacteria have highly conserved secondary and tertiary structures despite minimal homology in amino acid sequences among them (20). In Color Plate 2, the tertiary structure of SEA is shown as an example of standard SAgs. X-ray crystal structure analyses of SAgs have revealed that they share a common two-domain fold, the β-barrel globular domain (domain 1) and the globular domain (domain 2). Domain 1 features a long central α-helix resting against a sheet of four β-strands, constructing a motif known as the β-grasp that has been observed in many bacterial products. Domain 2 is a five-stranded β-barrel known as the oligonucleotide/oligosaccharide-binding fold and is found in many bacterial products. It has been speculated that SAgs evolved through recombination of the two smaller β-strand motifs (20).

A study on the tertiary structure of YPMa revealed the crystal and solution structures of YPMa (9). YPMa exists in the form of a jelly-roll fold comprising two β-sheets, each containing four antiparallel strands (Color Plate 2). In the YPMa molecule, sheet 1 contains strands A, H, C, and F, and sheet 2 contains strands B, G, D, and E. A stretch of polypeptide at the C terminus runs transverse to sheet 2 and contains a helix structure that is bound to strand B by two hydrogen bonds. The C terminus connects with strand 2 via a disulfide bond (Cys129-Cys32). Structural comparison analysis indicated that the closest structural similarities of YPMa are viral capsid proteins, including Satellite tobacco necrosis virus (STNV), and members of the tumor necrosis factor superfamily proteins, including adipocyte complement-related protein (ACRP) (9). No apparent sequence basis exists for the observed structural similarities between YPMa and any of these proteins. The structural analysis also indicated that YPMa forms a trimer in the crystal, but behaves as a monomer in solution. The authors pointed out the possibility that YPMa trimerization is important for its function, because such an assembly may occur when YPMa interacts with MHC class II molecules and TCR in the crowded cell–cell interface that makes up the immunological synapse (9).

T-CELL ACTIVATION BY YPMs

T-Cell Activation by YPMs and T-Cell-Dependent Toxic Effects of YPMa

At doses of 10 pg/ml or more in the presence of MHC class II+ APCs YPMa stimulates human T cells to proliferate and produce large amounts of cytokines (3, 35), but 100 to 1,000 times higher doses of YPMa are required to substantially activate mouse T cells (22). The T-cell stimulating activity of YPMa, however, is 100 to 1,000 times lower than that of other potent bacterial SAgs, such as TSST-1 (34). Investigation of the TCR Vβ repertoire of T cells reactive with YPMs has shown that both YPMa (3, 35) and YPMb (25) activate Vβ3+, Vβ9+, Vβ13.1+, Vβ13.2+ T cells in humans (Table 1). Later, one of the two research teams found that YPMa activates an additional T-cell fraction, Vβ13.3+ T cells (13). YPMa activates Vβ7+, Vβ8.1+, Vβ8.2+, and Vβ8.3+ T cells in mice (22). In terms of their

Table 1. TCR Vβ repertoires of YPMa-reactive T cells and their relative YPMa reactivity

Parameter	TCR Vβ repertoires	
	Human	Mouse
Vβ of YPMa-reactive T cells	Vβ3, Vβ9, Vβ13.1, Vβ13.2[a]	Vβ7, Vβ8.1, Vβ8.2, Vβ8.3[b]
Strength relative to YPM reactivity	Vβ3 > Vβ9, Vβ13.1, Vβ13.2[c]	Vβ7 > Vβ8.1, Vβ8.2, Vβ8.3[d]

[a]From reference 35.
[b]From reference 22.
[c]From reference 2.
[d]From reference 6.

amino acid sequences the human Vβ3 element corresponds to the mouse Vβ7 element, and the human Vβ13 elements correspond to the mouse Vβ 8 elements. As discussed in the next section, activation of several YPMa-reactive T-cell fractions is biased by YPMa. The magnitude of the response of human Vβ3+CD4+ T cells and mouse Vβ7+CD4+ T cells to YPMa is higher than that of other YPM-reactive T-cell fractions (Table 1). Mouse NK T cells express a restricted TCR repertoire composed of an invariant TCR α-chain (Vα14-Jα281) associated with Vβ2, Vβ7, and Vβ8 elements, indicating that YPMa is the major SAg activator of mouse NK T cells. Our research team found that thymic Vβ7+CD4+ NK T cells in mice are highly reactive to YPMa (37).

Bacterial SAgs induce various pathological changes based on multiple organ failures on animals. For example, combined injection of mice with SAgs and D-galactosamine (33) induces lethal effects in a T-cell-dependent manner. In combination with D-galactosamine, YPMa also has the capacity to induce lethal shock in mice (22). The majority of mice that had been depleted of CD4+ T cells or both YPM-reactive TCR Vβ7+ and Vβ8+ T cells survived the YPM-induced lethal shock, whereas the depletion of CD8+ T cells had no effect on lethality. Administration of monoclonal antibodies (MAbs) to either tumor necrosis factor alpha (TNF-α) or gamma interferon (IFN-γ) completely blocked induction of the lethal shock. The results strongly suggest that cytokines produced by YPMa-reactive CD4+ T cells are involved in the generation of the abnormal changes seen in patients with systemic *Y. pseudotuberculosis* infection.

Mode of the YPMa-Induced T-Cell-Response–Biased Prolonged Activation of a Particular T-Cell Fraction

Many experimental findings have shown that all T-cell fractions reactive to the stimulating SAg undergo uniform transient expansion for a short period after stimulation, irrespective of the TCR Vβ expressed and CD4/CD8 subsets (33). For example, in mice SEA-reactive Vβ3+ and Vβ11+ CD4+ or CD8+ T cells expand equally on day 2 of SEA injection, and the expanded T cells return to the baseline level 2 days later (17).

Questions, however, arose from clinical observations of the behavior of SAg-reactive T cells in SAg-induced diseases as to whether the response pattern in the mouse experiments actually reflects the pattern in patients with SAg-induced diseases, and, more fundamentally, whether the respective SAgs activate the reactive T-cell fractions equally without any bias toward some particular fraction. For example, as shown below in Fig. 5, in three of seven children with systemic *Y. pseudotuberculosis* infection, T-cell expansion was detected only in Vβ3+ T cells among the four YPM-reactive T-cell fractions in peripheral blood mononuclear cells (PBMs) within 20 days after the onset of symptoms (1, 2). In one of the three patients the expansion was seen 30 days after the onset (J. Abe, personal communication), suggesting a biased, prolonged expansion of Vβ3+ T cells in these patients. Prolonged expansion has been observed more clearly in patients with TSS (8, 18). For example, massive expansions of Vβ2+ CD4+ and Vβ2+CD4+ T cells have been seen in acute-phase patients, and the expanded state of Vβ2+ T cells gradually decreased to the control level over 40 to 50 days after the onset (18) (Fig. 2A). Quite interestingly, a different pattern of T-cell expansion was seen in neonatal NTED patients. Massive expansion of Vβ2+ T cells was seen in the acute phase, but their expanded state rapidly decreased to the baseline level within 1 week after the onset, and to less than 10% of the baseline level by 1 to 2 months later (29) (Fig. 2B). There are several possible explanations for the difference in expansion pattern between adult TSS patients and neonatal NTED patients. The T cells in neonates have been shown to be very immature compared with the T cells in adults (12, 28), and the amount of TSST-1 to which the patients were exposed may have been much higher in the TSS patients than in the NTED patients. These two factors may have acted synergistically to enhance the expansion of Vβ2+ T cells in adult patients, while mitigating the expansion in neonatal patients.

We reproduced the response patterns seen in patients with TSS and systemic *Y. pseudotuberculosis* infection in mouse experiments (6). Mice were implanted with a miniosmotic pump filled with 300 μg of YPMa or 10 μg of SEA, which delivered YPMa and SEA continuously for ~7 days, and splenic YPMa and SEA-reactive T-cell fractions were monitored thereafter (Fig. 3). A prolonged biased expansion was seen in a particular T-cell fraction in the YPMa experiments (6) (Fig. 3A). Vβ7+CD4+ T cells, corresponding to human Vβ3+CD4+ T cells, expanded from 2.7% to 12% by 10 days after implantation, and their expansion gradually decreased throughout the monitoring period. Other YPMa-reactive T-cell fractions exhibited transient expansion or no expansion at all. The biased prolonged expansion in particular reactive fractions seen in the YPM experiments was seen more prominently in the SEA experiments. Vβ3+CD4+ T cells exhibited high-level protracted expansion for more than 30 days after implantation (Fig. 3B). Moderate expansions of Vβ11+CD4+ T cells and transient expansion of Vβ3+CD8+ and Vβ11+CD8+ T cells were observed. These clinical findings and experimental findings in mice indicated that SAgs induce biased responses in the SAg-reactive T-cell fractions that range from high to low depending on the TCR Vβ elements expressed and on the CD4/CD8 subsets (22). We hypothesize that the biased expansion is based on different binding affinities of TCR Vβ-elements for the complex of SAg/MHC class II molecules. Experiments to support this hypothesis are underway.

PATHOGENIC MECHANISM OF SYSTEMIC
Y. PSEUDOTUBERCULOSIS INFECTION

General Description of TSS and NTED

TSS was reported in 1978 as a new disease entity caused by *S. aureus* and characterized by severe-illness conditions based on multiple organ failure, such as high-grade fever, severe hypotension, skin rash, profuse diarrhea, and mental confusion (32, 33); desquamation is

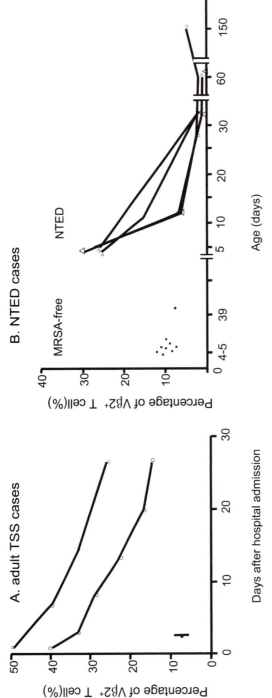

Figure 2. Different patterns of expansion of Vβ2+ T cells in adult TSS patients and neonatal NTED patients. Two adult TSS patients (A) (○, □) and four neonatal NTED patients (B) (○, □, ◇, △) were monitored for the percentage of Vβ2+ CD4+ T cells among PBMs. Data are expressed as functions of days after hospital admission (A) and the age of the patients (B). Symbols: ● in panel A, means ± standard deviation in seven healthy individuals; ◆ in panel B, one neonate at age 39 days; ■ in panel B, methicillin-resistant *S. aureus* (MRSA)-free neonates at age 5 days. The percentages of Vβ2+CD8+ T cells in adult TSS patients and neonatal NTED patients were similar to the percentages of Vβ2+CD4+ T cells. Data in panels A and B are from references 18 and 29, respectively.

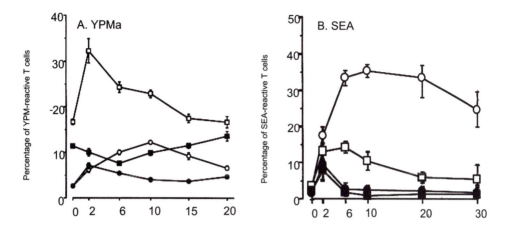

Figure 3. Expansion of YPMa-reactive and SEA-reactive T-cell fractions in mice implanted with osmotic pumps filled with YPMa or SEA. (A) C57Bl/6 mice implanted with an osmotic pump filled with 300 μg of YPMa were monitored for responses by Vβ7CD4+ (○), Vβ7CD8+ (●), Vβ8+CD4+ (□), and Vβ8+CD8+ (■) splenic T cells. (B) C57BL/6 mice implanted with an osmotic pump filled with 10 μg of SEA were monitored individually for responses by Vβ3CD4+ (○), Vβ3CD8+ (●), Vβ11+CD4+ (□), and Vβ11+CD8+ splenic T cells (■). Data are shown as percentages of the YPMa-reactive or SEA-reactive T cells. Data in panels A and B are from reference 6.

observed in the recovery phase. Direct evidence of involvement of TSST-1 in the pathogenic mechanism of TSS was obtained by the findings obtained in 1990 (8), one year after the proposal of the SAg concept, by reverse transcriptase (RT) PCR which showed expansion of Vβ2+ T cells in the acute phase. The results of the flow cytometric analysis of Vβ2+ T cells in TSS patients are shown in Fig. 2A.

NTED was reported in the middle 1990s as a new disease entity characterized by an exanthem, fever, low-positive serum C-reactive protein values, and thrombocytopenia within the first week of life. Desquamation does not occur. Direct evidence of involvement of TSST-1 in the disease was obtained in 1998 by flow cytometric analyses that showed expansion of Vβ2+ T cells in the acute phase (30), as shown in Fig. 2. Almost all term infants recover spontaneously within a week of the onset without active treatment. The clinical manifestations of many preterm infants are severe because of their physical immaturity.

General Description of Systemic *Y. pseudotuberculosis* Infection

Infections caused by *Y. pseudotuberculosis* are largely divided into two types: an acute and systemic type, which is mainly caused by YPMa, and a localized, gastrointestinal type. The latter type of infection has mainly been reported in Europe and North America (36, 38), and thus far there is no evidence that YPMs are involved in the development of this type of disease. Systemic *Y. pseudotuberculosis* infection has frequently been seen in Far Eastern countries, including Japan (10, 11, 26, 31, 36, 38), Korea (7), and the Russian Far East

(27). The active involvement of YPMa in the pathogenesis of this type of infectious disease is discussed in the next section. The clinical manifestations and laboratory data of most patients with this disease are not as severe as those of patients with TSS, and there have been hardly any fatalities. *Y. pseudotuberculosis* serotypes carrying YPMa genes are frequently isolated in Far Eastern countries but not frequently isolated in European countries or North America, which explains clearly the dichotomy in geographical distribution between systemic *Y. pseudotuberculosis* infection in the two regions (11, 36, 38) (Table 2).

A clinical study of the mass outbreak of infection by serotype 4b *Y. pseudotuberculosis* that affected more than 500 primary school children in Japan in 1986 (10) showed that the illness is characterized by fever (97%), skin rash (87%), generalized malaise (80%), straw-

Table 2. Examination for YPM production by 101 *Y. pseudotuberculosis* strains[a]

Serotype	Source[b]	YPM		
		Numbers	Gene	Production
O:1a	Animals	15	0	0
	n.d.	1	0	0
O:1b	Gastroenteritis	2	2	2
	Systemic	3	3	3
	n.d.	1	1	1
O:2a	Systemic	2	2	2
	n.d.	1	1	1
O:2b	Systemic	4	4	4
	n.d.	1	1	1
O:2c	Systemic	2	2	2
	n.d.	1	1	1
O:3	Systemic	5	3	3
	Animals	7	6	6
O:4a	Animals	8	8	8
	Mountain waters	3	3	3
	n.d.	4	4	4
O:4b	Gastroenteritis	2	2	2
	Systemic	11	11	11
O:5a	Gastroenteritis	1	1	1
	Systemic	4	4	4
	n.d.	1	1	1
O:5b	Gastroenteritis	2	2	2
	Systemic	8	8	8
	n.d.	1	1	1
O:6	Animals	2	2	2
O:7	Animals	3	1	1
	Mountain waters	1	0	0
O:9	Animals	1	1	1
O:10	Animals	1	1	1
	Mountain waters	1	1	1
O:11	Animals	1	1	1
O:12	Mountain waters	1	1	1

[a]Data from reference 36.
[b]Gastroenteritis, patients with gastroenteritis; systemic, patients with acute and generalized infection; n.d., not determined.

berry tongue (66% or more), abdominal pain (65%), vomiting (60%), headache (60%), diarrhea (50%), liver dysfunction (30%), dehydration (20%), arthralgia/chest-back pain (10 to 20%), and acute renal failure (8%). As shown in Fig. 4, the skin rash was quite variable: maculopapular, erythematous, scarlet-fever-like, urticaria-like, or erythema-multiform-like. Desquamation of the skin of the fingers and toes occurred during the recovery phase, 1 to 2 weeks after the onset (68%). No coronary aneurysms, which have infrequently been reported in other papers (16, 31), were detected in this study.

Exanthem in *Y. pseudotuberculosis* Infection

1. Incidence

Primary exanthem 87%   Secondary exanthem   12%

(30% of patients with 2-peak fever)

2. Timing of occurence

Primary exanthem

days after the onset			
1	2	3	unknown
26%	51%	15%	8%

3. Types

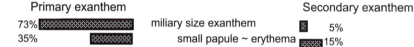

Primary exanthem		Secondary exanthem
73%	miliary size exanthem	5%
35%	small papule ~ erythema	15%

4. Sites

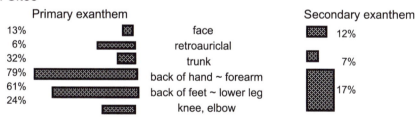

Primary exanthem		Secondary exanthem
13%	face	12%
6%	retroauriclal	
32%	trunk	7%
79%	back of hand ~ forearm	
61%	back of feet ~ lower leg	17%
24%	knee, elbow	

5. Desquamation

(+) 68%	(-) 10%	(unknown) 22%

6. Erythema nodosum

9 cases   6.5%

Figure 4. Skin rashes observed in patients with acute and systemic *Y. pseudotuberculosis* infection. The incidence of skin rashes, including primary and secondary exanthems, desquamation, and erythema nodosum in patients in the mass outbreak of systemic *Y. pseudotuberculosis* infection that occurred in Japan in 1986 (10) is shown. Data are from reference 10.

Pathogenic Mechanism of Systemic *Y. pseudotuberculosis* Infection

Patients with TSS and systemic *Y. pseudotuberculosis* infection exhibit overlapping clinical manifestations. All *Y. pseudotuberculosis* strains isolated from patients have produced YPMa, providing circumstantial strong evidence that YPMa is involved in the pathogenic mechanism of the disease. Direct evidence for active involvement of YPMa in the disease was the finding of expansion of YPMa-reactive Vβ3+ T cells in three of the seven patients in the acute phase of the illness (2) (Fig. 5). The level of expansion of Vβ3+ T cells in the three patients did not seem to be as high as the Vβ2+ T cell level in the TSS patients shown in Fig. 2A. These findings suggest that the level of activation of Vβ3+ T cells in patients with systemic *Y. pseudotuberculosis* infection is much lower than the level of activation of Vβ2+ T cells in TSS patients.

We think that the different level of activation of TSST-1-reactive T cells in the patients with TSS and NTED shown in Fig. 2 is closely related with the dichotomy in the severity of the illness caused by the two diseases. Our experiences seem to support the view above: TSS patients who were not diagnosed with TSS based on the clinical criteria for TSS because of their mild clinical manifestations showed mild expansion of Vβ2+ T cells (Y.

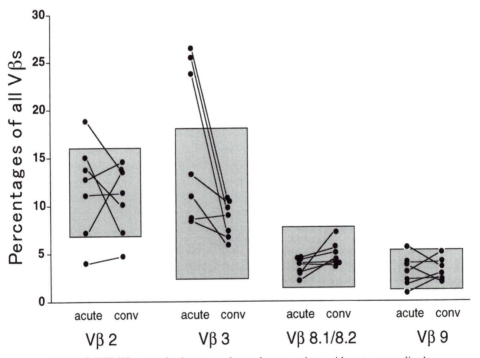

Figure 5. TCR Vβ expression in acute and convalescent patients with acute, generalized *Y. pseudotuberculosis* infection. T cells of patients with acute, generalized *Y. pseudotuberculosis* infection were examined for TCR Vβ expression by RT-PCR. Acute, within 20 days of the disease onset; conv (convalescent), later than 120 days after the disease onset. The original figure is provided by J. Abe in reference 2.

Matsuda, H. Kato, E. Ono, K. Kikuchi, K. Imanishi, M. Muraoka, K. Takagi, H. Ohta, and T. Uchiyama, submitted for publication), indicating that the illness really was TSS. An NTED patient with exceptionally severe clinical manifestations was found to have an adult-type massive, protracted expansion of Vβ2+ T cells (19). This evidence suggests that the mild activation of YPMa-reactive T cells is likely to be closely associated with the mild clinical manifestations in systemic *Y. pseudotuberculosis* infection.

Acknowledgments. This work was in part supported by Grants-in-Aid from the Ministry of Education, Culture, Sports, Science and Technology of Japan.

REFERENCES

1. **Abe, J.** 2004. Superantigens of *Yersinia pseudotuberculosis*, p. 193–213. *In* E. Carniel and B. J. Hinnebusch (ed.), *Yersinia—Molecular and Cellular Biology.* Horizon Bioscience, Norfolk, United Kingdom.
2. **Abe, J., M. Onimaru, S. Matsumoto, S. Noma, K. Baba, Y. Ito, T. Kohsaka, and T. Takeda.** 1997. Clinical role for a superantigen in *Yersinia pseudotuberculosis* infection. *J. Clin. Investig.* **99:**1823–1830.
3. **Abe, J., T. Takeda, Y. Watanabe, H. Nakao, N. Kobayashi, D. Y. Leung, and T. Kohsaka.** 1993. Evidence for superantigen production by *Yersinia pseudotuberculosis. J. Immunol.* **151:**4183–4188.
4. **Carnoy, C., S. Floquet, M. Marceau, F. Sebbane, S. Haentjens-Herwegh, A. Devalckenaere, and M. Simonet.** 2002. The superantigen gene ypm is located in an unstable chromosomal locus of *Yersinia pseudotuberculosis. J. Bacteriol.* **184:**4489–4499.
5. **Carnoy, C., and M. Simonet.** 1999. *Yersinia pseudotuberculosis* superantigenic toxins, p. 611–622. *In* J.E. Alouf and H. Freer (ed.), *Bacterial Protein Toxins: a Comprehensive Sourcebook,* 2nd ed. Academic Press, London, United Kingdom.
6. **Chen, L., M. Koyanagi, K. Fukada, K. Imanishi, J. Yagi, H. Kato, T. Miyoshi-Akiyama, R. Zhang, K. Miwa, and T. Uchiyama.** 2002. Continuous exposure of mice to superantigenic toxins induces a high-level protracted expansion and an immunological memory in the toxin-reactive CD4$^+$ T cells. *J. Immunol.* **168:** 3817–3824.
7. **Cheong, H. I., E. H. Choi, I. S. Ha, H. J. Lee, and Y. Choi.** 1995. Acute renal failure associated with *Yersinia pseudotuberculosis* infection. *Nephron* **70:**319–323.
8. **Choi, Y., J. A. Lafferty, J. R. Clements, J. K. Todd, E. W. Gelfand, J. Kappler, P. Marrack, and B. L. Kotzin.** 1990. Selective expansion of T cells expressing Vβ2 in toxic shock syndrome. *J. Exp. Med.* **172:**981–984.
9. **Donadini, R., C. W. Liew, A. H. Kwan, J. P. Mackay, and B. A. Fields.** 2004. Crystal and solution structures of a superantigen from *Yersinia pseudotuberculosis* reveal a jelly-roll fold. *Structure (Camb.)* **12:**145–156.
10. **Fukumoto, Y., M. Kaneko, Y. Yamazaki, H. Abe, F. Kurino, J. Masaoka, K. Aoyama, and M. Toyama.** 1987. Mas-infection of *Yersinia pseudotuberculosis* 4B in Shisui, Chiba (clinical report). *Kansenshogaku Zasshi* **61:**772–782.
11. **Fukushima, H., Y. Matsuda, R. Seki, M. Tsubokura, N. Takeda, F. N. Shubin, I. K. Paik, and X. B. Zheng.** 2001. Geographical heterogeneity between Far Eastern and Western Countries in prevalence of the virulence plasmid, the superantigen *Yersinia pseudotuberculosis*-derived mitogen, and the high-pathogenicity island among Yersinia pseudotuberculosis strains. *J. Clin. Microbiol.* **39:**3541–3547.
12. **Imanishi, K., K. Seo, H. Kato, T. Miyoshi-Akiyama, R. H. Zhang, Y. Takanashi, Y. Imai, and T. Uchiyama.** 1998. Post-thymic maturation of migrating human thymic single positive T cells: thymic CD1a$^-$ CD4$^+$ T cells are more susceptible to anergy induction by toxic shock syndrome toxin-1 than cord blood CD4$^+$ T cells. *J. Immunol.* **160:**112–119.
13. **Ito, Y., J. Abe, K.Yoshino, T. Takeda, and T. Kohsaka.** 1995. Sequence analysis of the gene for a novel superantigen produced by *Yersinia pseudotuberculosis* and expression of the recombinant protein. *J. Immunol.* **154:**5896–5906.
14. **Janeway, C. A., Jr., J. Yagi, P. J. Conrad, M. E. Katz, B. Jones, S. Vroegop, and S. Buxser.** 1989. T-cell responses to Mls and to bacterial proteins that mimic its behavior. *Immunol. Rev.* **107:**61–88.
15. **Kappler, J., B. Kotzin, L. Herron, E. W. Gellfand, R. D. Bigler, A. Boylston, S. Carrel, D. N. Posnett, Y. Choi, and P. Marrack.** 1989. Vβ specific stimulation of human T cells by staphylococcal toxins. *Science* **244:**811–813.

16. **Konishi, N., K. Baba, J. Abe, T. Maruko, K. Waki, N. Takeda, and M. Tanaka.** 1997. A case of Kawasaki disease with coronary artery aneurysms documenting *Yersinia pseudotuberculosis* infection. *Acta Paediatr.* **86:**661–664.

17. **Kuroda, K., J. Yagi, K. Imanishi, X. J. Yan, X. Y. Li, W. Fujimaki, H. Kato, T. Miyoshi-Akiyama, Y. Kumazawa, H. Abe, and T. Uchiyama.** 1996. Implantation of IL-2-containing osmotic pump prolongs the survival of superantigen-reactive T cells expanded in mice injected with bacterial superantigens. *J. Immunol.* **157:**1422–1431.

18. **Matsuda, Y., H. Kato, R. Yamada, H. Okano, H. Ohta, K. Imanishi, K. Kikuchi, K. Totsuka, and T. Uchiyama.** 2003. Early and definitive diagnosis of toxic shock syndrome by detection of marked expansion of T-cell-receptor Vb2-positive T cells. *Emerg. Infect. Dis.* **9:**387–389.

19. **Miki, M., T. Uchiyama, H. Kato, H. Nishida, and N. Takahashi.** 2006. A severe case of neonatal TSS-like exanthematous disease with superantigen-induced high T cell response. *Pediatr. Infect. Dis. J.* **25:**950.

20. **Mitchell, D. T., D. G. Levitt, P. M. Schlievert, and D. H. Ohlendorf.** 2000. Structural evidence for the evolution of pyrogenic toxin superantigens. *J. Mol. Evol.* **51:**520–531.

21. **Miyoshi-Akiyama, T., A. Abe, H. Kato, K. Kawahara, H. Narimatsu, and T. Uchiyama.** 1995. DNA sequencing of the gene encoding a bacterial superantigen, *Yersinia pseudotuberculosis*-derived mitogen (YPM), and characterization of the gene product, cloned YPM. *J. Immunol.* **154:**5228–5234.

22. **Miyoshi-Akiyama, T., W. Fujimaki, X.-J. Yan, J. Yagi, K. Imanishi, H. Kato, K. Tomonari, and T. Uchiyama.** 1997. Identification of murine T cells reactive with bacterial superantigen *Yersinia pseudotuberculosis*-derived mitogen (YPM) and factors involved in YPM-induced toxicity in mice. *Microbiol. Immunol.* **41:**345–352.

23. **Miyoshi-Akiyama, T., K. Imanishi, and T. Uchiyama.** 1993. Purification and partial characterization of a product from *Yersinia pseudotuberculosis* with the ability to activate human T cells. *Infect. Immun.* **61:**3922–3927.

24. **Proft, T., and J. D. Fraser.** 2003. Bacterial superantigens. *Clin. Exp. Immunol.* **133:**299–306.

25. **Ramamurthy, T., K. Yoshino, J. Abe, N. Ikeda, and T. Takeda.** 1997. Purification, characterization and cloning of a novel variant of the superantigen *Yersinia pseudotuberculosis*-derived mitogen. *FEBS Lett.* **413:**174–176.

26. **Sato, K., K. Ouchi, and M. Takai.** 1983. *Yersinia pseudotuberculosis* infection in children, resembling Izumi fever and Kawasaki syndrome. *Pediatr. Infect. Dis.* **2:**123–126.

27. **Somov, G. P., and I. L. Martinevsky.** 1973. New facts about pseudotuberculosis in the USSR. *Contrib. Microbiol. Immunol.* **2:**214–216.

28. **Takahashi, N., K. Imanishi, H. Nishida, and T. Uchiyama.** 1995. Evidence for immunologic immaturity of cord blood T cells. Cord blood T cells are susceptible to tolerance induction to in vitro stimulation with a superantigen. *J. Immunol.* **155:**5213–5219.

29. **Takahashi, N., H. Kato, K. Imanishi, K. Miwa, S. Yamanami, H. Nishida, and T. Uchiyama.** 2000. Immunopathophysiological aspects of an emerging neonatal infectious disease induced by a bacterial superantigen. *J. Clin. Investig.* **106:**1409–1415.

30. **Takahashi, N., H. Nishida, H. Kato, K. Imanishi, Y. Sakata, and T. Uchiyama.** 1998. Exanthematous disease induced by toxic shock syndrome toxin 1 in the early neonatal period. *Lancet* **351:**1614–1619.

31. **Takeda, N., M. Tanaka, and K. Notohara.** 1989. Clinopathological examinations of the Yersinia pseudotuberculosis infection. *Media Circle* **34:**273–279.

32. **Todd, J. K.** 1988. Toxic shock syndrome. *Clin. Microbiol. Rev.* **1:**432–446.

33. **Uchiyama, T., K. Imanishi, T. Miyoshi-Akiyama, and H. Kato.** 2005. Staphylococcal superantigens and diseases caused by them. *In* J. E. Alouf and M. R. Popoff (ed.), *The Comprehensive Sourcebook of Bacterial Protein Toxins,* 3rd ed. Elsevier, Oxford, United Kingdom.

34. **Uchiyama, T., Y. Kamagata, M. Wakai, M. Yoshioka, H. Fujikawa, and H. Igarashi.** 1986. Study of the biological activities of toxic shock syndrome toxin-1. I. Proliferative response and interleukin 2 production by T cells stimulated with the toxin. *Microbiol. Immunol.* **30:**469–483.

35. **Uchiyama, T., T. Miyoshi-Akiyama, H. Kato, W. Fujimaki, K. Imanishi, and X. J. Yan.** 1993. Superantigenic properties of a novel mitogenic substance produced by *Yersinia pseudotuberculosis* isolated from patients manifesting acute and systemic symptoms. *J. Immunol.* **151:**4407–4413.

36. **Ueshiba, H., H. Kato, T. Miyoshi-Akiyama, M. Tsubokura, T. Nagano, S. Kaneko, and T. Uchiyama.** 1998. Analysis of the superantigen-producing ability of *Yersinia pseudotuberculosis* strains of various

serotypes isolated from patients with systemic or gastroenteric infections, wildlife animals and natural environments. *Zentbl. Bakteriol.* **288:**277–291.

37. **Yagi, J., U. Dianzani, H. Kato, T. Okamoto, T. Katsurada, D. Buonfiglio, T. Miyoshi-Akiyama, and T. Uchiyama.** 1999. Identification of a new type of invariant Va14+ T cells and responsiveness to a superantigen, *Yersinia pseudotuberculosis*-derived mitogen. *J. Immunol.* **163:**3083–3091.

38. **Yoshino, K., T. Ramamurthy, G. B. Nair, H. Fukushima, Y. Ohtomo, N. Takeda, S. Kaneko, and T. Takeda.** 1995. Geographical heterogeneity between Far East and Europe in prevalence of *ypm* gene encoding the novel superantigen among *Yersinia pseudotuberculosis* strains. *J. Clin. Microbiol.* **33:**3356–3358.

Section II

SUPERANTIGEN STRUCTURE AND FUNCTION

Superantigens: Molecular Basis for Their Role in Human Diseases
Edited by Malak Kotb and John D. Fraser
© 2007 ASM Press, Washington, D.C.

Chapter 6

Superantigen Architecture: Functional Decoration on a Conserved Scaffold

Vickery L. Arcus and Edward N. Baker

INTRODUCTION

A defining and consistent feature of the bacterial superantigens from *Staphylococcus aureus* and *Streptococcus pyogenes* is their strongly conserved three-dimensional structure. Structural studies to date show that the array of more than 280 amino acid sequences known for superantigens (SAgs) and staphylococcal superantigen-like (SSL) proteins all have the same fold—a structure in which the same three-dimensional arrangement of α-helices and β-sheets is traced by each amino acid sequence, with the same topology (for recent reviews, see references 29 and 43). A typical SAg structure comprises two domains—an N-terminal β-barrel domain called an OB-fold (4, 25) and a C-terminal β-grasp domain in which a long α-helix packs on to a mixed parallel and antiparallel β-sheet. These two domains are traversed by an α-helix that lies at the N terminus of the protein and packs against the β-grasp domain, thus linking the N- and C-terminal domains.

In striking juxtaposition with the conserved architecture among SAgs is the myriad of functions that have been grafted on to the SAg fold. For example, SAgs bind to major histocompatibility class II molecules (MHC-II), in some cases via an N-terminal binding face (17, 18), and in other cases via a C-terminal binding face (24, 30). In the case of staphylococcal enterotoxin A (SEA), both binding faces are utilized, resulting in simultaneous binding and cross-linking of MHC-II molecules at the antigen-presenting-cell surface (2, 16, 44). Some SAgs mediate their binding to MHC-II via a zinc ion and some use their N-terminal binding faces for oligomerization (38). SAgs also bind to T-cell receptors (TCRs), and although the TCR binding surface is consistent in its location on the SAg fold among different members of the SAg family, variation in sequence allows selectivity in binding to differing cohorts of TCRs.

Vickery L. Arcus • AgResearch Protein Engineering Laboratory, Department of Biological Sciences, University of Waikato, Private Bag 3105, Hamilton, and Centre for Molecular Biodiscovery, School of Biological Sciences, University of Auckland, Private Bag 92-019, Auckland, New Zealand. *Edward N. Baker* • Centre for Molecular Biodiscovery, School of Biological Sciences, University of Auckland, Private Bag 92-019, Auckland, New Zealand.

Further variation has recently been seen for the staphylococcal superantigen-like proteins (SSLs) from the pathogenicity island SaInP2 (19, 47), which do not form complexes with the TCR and MHC-II molecules but instead interact with other components of the human immune system, apparently to dilute its ability to fight infection. Recently, members of this family have been shown to bind to immunoglobulin A (IgA) and complement C5 (20). Again, the conserved SAg fold has served as a scaffold for a diverse range of functions.

A logical extension of this theme is provided by the recently reported structures of the C5a receptor blocking domain (14) and the EAP domains (13), which are secreted staphylococcal virulence factors whose architecture comprises a single β-grasp domain. These proteins interact with the C5a receptor and extracellular host proteins, respectively. In a similar vein, the N-terminal SAg domain, the OB-fold, is well known as a "binding" domain capable of supporting an array of functions from binding to DNA, RNA, oligosaccharides, and proteins (4, 25).

An evolutionary story thus emerges for the SAg fold which suggests that this fold has arisen from the co-option of two versatile "binding" domains: the OB-fold and the β-grasp domain. These domains may then, through sequence variation, have adopted a wide range of binding modes to MHC-II molecules, the TCRs, and, in the case of the SSL proteins, a range of other components of the immune system. This is an evolutionary game of cat and mouse, as the toxicity of the SAgs would see them under heavy selection pressure to be eliminated by the immune system and, in return, the reciprocal pressure on SAgs is to vary widely and thus avoid the immune armory.

This chapter will first outline the details of the core three-dimensional structure of the SAgs and discuss precisely what is conserved among the family along with the evolutionary reasons for conservation. We will then discuss the variation that has been grafted onto the conserved structure, allowing different members of the family to bind to MHC-II and the TCR in many different configurations, with different affinities and, in the case of TCR binding, different specificities.

THE SUPERANTIGEN FOLD: A CONSERVED SCAFFOLD

The classic SAg fold is shown in Color Plate 3A using the structure of the streptococcal superantigen SMEZ-2 as an example (6). An N-terminal helix (at the top of the figure) packs into a groove between two structural domains. Following the N-terminal helix is the N-terminal domain, which is a five-stranded mixed β-barrel with Greek-key topology (48) and is called an OB-fold (25). This is connected to the C-terminal β-grasp domain by a large loop. The β-grasp domain is a mixed five-stranded β-sheet that packs onto a long α-helix. Each domain has a hydrophobic core at its center, and a smaller hydrophobic core is formed by packing the N-terminal helix onto one face of the β-grasp domain. In this sense, the folding of the SAg polypeptide chain for each domain, and for the protein as a whole, fits the classic paradigm for proteins, with a hydrophobic interior and a hydrophilic exterior. This also highlights and explains the conservation of residues along the central helix of the β-grasp domain, which constitutes the most highly conserved SAg sequence motif and defines this protein family (Color Plate 3, B and C). Most of these conserved residues are hydrophilic but are buried among hydrophobic residues as a result of the packing of the three major structural elements—the N-terminal helix, the OB-fold, and the β-grasp domain. Hydrophilic residues that form polar interactions (hydrogen bonding or charge–

charge pairing) in a buried hydrophobic environment are subject to tight evolutionary constraints. This is due to the large free-energy penalty that is paid should one residue of the pair be mutated in the course of evolution. If one residue of a pair that forms a buried polar interaction is lost, this leaves an unpaired charge or polar group in a hydrophobic environment and is energetically costly for the structure as a whole. This is in contrast to buried hydrophobic residues that, in most cases, can tolerate mutation to other hydrophobic residues with little energetic cost. Thus, the majority of residues that are highly conserved across the SAg family are buried polar or charged residues and their conservation reflects structural and not functional constraints.

The SAg N-terminal domain forms a β-barrel with the OB-fold topology, a fold that is ubiquitous in nature; OB-fold domains are found in archaea, bacteria, and eukaryotes and are one of the most prevalent structural architectures (35). The OB-fold was first named by Murzin as an "oligosaccharide/oligonucleotide binding" fold when he noted that different examples of this fold could bind different ligands on the same face of the protein (25). This led to the suggestion that the OB-fold architecture can support a binding face that is easily adapted to the binding of a range of different ligands. This original observation, based on just four structures, has been borne out by the more than 90 OB-fold structures that have been deposited in the Protein Data Bank (PDB). Among these structures are OB-fold domains that use their binding face to bind RNA (the anticodon binding domains of the Asp- and Lys-tRNA synthetases), single-stranded DNA (the telomere-end-binding proteins of eukaryotes and phage-derived gene V proteins), double-stranded DNA (cold-shock proteins), and oligosaccharides (bacterial AB_5 toxins). The OB-fold-binding face has even been adapted for catalysis in the inorganic pyrophosphatases (4).

The SAgs and SAg-like proteins use the binding face of their OB-fold domain as a protein–protein interaction domain. Even for this protein family, there is wide functional variation. A group of SAgs including SEB, SEC1-3, SSA, and SPE-A use the OB-fold binding face to bind to the α-chain of MHC-II (17, 28, 40). TSST-1 and TSST-2 use the same face to bind to the α-chain of MHC-II, but in a different orientation (18). In contrast, SPE-C uses this OB-fold binding face to oligomerize and form dimers (38). The OB-fold is sufficiently tolerant to mutation that there are just two short sequence motifs which define the SAg N-terminal OB-fold domain. These residues are buried at the interface between the two SAg domains and are conserved for structural rather than functional reasons.

The superantigen C-terminal β-grasp domain also presents a binding face at the surface of its mixed β-sheet. This binding face is used by, for example, SEA, SPE-C, SMEZ-2, SPE-G, SPE-J, and SEH to bind to the β-chain of MHC-II molecules (24, 26, 30, 33). The binding is zinc dependent; a zinc ion is ligated by two histidine side chains and an aspartic acid at this face. The recent three-dimensional structure of SPE-C in complex with MHC-II shows this interaction in detail (24). Upon complex formation, tetrahedral coordination of the Zn^{2+} ion is completed by His-81 from the β-chain of MHC-II.

The β-grasp domain is also very well represented in nature. Many examples of this architecture are intriguing in the light of SAg structure and activity. The β-grasp domains from streptococcal immunoglobulin-binding protein interact with IgG antibodies to subvert the immune response (10). The thrombolytic agents staphylokinase and streptokinase are also β-grasp protein-protein binding domains (36, 46). More recently, two other virulence factors from *Streptococcus* and *Staphylococcus* have been found to contain β-grasp domains with structural homology to the SAg C-terminal domain. The first of these is the extracellular adherence protein (EAP) domain from *S. aureus* (13). EAP is secreted by the bacteria and is thought to aid pathogenicity by interacting with host proteins such as fibrinogen, fibronectin, and vitronectin, which, in turn, leads to agglutination. The full-length protein is between 50 and 70 kDa and contains, in different bacterial strains, either four or six β-grasp domains. Notably, the EAP β-grasp domains have no recognizable sequence homology with SAg C-terminal domains (13).

The C5a receptor blocking domain of the chemotaxis inhibitory protein from *S. aureus* is also a pathogenicity factor and also a β-grasp domain (14). In this case, the secreted protein binds to the C5a receptor through its β-grasp domain and interferes with phagocyte responses.

The affinity for a range of ligands shown by these other β-grasp domains is consistent with our paradigm for SAgs, whereby adaptable binding scaffolds are utilized by secreted proteins in *Staphylococcus* and *Streptococcus* pathogenesis.

ALLELIC VARIATIONS IN SEQUENCE DECORATE THE SUPERANTIGEN FOLD

The variation among SAg sequences is a continuum from allelic variation where sequences from different strains differ by just a few amino acids (>98% identity), to pairwise sequence identities of less than 10%. In the case of allelic variation, the differences are almost universally found at the surface of the proteins and suggest that these are occurring under selection to vary epitopes that are targeted by the immune system. For example, the extraordinarily potent streptococcal superantigen, SMEZ, has 21 alleles that segregate with different M/emm types (34). Of the 31 amino acid positions that vary across the SMEZ sequence, 26 of these amino acids are surface exposed. Color Plate 3D maps these positions onto the structure of SMEZ-2. Similarly, five alleles of the SEC superantigen have been reported, including one from a strain of *S. aureus* isolated from a bovine infection. Once again, with just one exception, the variations are seen at the protein surface.

A similar phenomenon is seen for the SSL family of proteins, which share the SAg fold but bind other components of the immune response, and which are encoded on a pathogenicity island of *S. aureus* (19, 47). These 11 genes lie adjacent to one another and upstream from a putative transposase gene, suggesting a capacity for this island to be horizontally transferred. A survey of different *S. aureus* strains showed that all strains carry the pathogenicity island and that a subset of strains carries all 11 genes on the island; in other strains, up to four SSL genes have been deleted from the pathogenicity island (12). Allelic variation is seen for each of the SSL proteins (85 to 100% identity) and can be mapped on to the three-dimensional structures of the two SSLs for which structures are available, SSL-5 and SSL-7 (5, 20) (M. Chung, personal communication). The same theme of surface variation is continued for this family of immune interactors, such that in the case of SSL-5, 32 of the 37 positions that vary between alleles lie at the surface of the protein and the remaining 5 variants are buried hydrophobic residues (5).

The mosaic nature of the allelic variants for both SMEZ and SSL-5 has been cited as evidence that these alleles arise principally from recombination and not from point mutation (34). However, it is likely that a combination of both effects applies. Although the origins of this variation remain equivocal, the outcome is compelling—wide allelic variation at the surface of many SAgs and SSLs is most probably driven by the constant evolutionary pressure to escape host immune detection.

VARIATIONS ON SUPERANTIGEN BINDING TO MHC-II AND TCR

At one end of the spectrum of SAg variability lie the allelic variants (discussed above), which presumably retain the same functional determinants within a particular molecule. At the other end of the spectrum are SAgs that have not only disparate sequences but also altered functional modes of action. At the extreme end of this spectrum lie the SSLs, EAP, C5a, and IgG-binding proteins, all of which share clear structural relationships with the SAgs but target other protein components of the immune response.

The interactions between SAgs and their target MHC-II molecules and TCRs cover virtually all permutations of the following binding modes: MHC-II α-chain binding; MHC-II β-chain binding; TCR Vα binding and restriction; TCR Vβ binding and restriction; SAg oligomerization; MHC-II cross-linking. For the purposes of discussion we can loosely divide these variations into MHC-II α-chain binding and its associated TCR interactions, MHC-II β-chain binding and its associated TCR interactions, and SAg oligomerization and MHC-II cross-linking.

MHC-II α-Chain Binding

SAgs that bind to the α-chain of MHC-II molecules generally do so with low affinity (in the range 0.1 to 1.0 μM) (37). There are several three-dimensional structures of SAg/MHC-II complexes that show this interaction in molecular detail, epitomized by the SEB/MHC-II complex structure (see Color Plate 4A) (17). Loops that lie above and below the binding face of the OB-fold domain of SEB form both polar and hydrophobic interactions with residues from the MHC-II α-chain helix that flanks the peptide-binding groove. In addition, interactions are made between SEB and loops at the end of the β-sheet that forms the floor of the MHC-II peptide-binding groove. The small surface area that is buried on complex formation between SEB and MHC ($660 \, \text{Å}^2$) accounts in part for the low affinity of this interaction.

This SAg/MHC-II binding interface is conserved when the structures of the MHC-II complexes with SEB and SEC3 are compared (17, 42). Just two conservative mutations are at the MHC-II-binding interface when SEB is compared with SEC3, despite an overall sequence identity of 66% between the two SAgs. Other SAgs from both *S. aureus* and *S. pyogenes* that interact with MHC-II in this manner are SEC1, SEC2, SEG, SSA, and SPE-A.

The binding of this group of SAgs to the TCR has also been well defined by the experimentally determined structures of SEB, SEC2, SEC3, and SPE-A, each in complex with mouse TCR Vβ8.2 (11, 22, 41). Residues on the SAgs that are involved in binding lie on the face between the two domains and at the surface of the N-terminal α-helix. The regions involved on the TCR are primarily located on the CDR2 and HV4 loops and the adjacent FR3 regions (see Color Plate 5). From Color Plate 5A, it is evident that this is a weak protein-protein interaction with just three long hydrogen bonds between side chains of SEB and main-chain atoms of the TCR. Additionally, the buried interface is relatively small at $540 \, \text{Å}^2$.

The inferred functional complex for MHC-II/SEB/TCR can be constructed from the experimentally determined MHC-II/SEB and SPE-A/TCR binary complexes. This presents a picture of a circular, ternary complex where each of the components interacts with the other (Color Plate 6). Here, the SAg interferes with the normal MHC-II/TCR interaction by inserting the N-terminal OB-fold domain between the MHC-II α-chain and the TCR β-chain. The TCR now binds to both the SAg and the β-chain of MHC-II. It has been speculated that the cooperative set of interactions that form between TCR, MHC-II, and SAg in the complete complex may compensate for the low affinities that are seen in complexes between the pairs of protagonists (3, 37).

TSST is an enigma among MHC-II α-chain-binding SAgs. TSST binds to MHC-II in a different orientation when compared with SEB/MHC-II binding, lying across the α-helix that flanks the peptide-binding groove and making contacts with the displayed peptide (18, 45). It is not known what implications this alternative SAg/MHC-II interaction would have on the TSST/MHC-II/TCR complex, and no direct structural information is available on the mode of TSST/TCR interaction.

MHC-II β-Chain Binding

A second group of SAgs bind to the β-chain of MHC-II. The SAgs in this group (SPE-C, SPE-J, SMEZ, SED, SEH, and SEJ) are illustrated by SPE-C and SEH, for which the structures of SAg/MHC-II complexes have recently been reported (24, 30). At the center of the binding interface is a zinc ion that is tetrahedrally coordinated by three ligands from the SAg and a single histidine from MHC β-chain (His 81, see Color Plate 4B). The SAg/MHC-II binding has been shown to be zinc dependent in vivo, such that addition of the zinc-chelating agent EDTA abolishes T-cell activation (23, 33). The SAg interface covers residues on the MHC-II β-chain helix along with residues of the displayed peptide. In contrast to the binding between SEB and the α-chain of MHC-II, the affinity of the interaction between the SPE-C group SAgs and the β-chain of MHC is some three orders of magnitude greater (0.1 to 100 nM) (23, 26, 33). A comparison of the surface area buried by SEB binding to the α-chain of MHC-II with that buried by SPE-C binding to the β-chain of MHC-II shows that the surface areas are similar, and by implication, the binding affinities should also be comparable. However, the bonding that results from the involvement of a transition metal (zinc) bound with optimal tetrahedral geometry at the interface confers tighter binding on the SPE-C/MHC-II β-chain interaction.

This orientation of SPE-C in binding to the β-chain of MHC-II dictates that the TCR now binds to SPE-C at a distance from MHC-II, producing a more linear MHC-II/SAg/TCR complex (Color Plates 5B and 7A) (41). Although the TCR binding site on SPE-C is in the same region as that on SEB, some important differences exist in the detail of the SAg/TCR interactions. SPE-C has more extensive interactions with the TCR including the CDR1, CDR2, and CDR3 loops of the β-chain of the TCR, along with the HV4/FR3 components (41). The SPE-C/TCR interface also includes 9 hydrogen bonds that are in some cases mediated by side chains from both the SAg and TCR. Whereas the SEB interactions primarily involve hydrogen bonds with main-chain atoms of the TCR loops, and thus primarily discriminate between TCRs on the basis of the backbone conformations of these loops (22), the SPE-C interaction is highly specific. This is due to the more extensive range of interactions between SAg and TCR, and to the unique conformations of CDR loops of human Vβ2.1 due to amino acid insertions on CDR1 and CDR2 loops and an extended CDR3 loop (see Color Plate 5B). The affinity of the SPE-C/TCR interaction is also greater than that seen between SEB and TCR (21) and this is reflected in a significantly greater burial of surface area on complexation (810 Å^2).

The increased affinity of both the SPE-C/MHC-II and the SPE-C/TCR interactions may be required due to the linear configuration of the ternary complex, which precludes cooperativity of binding between the three components. The hypothesis is that stimulation of the T cells requires long residence times for the SAg to cross-connect TCR and MHC-II, and this can be achieved either by independent binding interactions of nanomolar affinity, in the case of the linear MHC-II/SPE-C/TCR complex, or by triangular, cooperative, binding to achieve nanomolar affinity in the circular MHC-II/SEB/TCR complex.

In the case of SEH, there is evidence for TCR Vα chain selectivity, although it is not clear how this is effected. It has been reported that there is upregulation of human TCR Vα10 T cells after SEH stimulation (31). SEH bridges the linear MHC-II/SAg/TCR complex and it is possible that the SEH/TCR interaction may include binding to the TCR Vα region (31). In addition a single report has demonstrated a role for TCR Vα interactions with SEA and SEE in the T-cell response to SAgs (9).

Cross-Linking MHC-II

Two SAgs have been demonstrated to cross-link MHC-II molecules at the antigen-presenting cell (APC) surface. SEA achieves this by simultaneously binding to the α-chain of MHC-II in an SEB-like manner (using the OB-fold binding face), and to the β-chain of MHC-II in a SPE-C-like manner (using the β-grasp binding face at the opposite end of the molecule) (1, 16, 32). The resulting complex at the APC/T-cell interface has a stoichiometry of MHC$_2$/SEA/TCR. Note that an MHC-II/SEA$_2$ complex could not bind to the TCR, as simultaneous binding of two SEA molecules to a single MHC at both α- and β-chains would occlude TCR binding in a triangular MHC-II/SEA/TCR complex (32). It has been proposed that rafting of MHC-II molecules at the cell surface facilitates the release of cytokines from the APC and that cross-linking by SEA may contribute to the overproduction of cytokines that is characteristic of toxic shock (16). By sequence homology, it is proposed that SED and SEE also cross-link MHC-II in a similar fashion.

A second variation is the cross-linking of MHC-II that can be effected by SAg dimers. Thus, SPE-C has been shown to form dimers through its OB-fold domain (23, 38), leaving the C-terminal β-grasp domain on each SPE-C monomer free to make its Zn-mediated interaction with MHC-II (24). This results in a proposed complex of the type (MHC/SPE-C/TCR)$_2$ (Color Plate 7B). SPE-C is a dimer both in solution and in the crystal structure, and the importance of the dimer for T-cell stimulation has been demonstrated, although this remains controversial. A second form of dimerization is shown by the streptococcal SAg SPE-J (7). In this case, the dimerization surface overlaps the TCR binding surface, implying that dimerization and TCR binding are mutually exclusive, but that SPE-J dimers could still function in MHC-II cross-linking.

SAg Oligomerization

The question of SAg oligomerization is controversial. Most SAgs appear to act as monomers, but some, such as SPE-C and SPE-J (discussed above), can form dimers, albeit at relatively high concentrations. Crystal structures of other SAgs, such as TSST-1 (27) and SPE-A (8), have also suggested oligomeric associations whose significance is unclear; given that these associations must be weak, their relevance in vivo will depend on local environments and local concentrations. An instructive example is provided by the SAg-like protein SSL-5 (formerly known as SET3). The dimer found in crystals of SSL-5 buries only a small surface and is not detected in solution (5). It may still be biologically relevant, however, where its binding partner(s) provide added stabilization, a suggestion given weight by the observation that a similar mode of dimerization is found for SSL-11 (H. Baker and M. Chung, manuscript in preparation).

CONCLUDING REMARKS

As secreted proteins from two highly adapted human pathogens, *S. aureus* and *S. pyogenes*, SAgs and the related SSLs must be subject to severe immune pressure due to their potent effects. This serves as an explanation for their defining structural characteristic—extensive surface sequence variability superimposed onto a highly conserved fold that is built from two promiscuous binding modules (the OB-fold and β-grasp domains). The result is a diversity of binding properties, in which many protein-protein interactions are weak. The challenge is to understand which interactions are of real physiological significance and which are not; only when cooperativity of binding occurs or specific features arise, such as the zinc site on the β-grasp domain, are high-affinity complexes formed, but other, more transient, associations may still be relevant in vivo. The implications for infection and disease are similar. Despite their notoriety, it is likely that, for the most part, the effects of SAg and SSL secretion are relatively benign, and that only when local concentrations rise, or synergistic relationships with other factors apply, do they trigger the severe invasive disease with which they are associated.

Acknowledgments. We gratefully acknowledge the Health Research Council of New Zealand for its support of our research on superantigen structure, John Fraser and Thomas Proft for many stimulating discussions, and Matthew Chung and Heather Baker for access to unpublished data.

REFERENCES

1. **Abrahmsen, L., M. Dohlsten, S. Segren, P. Bjork, E. Jonsson, and T. Kalland.** 1995. Characterization of two distinct MHC class II binding sites in the superantigen staphylococcal enterotoxin A. *EMBO J.* **14:**2978–2986.
2. **Al-Daccak, R., K. Mehindate, F. Damdoumi, P. Etongue-Mayer, H. Nilsson, P. Antonsson, M. Sundstrom, M. Dohlsten, R. P. Sekaly, and W. Mourad.** 1998. Staphylococcal enterotoxin D is a promiscuous superantigen offering multiple modes of interactions with the MHC class II receptors. *J. Immunol.* **160:**225–232.
3. **Andersen, P. S., P. M. Lavoie, R. P. Sekaly, H. Churchill, D. M. Kranz, P. M. Schlievert, K. Karjalainen, and R. A. Mariuzza.** 1999. Role of the T cell receptor alpha chain in stabilizing TCR-superantigen-MHC class II complexes. *Immunity* **10:**473–483.
4. **Arcus, V. L.** 2002. OB-fold domains: a snapshot of the evolution of sequence, structure and function. *Curr. Opin. Struct. Biol.* **12:**794–801.
5. **Arcus, V. L., R. Langley, T. Proft, J. D. Fraser, and E. N. Baker.** 2002. The three-dimensional structure of a superantigen-like protein, SET3, from a pathogenicity island of the *Staphylococcus aureus* genome. *J. Biol. Chem.* **277:**32274–32281.
6. **Arcus, V. L., T. Proft, J. A. Sigrell, H. M. Baker, J. D. Fraser, and E. N. Baker.** 2000. Conservation and variation in superantigen structure and activity highlighted by the three-dimensional structures of two new superantigens from *Streptococcus pyogenes. J. Mol. Biol.* **299:**157–168.
7. **Baker, H. M., T. Proft, P. D. Webb, V. L. Arcus, J. D. Fraser, and E. N. Baker.** 2004. Crystallographic and mutational data show that the streptococcal pyrogenic exotoxin J can use a common binding surface for T-cell receptor binding and dimerization. *J. Biol. Chem.* **279:**38571–38576.
8. **Baker, M. D., I. Gendlina, C. M. Collins, and K. R. Acharya.** 2004. Crystal structure of a dimeric form of streptococcal pyrogenic exotoxin A (SpeA1). *Protein Sci.* **13:**2285–2290.
9. **deAlba, Y. B., P. N. Marche, P. A. Cazenave, I. Cloutier, R. P. Sekaly, and J. Thibodeau.** 1997. V alpha domain modulates the multiple topologies of mouse T cell receptor V beta 20/staphylococcal enterotoxins A and E complexes. *Eur. J. Immunol.* **27:**92–99.

10. **Derrick, J. P., and D. B. Wigley.** 1994. The 3rd IgG-binding domain from Streptococcal protein-G—an analysis by X-ray crystallography of the structure alone and in a complex with Fab. *J. Mol. Biol.* **243:**906–918.

11. **Fields, B. A., E. L. Malchiodi, H. M. Li, X. Ysern, C. V. Stauffacher, P. M. Schlievert, K. Karjalainen, and R. A. Mariuzza.** 1996. Crystal structure of a T-cell receptor beta-chain complexed with a superantigen. *Nature* **384:**188–192.

12. **Fitzgerald, J. R., S. D. Reid, E. Ruotsalainen, T. J. Tripp, M. Y. Liu, R. Cole, P. Kuusela, P. M. Schlievert, A. Jarvinen, and J. M. Musser.** 2003. Genome diversification in *Staphylococcus aureus*: molecular evolution of a highly variable chromosomal region encoding the staphylococcal exotoxin-like family of proteins. *Infect. Immun.* **71:**2827–2838.

13. **Geisbrecht, B. V., B. Y. Hamaoka, B. Perman, A. Zemla, and D. J. Leahy.** 2005. The crystal structures of EAP domains from *Staphylococcus aureus* reveal an unexpected homology to bacterial superantigens. *FASEB J.* **19:**A313–A314.

14. **Haas, P. J., C. J. C. de Haas, M. Poppelier, K. P. M. van Kessel, J. A. G. van Strijp, K. Dijkstra, R. M. Scheek, H. Fan, J. A. W. Kruijtzer, R. M. J. Liskamp, and J. Kemmink.** 2005. The structure of the C5a receptor-blocking domain of chemotaxis inhibitory protein of *Staphylococcus aureus* is related to a group of immune evasive molecules. *J. Mol. Biol.* **353:**859–872.

15. **Hennecke, J., and D. C. Wiley.** 2002. Structure of a complex of the human alpha/beta T cell receptor (TCR) HA1.7, influenza hemagglutinin peptide, and major histocompatibility complex class II molecule, HLA-DR4 (DRA*0101 and DRB1*0401): Insight into TCR cross-restriction and alloreactivity. *J. Exp. Med.* **195:**571–581.

16. **Hudson, K. R., R. E. Tiedemann, R. G. Urban, S. C. Lowe, J. L. Strominger, and J. D. Fraser.** 1995. Staphylococcal-enterotoxin-A has 2 cooperative binding-sites on major histocompatibility complex class-II. *J. Exp. Med.* **182:**711–720.

17. **Jardetzky, T. S., J. H. Brown, J. C. Gorga, L. J. Stern, R. G. Urban, Y. I. Chi, C. Stauffacher, J. L. Strominger, and D. C. Wiley.** 1994. 3-Dimensional structure of a human class-II histocompatibility molecule complexed with superantigen. *Nature* **368:**711–718.

18. **Kim, J. S., R. G. Urban, J. L. Strominger, and D. C. Wiley.** 1994. Toxic shock syndrome toxin-1 complexed with a class-II major histocompatibility molecule HLA-DR1. *Science* **266:**1870–1874.

19. **Kuroda, M., T. Ohta, I. Uchiyama, T. Baba, H. Yuzawa, I. Kobayashi, L. Cui, A. Oguchi, K. Aoki, Y. Nagai, J. Lian, T. Ito, M. Kanamori, H. Matsumaru, A. Maruyama, H. Murakami, A. Hosoyama, Y. Mizutani-Ui, N. K. Takahashi, T. Sawano, R. Inoue, C. Kaito, K. Sekimizu, H. Hirakawa, S. Kuhara, S. Goto, J. Yabuzaki, M. Kanehisa, A. Yamashita, K. Oshima, K. Furuya, C. Yoshino, T. Shiba, M. Hattori, N. Ogasawara, H. Hayashi, and K. Hiramatsu.** 2001. Whole genome sequencing of meticillin-resistant *Staphylococcus aureus*. *Lancet* **357:**1225–1240.

20. **Langley, R., B. Wines, N. Willoughby, I. Basu, T. Proft, and J. D. Fraser.** 2005. The staphylococcal superantigen-like protein 7 binds IgA and complement C5 and inhibits IgA-Fc alpha RI binding and serum killing of bacteria. *J. Immunol.* **174:**2926–2933.

21. **Leder, L., A. Llera, P. M. Lavoie, M. I. Lebedeva, H. M. Li, R. P. Sekaly, G. A. Bohach, P. J. Gahr, P. M. Schlievert, K. Karjalainen, and R. A. Mariuzza.** 1998. A mutational analysis of the binding of staphylococcal enterotoxins B and C3 to the T cell receptor beta chain and major histocompatibility complex class II. *J. Exp. Med.* **187:**823–833.

22. **Li, H. M., A. Llera, D. Tsuchiya, L. Leder, X. Ysern, P. M. Schlievert, K. Karjalainen, and R. A. Mariuzza.** 1998. Three-dimensional structure of the complex between a T cell receptor beta chain and the superantigen staphylococcal enterotoxin B. *Immunity* **9:**807–816.

23. **Li, P. L., R. E. Tiedemann, S. L. Moffat, and J. D. Fraser.** 1997. The superantigen streptococcal pyrogenic exotoxin C (SPE-C) exhibits a novel mode of action. *J. Exp. Med.* **186:**375–383.

24. **Li, Y. L., H. M. Li, N. Dimasi, J. K. McCormick, R. Martin, P. Schuck, P. M. Schlievert, and R. A. Mariuzza.** 2001. Crystal structure of a superantigen bound to the high-affinity, zinc-dependent site on MHC class II. *Immunity* **14:**93–103.

25. **Murzin, A. G.** 1993. OB (Oligonucleotide Oligosaccharide Binding)-fold—common structural and functional solution for nonhomologous sequences. *EMBO J.* **12:**861–867.

26. **Nilsson, H., P. Bjork, M. Dohlsten, and P. Antonsson.** 1999. Staphylococcal enterotoxin H displays unique MHC class II-binding properties. *J. Immunol.* **163:**6686–6693.

27. **Papageorgiou, A. C., R. D. Brehm, D. D. Leonidas, H. S. Tranter, and K. R. Acharya.** 1996. The refined crystal structure of toxic shock syndrome toxin-1 at 2.07 angstrom resolution. *J. Mol. Biol.* **260:**553–569.

28. **Papageorgiou, A. C., C. M. Collins, D. M. Gutman, J. B. Kline, S. M. O'Brien, H. S. Tranter, and K. R. Acharya.** 1999. Structural basis for the recognition of superantigen streptococcal pyrogenic exotoxin A (SpeA1) by MHC class II molecules and T-cell receptors. *EMBO J.* **18:**9–21.

29. **Petersson, K., G. Forsberg, and B. Walse.** 2004. Interplay between superantigens and immunoreceptors. *Scand. J. Immunol.* **59:**345–355.

30. **Petersson, K., M. Hakansson, H. Nilsson, G. Forsberg, L. A. Svensson, A. Liljas, and B. Walse.** 2001. Crystal structure of a superantigen bound to MHC class II displays zinc and peptide dependence. *EMBO J.* **20:**3306–3312.

31. **Petersson, K., H. Pettersson, N. J. Skartved, B. Walse, and G. Forsberg.** 2003. Staphylococcal enterotoxin H induces V alpha-specific expansion of T cells. *J. Immunol.* **170:**4148–4154.

32. **Petersson, K., M. Thunnissen, G. Forsberg, and B. Walse.** 2002. Crystal structure of a SEA variant in complex with MHC class II reveals the ability of SEA to crosslink MHC molecules. *Structure* **10:**1619–1626.

33. **Proft, T., S. L. Moffatt, C. J. Berkahn, and J. D. Fraser.** 1999. Identification and characterization of novel superantigens from *Streptococcus pyogenes*. *J. Exp. Med.* **189:**89–101.

34. **Proft, T., S. L. Moffatt, K. D. Weller, A. Paterson, D. Martin, and J. D. Fraser.** 2000. The streptococcal superantigen SMEZ exhibits wide allelic variation, mosaic structure, and significant antigenic variation. *J. Exp. Med.* **191:**1765–1776.

35. **Qian, J., B. Stenger, C. A. Wilson, J. Lin, R. Jansen, S. A. Teichmann, J. Park, W. G. Krebs, H. Y. Yu, V. Alexandrov, N. Echols, and M. Gerstein.** 2001. PartsList: a web-based system for dynamically ranking protein folds based on disparate attributes, including whole-genome expression and interaction information. *Nucleic Acids Res.* **29:**1750–1764.

36. **Rabijns, A., H. L. DeBondt, and C. DeRanter.** 1997. Three-dimensional structure of staphylokinase, a plasminogen activator with therapeutic potential. *Nat. Struct. Biol.* **4:**357–360.

37. **Redpath, S., S. M. Alam, C. M. Lin, A. M. O'Rourke, and N. R. J. Gascoigne.** 1999. Cutting edge: Trimolecular interaction of TCR with MHC class II and bacterial superantigen shows a similar affinity to MHC:peptide ligands. *J. Immunol.* **163:**6–10.

38. **Roussel, A., B. F. Anderson, H. M. Baker, J. D. Fraser, and E. N. Baker.** 1997. Crystal structure of the streptococcal superantigen SPE-C: dimerization and zinc binding suggest a novel mode of interaction with MHC class II molecules. *Nat. Struct. Biol.* **4:**635–643.

39. **Schuster-Boeckler, B., J. Schultz, and S. Rahmann.** 2004. HMM logos for visualization of protein families. *BMC Bioinformatics* **5:**7.

40. **Sundberg, E., and T. S. Jardetzky.** 1999. Structural basis for HLA-DQ binding by the streptococcal superantigen SSA. *Nat. Struct. Biol.* **6:**123–129.

41. **Sundberg, E. J., H. M. Li, A. S. Llera, J. K. McCormick, J. Tormo, P. M. Schlievert, K. Karjalainen, and R. A. Mariuzza.** 2002. Structures of two streptococcal superantigens bound to TCR beta chains reveal diversity in the architecture of T cell signaling complexes. *Structure* **10:**687–699.

42. **Sundberg, E. J., P. S. Andersen, P. M. Schlievert, K. Karjalainen, and R. A. Mariuzza.** 2003. Structural, energetic, and functional analysis of a protein-protein interface at distinct stages of affinity maturation. *Structure* **11:**1151–1161.

43. **Sundberg, E. J., Y. L. Li, and R. A. Mariuzza.** 2002. So many ways of getting in the way: diversity in the molecular architecture of superantigen-dependent T-cell signaling complexes. *Curr. Opin. Immunol.* **14:**36–44.

44. **Tiedemann, R. E., and J. D. Fraser.** 1996. Cross-linking of MHC class II molecules by staphylococcal enterotoxin A is essential for antigen-presenting cell and T cell activation. *J. Immunol.* **157:**3958–3966.

45. **Vonbonin, A., S. Ehrlich, G. Malcherek, and B. Fleischer.** 1995. Major histocompatibility complex class II-associated peptides determine the binding of the superantigen toxic shock syndrome toxin-1. *Eur. J. Immunol.* **25:**2894–2898.

46. **Wang, X. Q., X. L. Lin, J. A. Loy, J. Tang, and X. J. C. Zhang.** 1998. Crystal structure of the catalytic domain of human plasmin complexed with streptokinase. *Science* **281:**1662–1665.

47. **Williams, R. J., J. M. Ward, B. Henderson, S. Poole, B. P. O'Hara, M. Wilson, and S. P. Nair.** 2000. Identification of a novel gene cluster encoding staphylococcal exotoxin-like proteins: characterization of the prototypic gene and its protein product, SET1. *Infect. Immun.* **68:**4407–4415.

48. **Zhang, C., and S. H. Kim.** 2000. A comprehensive analysis of the Greek key motifs in protein beta-barrels and beta-sandwiches. *Proteins-Struct. Func. Genet.* **40:**409–419.

Superantigens: Molecular Basis for Their Role in Human Diseases
Edited by Malak Kotb and John D. Fraser
© 2007 ASM Press, Washington, D.C.

Chapter 7

Structural Evidence for Zinc and Peptide Dependence in Superantigen-Major Histocompatibility Complex Class II Interaction

Björn Walse

Bacterial superantigens (SAgs) (13) are small, highly mitogenic proteins that cross-link antigen-presenting cells (APCs) and T cells by binding simultaneously to the immunoreceptors major histocompatibility complex (MHC) class II (35, 37, 38) and the T-cell receptors (TCRs) (36, 52, 112) leading to the stimulation of large numbers of T cells (61). The SAgs are absorbed by the intestinal/gastric epithelium as intact proteins (45) and, in contrast to conventional antigens, SAgs are not processed and presented as short peptides. Instead, they bind directly to the MHC molecules outside the peptide-binding groove (23, 47, 94). The oligoclonal T-cell stimulation (up to 20% of all T cells) results in high systemic levels of the proinflammatory cytokines interleukin-2 (IL-2), tumor necrosis factor alpha (TNF-α), and gamma interferon (IFN-γ) being released from T cells, and IL-1 and TNF-α being released from APCs (27, 36, 61, 80). In contrast, a conventional peptide antigen activates about 0.001% of all T cells. SAgs activate T cells by binding to the variable part of the TCR β-chain (TCR Vβ) (18). In addition to cytokine production and T-cell proliferation, SAgs are also capable of inducing cytotoxicity toward target cells (26). This extensive activation of T cells results in diseases such as food poisoning, hypotension, fever and toxic shock, which may lead to death of the host (25, 56, 66). The advantages for microbes of secreting SAgs are not very well understood, but apart from disturbing the normal immune response they might prolong survival by promoting local inflammation, thereby increasing the blood and nutrient supply (39, 67). SAgs are produced mainly by the gram-positive bacteria *Staphylococcus aureus* and *Streptococcus pyogenes,* but genes encoding SAg-like proteins have also been discovered in other closely related strains such as *Streptococcus equi* (8) and *Streptococcus dysgalactiae* (71). In addition, other bacteria such as *Mycoplasma arthritidis* and *Yersinia pseudotuberculosis* have been reported to secrete mitogens with superantigenic properties (19, 70).

Björn Walse • SARomics AB, SE-220 07 Lund, Sweden.

THE STAPHYLOCOCCAL AND STREPTOCOCCAL SUPERANTIGEN FAMILY

The most studied bacterial SAgs are those produced by the gram-positive bacteria *S. aureus* and *S. pyogenes*. *S. aureus* secretes more than 15 different SAgs (Table 1), named staphylococcal enterotoxins (SEs) A, B, C1–3, D, E, G, H, I, J, K, L, M, and toxic shock syndrome toxin-1 (TSST-1) (25). The SAgs secreted by several strains of *S. pyogenes* include the classic pyrogenic exotoxins (SPEs) A1–4 and C, and the more recently identified pyrogenic toxins G, H, I, J, L, M, the streptococcal mitogenic exotoxins (SMEZ) 1–24, and the streptococcal superantigen (SSA) (see Table 1) (89–92). The SAgs described here are the most well characterized, but new allelic variants are continuously being discovered in different strains of *Staphylococcus* and *Streptococcus* following whole-genome-sequencing campaigns (33, 60). The different SAgs display a high degree of variability between their primary peptide sequences. Some SAgs are very similar with an amino acid identity up to 83% for SEA and SEE, while some are less similar, such as SEH and SEC1 with an amino acid identity of only 20.7%. Approximately 15% of the residues are entirely conserved throughout the known SAgs. Most of these residues are located either centrally or at the C terminus (Fig. 1). In addition, proteins with high structural similarity to SAgs have recently been identified in *S. aureus* (6). These proteins, termed staphylococcal superantigen-like proteins (SSLs) have no functional similarity to SAgs.

Based on amino acid sequence alignment, SAgs can be divided into four major groups (90) (Fig. 2). SMEZn, SPE-C, SPE-G, SPE-J, SPE-L, and SPE-M belong to group A; SEB, SECn, SEG, SSA, and SPE-A belong to group B; SEA, SED, SEE, SEH, and SEJ belong to group C; and SEI, SEK, SEL, SEM, and SPE-I belong to group D. TSST-1, which has approximately 25 to 30% homology with other SAgs, can not be classified in any of these groups. The same is true for SPE-H.

The bacterial SAgs (Table 1) comprise proteins that range from 22 to 28 kDa and vary between 194 and 242 amino acids in length (4, 73). Despite the fact that some SAgs display a sequence identity as low as 20% they adopt remarkably similar three-dimensional folds (Table 1 and references therein). They have a conserved two-domain architecture where the amino- and carboxy-terminal domains are divided by a long α-helix spanning the center of the molecule. The amino-terminal domain consists of a Greek-key β-barrel, which is structurally homologous to the oligosaccharide/oligonucleotide-binding (OB) fold common to staphylococcal nuclease and several other exotoxins, such as cholera toxin, pertussis toxin, and vero toxin (68). The domain contains several solvent-exposed hydrophobic residues and a characteristic flexible disulfide-bonded loop at the end. The loop varies in length between the different SAgs and some SAgs, such as TSST-1, SPE-C, and SMEZ-2, actually lack the disulfide bond (Fig. 1). The carboxy-terminal domain adopts a β-grasp motif composed of a five-stranded, antiparallel β-sheet wall that has high structural similarity to the immunoglobulin (Ig)-binding motifs of the streptococcal proteins G and L (42, 113). The structural similarities between SAgs and other bacterial proteins suggest that SAgs have evolved through the recombination of these two smaller subunits (69).

SUPERANTIGEN INTERACTION WITH MHC CLASS II MOLECULES

It has been known for a long time that SAgs can interact with the immunoreceptor MHC class II (35, 37, 38). The ability of SAgs to activate the immune system systemically became clear when evidence was presented that the interaction took place outside the antigen

Table 1. Crystal structures of bacterial SAgs and their complexes

SAg	Crystal structure PDB codes (references)	Zinc site	Binding to MHC α/β-chain	Crystal structure of SAg-MHC complex PDB codes (references)	Crystal structure of SAg-TCR complex PDB codes (references)
S. aureus					
SEA	1ESF (96), 1SXT (103), 1I4G (43), 1I4H (43), 1DYQ (58)	C-term	+/+	1LO5 (84)	–
SEB	1SE3 (104), 1SE4 (104), 3SEB (79), 1GOZ (12)	–	+/–	1SEB (50), 2SEB (24), 1D5M (14), 1D5X (14), 1D5Z (14), 1D6E (14)	1SBB (63)
SEC₁	–	cleft	+/–	–	–
SEC₂	1SE2 (105), 1STE (74), 1CQV (59), 1I4P (59), 1I4Q (59), 1I4R (59), 1I4X (59), 1UNS (75)	cleft	+/–	1KLG (101), 1KLU (101), 1JWM (98), 1JWS (98), 1JWU (98), 1PYW (117), 1SJE (116), 1SJH (116), 1T5X (115)	Not deposited (34)
SEC₃	1CK1 (17)	cleft	+/–	–	1JCK (34)
SED	Not deposited (102)	C-term, cleft	+/+	–	–
SEE	–	C-term	+/+	–	–
SEG	–	–	+/–	–	–
SEH	1ENF (44), 1EWC (44), 1F77 (44)	C-term	–/+	1HXY (82)	–
SEI	–	C-term	–/+	–	–
SEJ	–	C-term?	+/+	–	–
SEK	–	C-term?	+/+	–	–
SEL	–	C-term?	+/+	–	–
SEM	–	C-term?	+/+	–	–
TSST-1	2-5TSS (87, 88), 1QIL (78), 2QIL (76), 1TS2-5 (29), 1AW7 (29)	–	+/–	Not deposited (55)	–
S. pyogenes					
SPE-A	1B1Z (77), 1FNU (30), 1FNV (30), 1FNW (30), 1HA5 (11), 1UUP (10)	cleft	+/–	–	1LOX (99), 1L0Y (99)
SPE-C	1AN8 (93)	C-term	–/+	1HQR (64)	1KTK (99)
SPE-G	–	C-term	–/+	–	–
SPE-H	1ET9 (7), 1EU4 (7)	C-term	–/+	–	–
SPE-I	–	C-term?	–/+	–	–
SPE-J	1TY0 (9), 1TY2 (9)	C-term	–/+	–	–
SPE-L	–	C-term?	–/+	–	–
SPE-M	–	C-term?	–/+	–	–
SSA	1BXT (97)	–	+/–	–	–
SMEZ	–	C-term	–/+	–	–
SMEZ-2	1ET6 (7), 1EU3 (7)	C-term	–/+	–	–

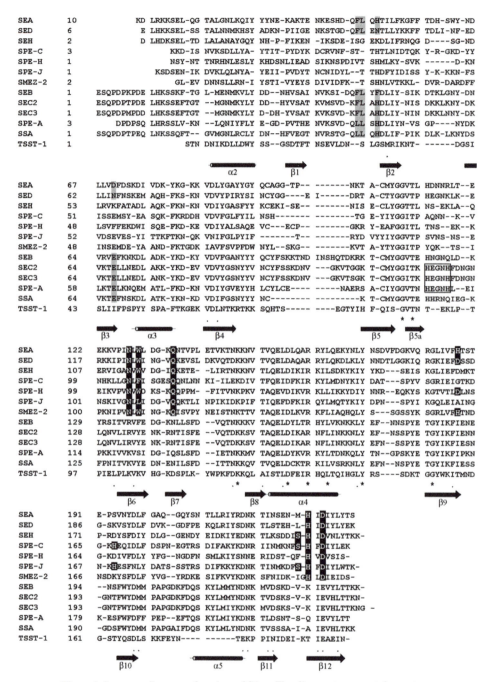

Figure 1. Sequence alignment of a subset of SAgs. The alignment was created as a structural alignment by superpositioning different SAg structures. Secondary structural elements for SEA are indicated below the sequences. Residues involved in the zinc-dependent high-affinity interaction with the β-chain of MHC class II are indicated with black boxes and residues involved in the low-affinity interaction with the α-chain of MHC class II are indicated with gray boxes. The HExxH motif in SEC2, SEC3, and SPE-A is outlined with black lines.

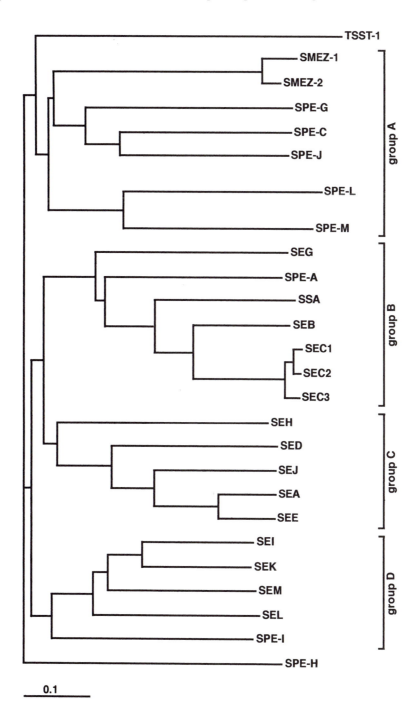

Figure 2. Family tree of streptococcal and staphylococcal SAgs. The tree was created using ClustalW (106).

groove (23). This explained why the SAgs had such potent effects on cells of the immune system and the fact that they were independent of the type of antigenic peptide that was bound to MHC. The first structural evidence of a SAg-MHC interaction was the binding of the SAg SEB to invariant regions of the α-chain on the side of MHC outside the peptide-binding groove (50) (Color Plate 8A). A hydrophobic cleft at the amino-terminal domain of SEB accounted for most of this relatively weak interaction (0.4 to 0.7 μM). Subsequent crystallization of SEC and later SEB in complex with the TCR β-chain (34, 63) made it possible to model the MHC-SEB-TCR interaction. This showed that at least some interactions were allowed between the TCR and the peptide-MHC complex. The structure of the complex between TSST-1 and MHC was elucidated at about the same time as that of SEB-MHC (55). In contrast to SEB, TSST-1 did show interactions with the antigenic peptide (Color Plate 8B). Although the interaction, in principle, involves the same sites on the SAg and the MHC molecule as in the SEB complex, the C-terminal domain in TSST-1 extends above the putative MHC-peptide-TCR-binding groove occluding many of the contact sites between the MHC and the TCR. Crystal structures of complexes between MHC and the SAgs SEA (84) and SEC3 (98, 101) have since been determined showing the same binding mode as SEB, indicating that this binding mode is the more generic of the two. Sequence comparison suggests that in addition to SEB, SEA, SEC, and TSST-1, also SED, SEE, SEG, SEJ, SEK, SEL, SEM, SSA, and SPE-A interact with the α-chain of MHC through the binding site at the amino-terminal domain (Table 1, Fig. 1).

Soon after the discovery that an interaction was required between SAgs and MHC to activate T cells it was shown that MHC hosted two different binding sites for the SAgs TSST-1 and SEA. In fact, it was shown that SEA had multiple binding sites, one of which overlapped that for TSST-1 and one involving the β-chain of MHC (86). In addition to the generic binding site on the α-chain of MHC the residue His81 on the β-chain was identified as a critical hot spot on HLA-DR1 for binding to SEA (47, 53, 94). However, the exact role of this residue did not become apparent until it was demonstrated that zinc regulated the binding of SEA to MHC class II (40). In contrast to SEB and TSST-1, the binding of SEA (and also SEE) was shown to be strictly zinc dependent. Mutational and structural studies showed that residues His187, His225, and Asp227 on the carboxy-terminal domain of SEA have a major influence on MHC class II binding and are involved in Zn^{2+} coordination (1, 49, 96, 103). The affinity for this zinc-dependent β-chain interaction was approximately three orders of magnitude stronger than for the generic α-chain interaction. The residue His81 is widely conserved in different MHC class II alleles in the otherwise polymorphic β-chain, and it was therefore proposed that His81 contributed the fourth coordination residue to Zn^{2+} upon binding to SEA (1, 40, 49, 57). It was not until several years later that structural evidence was established for this zinc-dependent interaction between MHC and the SAgs SPE-C (Color Plate 8C) and SEH (Color Plate 8D) (64, 82).

SEA is an interesting SAg because it can interact with both the generic site on the α-chain of MHC class II and the zinc-dependent site on the β-chain of MHC class II (1, 49, 57). This means that different SAgs can be presented by MHC class II in three distinct ways despite their homologous three-dimensional fold (73, 81, 100). Because of this ability to interact with MHC class II, SAgs may be divided into three groups. They may be single α-chain-binding SAgs (e.g., SEB; Color Plate 8A) (50), single β-chain-binding SAgs (e.g., SEH; Color Plate 8D) (82), or they may be capable of binding two MHC molecules. In the latter case, where the SAg cross-links two MHC molecules, they either possess both the amino- and carboxy-terminal binding sites and bind one α-chain and one β-chain (e.g., SEA; see Color Plate 10) (84, 107, 108), or they are able to produce two binding sites through dimerization, and either bind two α-chains (e.g., SED) (3, 102) or two β-chains (e.g., SPE-C) (93).

ZINC-BINDING STAPHYLOCOCCAL
AND STREPTOCOCCAL SUPERANTIGENS

Several SAgs depend on zinc to be functional and to interact with MHC molecules. Several of these have been crystallized and their three-dimensional structures elucidated (Table 1). The structures show that the different SAgs have rather diverse ways of binding zinc. SEA, SED, SEH, SPE-C, SPE-H, SPE-J, and SMEZ-2 bind zinc ions with conserved residues located at the antiparallel β-sheet wall in the carboxy-terminal domain, SEC2 and SPE-A bind zinc in the cleft between the two domains, while SED uses the Zn^{2+} to form homodimers. Crystal structures of some of these SAgs in complex with MHC show that zinc is important for the high-affinity interaction to MHC (64, 82). In addition, the zinc ion is important for the three-dimensional stability of the SAg itself (15, 16). Of the SAgs whose structures have not yet been determined, a carboxy-terminal Zn^{2+}-binding site can be predicted for SEE, SEI, SEJ, SEK, SEL, SEM, SPE-G, SPE-I, SPE-L, SPE-M, and SMEZ based on sequence comparisons. Accordingly, for most of these SAgs a zinc-dependent interaction with MHC class II has been confirmed by biochemical or cell-based experiments (1, 32, 89, 90, 92).

A more detailed analysis of the Zn^{2+}-binding site in the carboxy-terminal domain shows that the residues responsible for Zn^{2+} binding are completely conserved in several SAgs (Fig. 1). The histidine, His225, and the aspartate, Asp227, that interact with Zn^{2+} in SEA (96, 103) are preserved as Zn^{2+}-coordinating residues in the structures of SED (102), SEH (44), SPE-C (93), SPE-H (7), SPE-J (9), and SMEZ-2 (7). The third coordinating residue varies, however, in the different SAgs. A histidine or an aspartate on the β9-strand coordinates Zn^{2+} in SEA (His187), SED (Asp182), SPE-H (Asp160), and SMEZ-2 (His162). SPE-C and SPE-J have a glycine (Gly161) and an alanine (Ala163), respectively, at the corresponding position, and the third coordinating residue is a histidine from the neighboring β10-strand (His167 in SPE-C and His169 in SPE-J). The side chain of this histidine is positioned at approximately the same location as the Zn^{2+}-coordinating side chain on the β9-strand of the other SAgs. It has been shown that the relative contributions of the individual SEA residues to Zn^{2+} coordination are in the order: Asp227 > His225 > His187 (1, 49), and that the last of these three residues has less importance for MHC class II interaction. SEH displays a slightly different Zn^{2+} binding. The zinc ion is coordinated only by the two conserved histidine and aspartate residues on the β9-strand (His206 and Asp208) (44). The position of the zinc ion is altered by approximately 2.5 Å due to structural dissimilarities of the β12-strand, and both Asp167 and Asp173 are thus too far away to interact with the zinc ion.

Although SED binds Zn^{2+} using the same conserved residues in the carboxy-terminal domain it behaves in a different way. The crystal structure shows that SED forms homodimers where two carboxy-terminal β-sheets from two SED molecules are packed against each other burying a large solvent-inaccessible area (102). Two zinc ions are symmetrically coordinated at the homodimer interface and each is tetrahedrally coordinated by His218 from one SED molecule and Asp182, His 220, and Asp222 from the other, and vice versa. The latter ligands are in the same position as the corresponding Zn^{2+} ligands in SEA. The SED homodimer is also present in solution, as gel filtration experiments have shown that in the presence and absence of Zn^{2+} the protein eluted as a dimer and a monomer, respectively (102). A second Zn^{2+}-binding site was also detected in the structure located at the inter-domain interface. The zinc ion is coordinated by two ligands from one molecule, His8 and Glu12, and another two, His109 and Lys113, from a second molecule in the asymmetric unit. It is still not clear whether this second metal-binding site is a functionally specific Zn^{2+}-binding site or whether it is induced by the crystallization conditions.

SEC2 and SPE-A, which lack the conserved residues for high-affinity Zn^{2+} binding to the carboxy-terminal domain, bind Zn^{2+} in the cleft at the interdomain interface, similar to SED (59, 74, 77). In the SEC2 structure the zinc ion is tetrahedrally coordinated to Asp83, His118, and His122 from one molecule, and to Asp9 from a symmetry-related molecule in the crystal lattice. No zinc could be found in this position in SEC2 crystallized in a different crystal form (105). The loop where the two histidines reside forms a classical His-Glu-x-x-His motif (Fig. 1), which is well known as a zinc-binding site in thermolysin-like met-alloproteases such as endopeptidases, and in other proteins (51). SPE-A also possesses this motif and binds a zinc ion by the corresponding residues Glu33, Asp77, His106, and His110, according to the crystal structure (11, 30, 77). In addition, it has been shown that if crystals of SEA are soaked in high concentrations of $ZnCl_2$ (10 mM) an additional SEC2-like zinc-binding site could be detected (95). Three of the zinc ligands are structurally equivalent to those in SPE-A (Glu39, Asp86, and His114) with a water molecule replacing the second histidine residue. No biological function has been attributed to this additional zinc site in SEA because it is unlikely that local zinc concentrations in vivo can be high enough to facilitate binding.

It has been speculated that this additional zinc-binding site in SEC2 and SPE-A is involved in interactions at the same site on the β-chain of MHC class II as SEA, SEH, and SPE-C (11, 74, 77). In addition, functional studies with mutants of SED indicate that this secondary zinc site may mediate binding to the β-chain of MHC class II (3). The latter study showed that if the high-affinity zinc-dependent site was involved in homodimeriza-tion, and if the generic SEB-like site was destroyed by mutation, SED was still able to cross-link two MHC molecules, indicating that another site on the molecule interacted with the β-chain of MHC class II. However, it cannot be excluded whether the secondary zinc site induces homodimerization or whether SED forms SPE-C-like homodimers. In fact, it has recently been shown that SEC3 dimerizes using the zinc ion at the secondary zinc site (17). Furthermore, mutagenesis studies of SEC2 have shown that even when the secondary zinc site is totally abrogated, the SAg has unaffected T-cell activation proper-ties, which would lead to the conclusion that the zinc ion is not involved in the MHC class II interactions (17, 75). In addition, SEC3 (which also has the HExxH motif) has been crystallized in complex with both MHC (98, 101) and a TCR Vβ-chain (34), displaying no zinc-dependent interaction with MHC class II. Rather, it shows the same generic MHC and TCR binding characteristics as SEB (50, 63). Moreover, MHC class II binding to SPE-A is sensitive to polymorphism on the α-chain of HLA-DQ, indicating that SPE-A interacts with MHC in the same manner as SEB (65). Thus, more evidence is needed before this zinc site in the cleft between the two domains can be established as anything other than a nonfunctional heavy atom.

A recent study on crystallization of SEC2 at high zinc concentration has revealed yet another zinc-binding site in the molecule. This site involves two ligands from one molecule, His47 and Glu71, and two from a symmetry-related molecule, Glu119 and Glu80 (75). More studies are needed to elucidate the importance of this site. It is currently not clear whether this zinc site is a crystallization artifact or if it is present under physiological conditions.

At high concentrations the streptococcal SAg SPE-C has the ability to cross-link two MHC molecules through a high-affinity, zinc-dependent interaction with the β-chain due to homodimer formation using residues in its amino-terminal domain (SPE-C probably binds MHC as a monomer under physiological conditions) (64, 93). However, a structure solved after soaking the crystal in 50 mM zinc acetate solution revealed two zinc-binding sites (93). In addition to the high-affinity site, SPE-C bound a second zinc ion located in the dimer interface. The authors concluded that this zinc ion adds stability to the dimer, but is not essential for dimerization as dimer association is seen regardless of whether this site is occupied or not.

The recently discovered *S. dysgalactiae*-derived mitogen (SDM), which is homologous to SPE-L and SPE-M (58% and 97% sequence identity, respectively), appears to belong to a group separate from the other well-established SAgs (71). SDM is predicted to be similar in structure to SPE-C (32% sequence identity) and possesses the same conserved zinc-binding residues, Asp173, His200, and Asp202. It contains less hydrophobic residues in the generic SEB-like MHC class II binding site and is thus predicted to interact in a zinc-dependent manner with the β-chain of MHC class II.

ZINC-DEPENDENT INTERACTION WITH THE β-CHAIN OF MHC CLASS II MOLECULES

The structural basis for SAg binding to the high-affinity, zinc-dependent site on MHC was recently revealed. The crystal structures of SPE-C in complex with HLA-DR2a (64) and SEH in complex with HLA-DR1 (82) were solved almost simultaneously. In both the SPE-C–HLA-DR2a and SEH–HLA-DR1 complexes, the carboxy-terminal domain of the SAg binds on top of MHC to the β-chain (Color Plate 8C, D). This is in contrast to the α-chain-binding SAgs that bind from the side. SPE-C and SEH use their carboxy-terminal antiparallel β-sheet wall (strands β6, β7, and β12) to interact with the carboxy-terminal portion of the α-helix in the β1-domain of MHC as well as the amino-terminal half of the antigenic peptide presented in the cleft. The interaction buries in total between 1,500 and 1,600 Å^2 of surface area comparable to ordinary TCR-MHC class I and II complexes (41, 46). Approximately two-thirds of the buried surface area is contributed by interaction with the β1-helix on MHC and one-third by the antigenic peptide, strongly implying that the peptide plays an important role in binding the SAg. There are no direct contacts with the MHC α1-domain. The zinc ion is located almost at the center of the contacting surface and cross-links the two molecules through the conserved His81 residue on MHC; His167, His201, and Asp203 on SPE-C; and His206 and Asp208 on SEH (64, 82) (Color Plate 9A). Overall, the two structures are quite similar. The central regions of the β6-, β7-, and β12-strands are in the same position in the two complexes. However, because of an approximately 20-degree tilt of SPE-C away from MHC class II compared with SEH, the loop between the β9- and β10-strands in SPE-C is located closer to residues in the β-chain of HLA-DR2a (Color Plate 8C, D). The third zinc ligand in SPE-C, His167, is located on the β10-strand and its involvement in the binding causes this part of the molecule to be closer to the interaction site.

The residues Asn113 and Ser205 in SEH mediate additional interactions to MHC around the zinc site (Color Plate 9A). They correspond to the residues Asn105 and Ser200 in SPE-C, and residues at similar positions are conserved in many other SAgs. The serine forms a hydrogen bond with the side-chain carboxyl group of Asp76 in MHC and the asparagine forms a hydrogen bond with the main-chain carbonyl of Thr77. Trp115 (which corresponds to Phe107 in SPE-C) contributes to the stabilization of the interaction by making van der Waals interactions with His81 on MHC class II. This tryptophan is conserved in almost all zinc-binding SAgs, indicating its importance.

An interesting feature in these structures is that the side chains of the zinc-interacting residues are hydrogen bonded to nearby residues, creating a network of hydrogen bonds that stabilize the zinc-interacting area (Color Plate 9A). For example, Asp208 in SEH forms a hydrogen bond to Asn113, which also interacts with Thr77 on HLA-DR1. His206 forms a hydrogen bond with Ser205, which in turn is hydrogen bonded to Asp76 on HLA-DR1. The network is then extended further with the side chain of Asp76 interacting with the side chain of Arg80 in the same molecule. This hydrogen bond network is also seen in the SPE-C–HLA-DR2a complex (64) and (excluding the HLA-DR1 residues) in the uncomplexed SEH structure (44). In other zinc-binding proteins such hydrogen bond networks in the metal-binding sites have been shown to enhance zinc affinity (54). In addition, a general motif between zinc ligands and protein residues in which zinc-bound histidine makes hydrogen bonds to an oxygen atom from a protein residue or water has been observed in numerous protein crystal structures (2). For example, a carboxylate-His hydrogen bond is believed to increase the basicity and ligand strength of the histidine and arrange it correctly for interaction with the metal (2). The zinc-binding histidines in both the SPE-C–HLA-DR2a and SEH–HLA-DR1 complexes undergo such interactions. In the SEH–HLA-DR1 complex His206 on SEH forms a hydrogen bond to the side-chain oxygen of Ser205, and His81 on HLA-DR1 forms a hydrogen bond to the carbonyl oxygen of Lys307 (P-1) in the hemagglutinin (HA) peptide. Thus, there is reason to believe that this motif is common to all other SAgs interacting with MHC in a high-affinity zinc-dependent way.

Despite the fact that the zinc ion is tetrahedrally coordinated with amino acid side chains in the SPE-C–HLA-DR2a complex, compared with the SEH–HLA-DR1 complex the interaction is slightly weaker. In the SEH–HLA-DR1 complex the fourth ligand is presumably water (82). The affinity for interaction with MHC is 0.5 nM for SEH and 70 nM for SPE-C (72, 90). These affinities are three to four orders of magnitude stronger than binding affinities for SAgs interacting with the α-chain of MHC class II. It is difficult to speculate which interactions differ in the two complexes and account for the relatively large difference in affinity. It may be the larger van der Waals surface contributed by Trp115 in SEH compared with Phe107 in SPE-C, or the hydrogen bond between Arg127 on the β7-strand in SEH and Glu69 in HLA-DR, that contributes to the higher affinity. This latter interaction has not been observed in the SPE-C–HLA-DR2a complex.

INTERACTIONS WITH THE ANTIGENIC PEPTIDE

A striking feature observed in both the SPE-C–HLA-DR2a and SEH–HLA-DR1 complexes is the extensive contact with the antigenic peptide (myelin-basic-protein-derived peptide MBP$_{89\text{-}101}$ in the SPE-C complex and hemagglutinin-derived peptide HA$_{306\text{-}318}$ in the SEH complex). In both cases the SAg is in contact with the amino-terminal portion of the peptide, from P-3 to P3 of MBP_{89-101} and from P-1 to P3 of $HA_{306-318}$ (P1 is the first anchor residue) (Color Plate 9B). This is in contrast to TCR, which binds more centrally around the P5 position (41, 46). In the SEH–HLA-DR1 complex these contacts involve mainly the loop between the β6- and β7-strands. Gln120, which is located on that loop, forms a bidentate hydrogen bond with the backbone of Lys310 (P3) on the HA peptide and Trp115 makes van der Waals interactions with Val309 (P2) (Color Plate 9B). Other contacts between SEH and the peptide involve the side chain of Asn210, which forms a hydrogen bond with the side chain of Lys307 (P-1) that extends out from the peptide. Gln113 in SPE-C, which is the corresponding residue to Gln120 in SEH, forms similar bonds with the backbone of the MBP peptide, indicating that both SAgs bind the peptides in similar ways although different peptides are present (Color Plate 9B). This backbone interaction with the peptide indicates that SEH and SPE-C are able to interact with any peptide presented. Overlaying the three-dimensional structures of the SEH–HLA-DR1 complex and three other peptide-HLA-DR complexes (with a collagen II-peptide, an MBP-peptide, and an endogenous peptide) shows that, although the peptide sequences vary, the SEH molecule does not overlap any of the peptide side chains (82). Thus, despite the fact that the antigenic peptide plays an important role in the complex interaction, the sequence variability of the peptide is probably not important for SAg binding, since the major interaction is with the backbone of the peptide. However, different peptides presented on MHC class II may modulate the affinity for the SAg (48, 57). More studies with different peptides must be performed to elucidate how this will affect SAg activity.

In contrast to the zinc family of SAgs, a peptide-specific T-cell response has been suggested for TSST-1 (48, 110, 111). The structure of the TSST-1–HLA-DR1 complex revealed several contacts with the carboxy-terminal portion of the antigenic peptide and the SAg (55), thus explaining the specificity for different peptides (Color Plate 8B). It has been suggested that this type of peptide dependence may allow SAgs to distinguish between different types of APCs, which are likely to display distinct arrays of peptides (114).

The glutamine responsible for the interaction with the antigenic peptide is almost completely conserved in the other β-chain-binding SAgs (Fig. 1). In addition, the amino-terminal parts of peptides bound to MHC show less structural variability than their carboxy-terminal parts (41, 46). Hence, together with the zinc-dependent interaction with the conserved His81 residue, this shows how this subclass of SAgs has evolved to circumvent the polymorphism that exists on the β-chain of MHC class II. The HLA molecules show the most genetic variability in the human genome (109). Although some SAgs have evolved to avoid this heterogeneity, it has been observed that HLA polymorphism strongly affects both quantitative and qualitative differences in the SAg response (65). This suggests that for bacteria to avoid host immune responses they display an array of extensive SAg diversity.

OTHER ZINC-BINDING BACTERIAL SUPERANTIGENS

M. arthritidis-derived mitogen (MAM) is a superantigen produced by *M. arthritidis* (19). Although MAM functions as a conventional SAg and interacts with both MHC class II and TCR Vβ it does not share significant global sequence homology with other SAgs (20). MAM has a novel fold composed of two α-helical domains and represents a new family of SAgs (118). It has been reported that zinc ions are required to induce MAM/MAM dimer formation necessary for MHC binding and efficient T-cell activation (62). However, no zinc could be located in the HLA-DR1–MAM structure (118). The binding site of MAM on the HLA-DR1 molecule is most similar to that for TSST-1 but a much larger surface is buried in the complex. MAM interacts with the central region of the antigenic peptide, similar to TCR, which is in contrast to other SAgs, in which TSST-1, SPE-C, or SEH binds either to the carboxy-terminal or to the amino-terminal region of the bound peptides (55, 64, 82). Thus, MAM mimics the peptide dependence seen in conventional antigen presentation, and different antigenic peptides influence MAM presentation (31, 118).

CONSEQUENCES FOR TCR INTERACTION AND ACTIVATION

Unlike the way in which SEB and TSST-1 interact with the α-chain of MHC and allow partial contacts with the Vβ-chain of TCR (5, 21 50, 55), SEH and SPE-C act as a bridge between the MHC and TCR molecules and prohibit direct contact (81, 99, 100). A model of the MHC-SAg-TCR ternary complex (Color Plate 10) that supports this view has been suggested based on the crystal structures of the SPE-C–HLA-DR2a complex and the recently determined structure of the SPE-C–TCR Vβ chain complex (99). In addition, T-cell stimulation studies with the zinc-dependent SAg SEA have shown that, upon binding to MHC, SEA limits access to those residues of MHC and peptide that normally interact with TCR, further supporting this view (28). Thus, the zinc-dependent presentation of SAgs on the β-chain of MHC defines new conditions for interactions with TCR. SPE-C interacts with human Vβ2.1 in a much more extensive and specific manner than α-chain-binding SAgs like SEB and SPE-A, and SEH has even been suggested to interact solely with the Vβ-chain of TCR (83). Moreover, this way of forming ternary complexes might explain the much higher affinity for the interaction with the β-chain compared with the α-chain of MHC. Because direct interaction between MHC and TCR is precluded in both the SEH- and the SPE-C–MHC complexes, sufficient stabilization must be achieved through interactions with MHC alone. Recent findings in support of this show that zinc-dependent SAgs remained at the surface of human B cells for at least 40 hours (85). This extended T-cell exposure thus contributes to the potency of SAgs as T-cell activators.

Today, almost forty years after the first characterization of bacterial SAgs, new features of these molecules are still being discovered. The numbers of new members of the different SAg families are constantly growing and there is no doubt that more studies are needed if we are to completely understand the role played by SAgs in the bacterial evasion of the host immune response.

Acknowledgments. I thank Maria Hånkansson and Marjolein Thunnissen at the Department of Molecular Biophysics, Lund University, for fruitful collaboration. In addition, I thank all past and present employees at Active Biotech Research AB involved in SAg-related research, especially Göran Forsberg. Finally, I express my gratitude to Karin (Petersson) Lindqvist. If it were not for her enthusiastic work we would not have known as much about these molecules.

REFERENCES

1. **Abrahmsén, L., M. Dohlsten, S. Segren, P. Bjork, E. Jonsson, and T. Kalland.** 1995. Characterization of two distinct MHC class II binding sites in the superantigen staphylococcal enterotoxin A. *EMBO J.* **14**(13):2978–2986.

2. **Alberts, I. L., K. Nadassy, and S. J. Wodak.** 1998. Analysis of zinc binding sites in protein crystal structures. *Protein Sci.* **7**(8):1700–1716.

3. **Al-Daccak, R., K. Mehindate, F. Damdoumi, P. Etongue-Mayer, H. Nilsson, P. Antonsson, M. Sundstrom, M. Dohlsten, R. P. Sekaly, and W. Mourad.** 1998. Staphylococcal enterotoxin D is a promiscuous superantigen offering multiple modes of interactions with the MHC class II receptors. *J. Immunol.* **160**(1):225–232.

4. **Alouf, J. E., and H. Muller-Alouf.** 2003. Staphylococcal and streptococcal superantigens: molecular, biological and clinical aspects. *Int. J. Med. Microbiol.* **292**(7–8):429–440.

5. **Andersen, P. S., P. M. Lavoie, R. P. Sekaly, H. Churchill, D. M. Kranz, P. M. Schlievert, K. Karjalainen, and R. A. Mariuzza.** 1999. Role of the T cell receptor alpha chain in stabilizing TCR-superantigen-MHC class II complexes. *Immunity* **10**(4):473–483.

6. **Arcus, V. L., R. Langley, T. Proft, J. D. Fraser, and E. N. Baker.** 2002. The three-dimensional structure of a superantigen-like protein, SET3, from a pathogenicity island of the Staphylococcus aureus genome. *J. Biol. Chem.* **277**(35):32274–32281.

7. **Arcus, V. L., T. Proft, J. A. Sigrell, H. M. Baker, J. D. Fraser, and E. N. Baker.** 2000. Conservation and variation in superantigen structure and activity highlighted by the three-dimensional structures of two new superantigens from Streptococcus pyogenes. *J. Mol. Biol.* **299**(1):157–168.

8. **Artiushin, S. C., J. F. Timoney, A. S. Sheoran, and S. K. Muthupalani.** 2002. Characterization and immunogenicity of pyrogenic mitogens SePE-H and SePE-I of Streptococcus equi. *Microb. Pathog.* **32**(2):71–85.

9. **Baker, H. M., T. Proft, P. D. Webb, V. L. Arcus, J. D. Fraser, and E. N. Baker.** 2004. Crystallographic and mutational data show that the streptococcal pyrogenic exotoxin j can use a common binding surface for T-cell receptor binding and dimerization. *J. Biol. Chem.* **279**:38571–38576.

10. **Baker, M. D., I. Gendlina, C. M. Collins, and K. R. Acharya.** 2004. Crystal structure of a dimeric form of streptococcal pyrogenic exotoxin a (Spea1) *Protein Sci.* **13**:2285–2290.

11. **Baker, M. D., D. M. Gutman, A. C. Papageorgiou, C. M. Collins, and K. R. Acharya.** 2001. Structural features of a zinc binding site in the superantigen strepococcal pyrogenic exotoxin A (SpeA1): implications for MHC class II recognition. *Protein Sci.* **10**(6):1268–1273.

12. **Baker, M. D., A. C. Papageorgiou, R. W. Titball, J. Miller, S. White, B. Lingard, J. J. Lee, D. Cavanagh, M. A. Kehoe, J. H. Robinson, and K. R. Acharya.** 2002. Structural and functional role of threonine 112 in a superantigen Staphylococcus aureus enterotoxin B. *J. Biol. Chem.* **277**:2756–2762.

13. **Bergdoll, M. S.** 1970. Enterotoxins, p. 265–326. *In* T. C. Montie, S. Kadio, and S. J. Ajil (ed.), *Microbial Toxins*. Academic Press Inc., New York, N.Y.

14. **Bolin, D. R., A. L. Swain, R. Sarabu, S. J. Berthel, P. Gillespie, N. J. Huby, R. Makofske, L. Orzechowski, A. Perrotta, K. Toth, J. P. Cooper, N. Jiang, F. Falcioni, R. Campbell, D. Cox, D. Gaizband, C. J. Belunis, D. Vidovic, K. Ito, R. Crowther, U. Kammlott, X. Zhang, R. Palermo, D. Weber, J. Guenot, Z. Nagy, and G. L. Olson.** 2000. Peptide and peptide mimetic inhibitors of antigen presentation by HLA-DR class II MHC molecules. Design, structure-activity relationships, and X-ray crystal structures. *J. Med. Chem.* **43**:2135–2148.

15. **Cavallin, A., H. Arozenius, K. Kristensson, P. Antonsson, D. E. Otzen, P. Bjork, and G. Forsberg.** 2000. The spectral and thermodynamic properties of staphylococcal enterotoxin A, E, and variants suggest that structural modifications are important to control their function. *J. Biol. Chem.* **275**(3):1665–1672.

16. **Cavallin, A., K. Petersson, and G. Forsberg.** 2003. Spectrophotometric methods for the determination of superantigen structure and stability. *Methods Mol. Biol.* **214**:55–63.

17. **Chi, Y. I., I. Sadler, L. M. Jablonski, S. D. Callantine, C. F. Deobald, C. V. Stauffacher, and G. A. Bohach.** 2002. Zinc-mediated dimerization and its effect on activity and conformation of staphylococcal enterotoxin type C. *J. Biol. Chem.* **277**(25):22839–22846.

18. **Choi, Y. W., A. Herman, D. DiGiusto, T. Wade, P. Marrack, and J. Kappler.** 1990. Residues of the variable region of the T-cell-receptor beta-chain that interact with S. aureus toxin superantigens. *Nature* **346**(6283):471–473.

19. **Cole, B. C., and C. L. Atkin.** 1991. The Mycoplasma arthritidis T-cell mitogen, MAM: a model superantigen. *Immunol. Today* **12**(8):271–276.

20. **Cole, B. C., K. L. Knudtson, A. Oliphant, A. D. Sawitzke, A. Pole, M. Manohar, L. S. Benson, E. Ahmed, and C. L. Atkin.** 1996. The sequence of the Mycoplasma arthritidis superantigen, MAM: identification of

functional domains and comparison with microbial superantigens and plant lectin mitogens. *J. Exp. Med.* **183**(3):1105–1110.

21. **Deckhut, A. M., Y. Chien, M. A. Blackman, and D. L. Woodland.** 1994. Evidence for a functional interaction between the beta chain of major histocompatibility complex class II and the T cell receptor alpha chain during recognition of a bacterial superantigen. *J. Exp. Med.* **180**(5):1931–1935.

22. **DeLano, W. L.** 2002. The PyMOL Molecular Graphics System (2002) on World Wide Web. @http://www.pymol.org.

23. **Dellabona, P., J. Peccoud, J. Kappler, P. Marrack, C. Benoist, and D. Mathis.** 1990. Superantigens interact with MHC class II molecules outside of the antigen groove. *Cell* **62**(6):1115–1121.

24. **Dessen, A., C. M. Lawrence, S. Cupo, D. M. Zaller, and D. C. Wiley.** 1997. X-ray crystal structure of HLA-DR4 (DRA*0101, DRB1*0401) complexed with a peptide from human collagen II. *Immunity* **7**(4):473–481.

25. **Dinges, M. M., P. M. Orwin, and P. M. Schlievert.** 2000. Exotoxins of Staphylococcus aureus. *Clin. Microbiol. Rev.* **13**(1):16–34.

26. **Dohlsten, M., G. Hedlund, and T. Kalland.** 1991. Staphylococcal-enterotoxin-dependent cell-mediated cytotoxicity. *Immunol. Today* **12**(5):147–150.

27. **Dohlsten, M., G. Hedlund, H. O. Sjogren, and R. Carlsson.** 1988. Two subsets of human CD4+ T helper cells differing in kinetics and capacities to produce interleukin 2 and interferon-gamma can be defined by the Leu-18 and UCHL1 monoclonal antibodies. *Eur. J. Immunol.* **18**(8):1173–1178.

28. **Dowd, J. E., R. W. Karr, and D. R. Karp.** 1996. Functional activity of staphylococcal enterotoxin A requires interactions with both the alpha and beta chains of HLA-DR. *Mol. Immunol.* **33**(16):1267–1274.

29. **Earhart, C. A., D. T. Mitchell, D. L. Murray, D. M. Pinheiro, M. Matsumura, P. M. Schlievert, and D. H. Ohlendorf.** 1998. Structures of five mutants of toxic shock syndrome toxin-1 with reduced biological activity. *Biochemistry* **37**:7194–7202.

30. **Earhart, C. A., G. M. Vath, M. Roggiani, P. M. Schlievert, and D. H. Ohlendorf.** 2000. Structure of streptococcal pyrogenic exotoxin A reveals a novel metal cluster. *Protein Sci.* **9**(9):1847–1851.

31. **Etongue-Mayer, P., M. A. Langlois, M. Ouellette, H. Li, S. Younes, R. Al-Daccak, and W. Mourad.** 2002. Involvement of zinc in the binding of Mycoplasma arthritidis-derived mitogen to the proximity of the HLA-DR binding groove regardless of histidine 81 of the beta chain. *Eur. J. Immunol.* **32**(1):50–58.

32. **Fernandez, M. M., M. C. De Marzi, P. Berguer, D. Burzyn, R. J. Langley, I. Piazzon, R. A. Mariuzza, and E. L. Malchiodi.** 2006. Binding of natural variants of staphylococcal superantigens SEG and SEI to TCR and MHC class II molecule. *Mol. Immunol.* **43**(7):927–938.

33. **Ferretti, J. J., W. M. McShan, D. Ajdic, D. J. Savic, G. Savic, K. Lyon, C. Primeaux, S. Sezate, A. N. Suvorov, S. Kenton, H. S. Lai, S. P. Lin, Y. Qian, H. G. Jia, F. Z. Najar, Q. Ren, H. Zhu, L. Song, J. White, X. Yuan, S. W. Clifton, B. A. Roe, and R. McLaughlin.** 2001. Complete genome sequence of an M1 strain of Streptococcus pyogenes. *Proc. Natl. Acad. Sci. USA* **98**(8):4658–4663.

34. **Fields, B. A., E. L. Malchiodi, H. Li, X. Ysern, C. V. Stauffacher, P. M. Schlievert, K. Karjalainen, and R. A. Mariuzza.** 1996. Crystal structure of a T-cell receptor beta-chain complexed with a superantigen. *Nature* **384**(6605):188–192.

35. **Fischer, H., M. Dohlsten, M. Lindvall, H. O. Sjogren, and R. Carlsson.** 1989. Binding of staphylococcal enterotoxin A to HLA-DR on B cell lines. *J. Immunol.* **142**(9):3151–3157.

36. **Fleischer, B., and H. Schrezenmeier.** 1988. T cell stimulation by staphylococcal enterotoxins. Clonally variable response and requirement for major histocompatibility complex class II molecules on accessory or target cells. *J. Exp. Med.* **167**(5):1697–1707.

37. **Fleischer, B., H. Schrezenmeier, and P. Conradt.** 1989. T lymphocyte activation by staphylococcal enterotoxins: role of class II molecules and T cell surface structures. *Cell. Immunol.* **120**:92–101.

38. **Fraser, J. D.** 1989. High-affinity binding of staphylococcal enterotoxins A and B to HLA-DR. *Nature* **339**(6221):221–223.

39. **Fraser, J. D., V. L. Arcus, E. N. Baker, and T. Proft.** 2003. Bacterial superantigens and immune evasion, p. 171–200. *In* B. Henderson and P. C. F. Oyston (ed.), *Bacterial Evasion of Host Immune Responses*. Cambridge University Press, Cambridge, United Kingdom.

40. **Fraser, J. D., R. G. Urban, J. L. Strominger, and H. Robinson.** 1992. Zinc regulates the function of two superantigens. *Proc. Natl. Acad. Sci. USA* **89**(12):5507–5511.

41. **Garcia, K. C., L. Teyton, and I. A. Wilson.** 1999. Structural basis of T cell recognition. *Annu. Rev. Immunol.* **17**:369–397.

42. **Gronenborn, A. M., D. R. Filpula, N. Z. Essig, A. Achari, M. Whitlow, P. T. Wingfield, and G. M. Clore.** 1991. A novel, highly stable fold of the immunoglobulin binding domain of streptococcal protein G. *Science* **253**(5020):657–661.

43. **Håkansson, M., P. Antonsson, P. Björk, and L. A. Svensson.** 2001. Cooperative zinc binding in a staphylococcal enterotoxin A mutant mimics the SEA-MHC class II interaction *J. Biol. Inorg. Chem.* **6:**757–762.

44. **Håkansson, M., K. Petersson, H. Nilsson, G. Forsberg, P. Bjork, P. Antonsson, and L. A. Svensson.** 2000. The crystal structure of staphylococcal enterotoxin H: implications for binding properties to MHC class II and TcR molecules. *J. Mol. Biol.* **302**(3):527–537.

45. **Hamad, A. R., P. Marrack, and J. W. Kappler.** 1997. Transcytosis of staphylococcal superantigen toxins. *J. Exp. Med.* **185**(8):1447–1454.

46. **Hennecke, J., and D. C. Wiley.** 2001. T cell receptor-MHC interactions up close. *Cell* **104**(1):1–4.

47. **Herman, A., N. Labrecque, J. Thibodeau, P. Marrack, J. W. Kappler, and R. P. Sekaly.** 1991. Identification of the staphylococcal enterotoxin A superantigen binding site in the beta 1 domain of the human histocompatibility antigen HLA-DR. *Proc. Natl. Acad. Sci. USA* **88**(22):9954–9958.

48. **Hogan, R. J., J. VanBeek, D. R. Broussard, S. L. Surman, and D. L. Woodland.** 2001. Identification of MHC class II-associated peptides that promote the presentation of toxic shock syndrome toxin-1 to T cells. *J. Immunol.* **166**(11):6514–6522.

49. **Hudson, K. R., R. E. Tiedemann, R. G. Urban, S. C. Lowe, J. L. Strominger, and J. D. Fraser.** 1995. Staphylococcal enterotoxin A has two cooperative binding sites on major histocompatibility complex class II. *J. Exp. Med.* **182**(3):711–720.

50. **Jardetzky, T. S., J. H. Brown, J. C. Gorga, L. J. Stern, R. G. Urban, Y. I. Chi, C. Stauffacher, J. L. Strominger, and D. C. Wiley.** 1994. Three-dimensional structure of a human class II histocompatibility molecule complexed with superantigen. *Nature* **368**(6473):711–718.

51. **Jiang, W., and J. S. Bond.** 1992. Families of metalloendopeptidases and their relationships. *FEBS Lett.* **312:**110–114.

52. **Kappler, J., B. Kotzin, L. Herron, E. W. Gelfand, R. D. Bigler, A. Boylston, S. Carrel, D. N. Posnett, Y. Choi, and P. Marrack.** 1989. V beta-specific stimulation of human T cells by staphylococcal toxins. *Science* **244**(4906):811–813.

53. **Karp, D. R., and E. O. Long.** 1992. Identification of HLA-DR1 beta chain residues critical for binding staphylococcal enterotoxins A and E. *J. Exp. Med.* **175**(2):415–424.

54. **Kiefer, L. L., S. A. Paterno, and C. A. Fierke.** 1995. Hydrogen bond network in the metal binding site of carbonic anhydrase enhances zinc affinity and catalytic efficiency. *J. Am. Chem. Soc.* **117:**6831–6837.

55. **Kim, J., R. G. Urban, J. L. Strominger, and D. C. Wiley.** 1994. Toxic shock syndrome toxin-1 complexed with a class II major histocompatibility molecule HLA-DR1. *Science* **266**(5192):1870–1874.

56. **Kotzin, B. L., D. Y. Leung, J. Kappler, and P. Marrack.** 1993. Superantigens and their potential role in human disease. *Adv. Immunol.* **54:**99–166.

57. **Kozono, H., D. Parker, J. White, P. Marrack, and J. Kappler.** 1995. Multiple binding sites for bacterial superantigens on soluble class II MHC molecules. *Immunity* **3**(2):187–196.

58. **Krupka, H. I., B. W. Segelke, R. G. Ulrich, S. Ringhofer, M. Knapp, and B. Rupp.** 2002. Structural basis for abrogated binding between staphylococcal enterotoxin A superantigen vaccine and MHC-IIalpha. *Protein Sci.* **11:**642–651.

59. **Kumaran, D., S. Eswaramoorthy, W. Furey, M. Sax, and S. Swaminathan.** 2001. Structure of staphylococcal enterotoxin C2 at various pH levels. *Acta Crystallogr. D Biol. Crystallogr.* **57:**1270–1275.

60. **Kuroda, M., T. Ohta, I. Uchiyama, T. Baba, H. Yuzawa, I. Kobayashi, L. Cui, A. Oguchi, K. Aoki, Y. Nagai, J. Lian, T. Ito, M. Kanamori, H. Matsumaru, A. Maruyama, H. Murakami, A. Hosoyama, Y. Mizutani-Ui, N. K. Takahashi, T. Sawano, R. Inoue, C. Kaito, K. Sekimizu, H. Hirakawa, S. Kuhara, S. Goto, J. Yabuzaki, M. Kanehisa, A. Yamashita, K. Oshima, K. Furuya, C. Yoshino, T. Shiba, M. Hattori, N. Ogasawara, H. Hayashi, and K. Hiramatsu.** 2001. Whole genome sequencing of meticillin-resistant Staphylococcus aureus. *Lancet* **357**(9264):1225–1240.

61. **Langford, M. P., G. J. Stanton, and H. M. Johnson.** 1978. Biological effects of staphylococcal enterotoxin A on human peripheral lymphocytes. *Infect. Immun.* **22**(1):62–68.

62. **Langlois, M. A., Y. El Fakhry, and W. Mourad.** 2003. Zinc-binding sites in the N terminus of Mycoplasma arthritidis-derived mitogen permit the dimer formation required for high affinity binding to HLA-DR and for T cell activation. *J. Biol. Chem.* **278**(25):22309–22315.

63. **Li, H., A. Llera, D. Tsuchiya, L. Leder, X. Ysern, P. M. Schlievert, K. Karjalainen, and R. A. Mariuzza.** 1998. Three-dimensional structure of the complex between a T cell receptor beta chain and the superantigen staphylococcal enterotoxin B. *Immunity* **9**(6):807–816.

64. **Li, Y., H. Li, N. Dimasi, J. K. McCormick, R. Martin, P. Schuck, P. M. Schlievert, and R. A. Mariuzza.** 2001. Crystal structure of a superantigen bound to the high-affinity, zinc-dependent site on MHC class II. *Immunity* **14**(1):93–104.

65. **Llewelyn, M., S. Sriskandan, M. Peakman, D. R. Ambrozak, D. C. Douek, W. W. Kwok, J. Cohen, and D. M. Altmann.** 2004. HLA class II polymorphisms determine responses to bacterial superantigens. *J. Immunol.* **172**(3):1719–1726.

66. **Manders, S. M.** 1998. Toxin-mediated streptococcal and staphylococcal disease. *J. Am. Acad. Dermatol.* **39**(3):383–398.

67. **Marrack, P., and J. Kappler.** 1990. The staphylococcal enterotoxins and their relatives. *Science* **248**(4956):705–711.

68. **Merritt, E. A., and W. G. Hol.** 1995. AB5 toxins. *Curr. Opin. Struct. Biol.* **5**(2):165–171.

69. **Mitchell, D. T., D. G. Levitt, P. M. Schlievert, and D. H. Ohlendorf.** 2000. Structural evidence for the evolution of pyrogenic toxin superantigens. *J. Mol. Evol.* **51**(6):520–531.

70. **Miyoshi-Akiyama, T., K. Imanishi, and T. Uchiyama.** 1993. Purification and partial characterization of a product from Yersinia pseudotuberculosis with the ability to activate human T cells. *Infect. Immun.* **61**(9):3922–3927.

71. **Miyoshi-Akiyama, T., J. Zhao, H. Kato, K. Kikuchi, K. Totsuka, Y. Kataoka, M. Katsumi, and T. Uchiyama.** 2003. Streptococcus dysgalactiae-derived mitogen (SDM), a novel bacterial superantigen: characterization of its biological activity and predicted tertiary structure. *Mol. Microbiol.* **47**(6):1589–1599.

72. **Nilsson, H., P. Bjork, M. Dohlsten, and P. Antonsson.** 1999. Staphylococcal enterotoxin H displays unique MHC class II-binding properties. *J. Immunol.* **163**(12):6686–6693.

73. **Papageorgiou, A. C., and K. R. Acharya.** 2000. Microbial superantigens: from structure to function. *Trends Microbiol.* **8**(8):369–375.

74. **Papageorgiou, A. C., K. R. Acharya, R. Shapiro, E. F. Passalacqua, R. D. Brehm, and H. S. Tranter.** 1995. Crystal structure of the superantigen enterotoxin C2 from Staphylococcus aureus reveals a zinc-binding site. *Structure* **3**(8):769–779.

75. **Papageorgiou, A. C., M. D. Baker, J. D. McLeod, S. K. Goda, C. N. Manzotti, D. M. Sansom, H. S. Tranter, and K. R. Acharya.** 2004. Identification of a secondary zinc-binding site in staphylococcal enterotoxin C2. Implications for superantigen recognition. *J. Biol. Chem.* **279**(2):1297–1303.

76. **Papageorgiou, A. C., R. D. Brehm, D. D. Leonidas, H. S. Tranter, and K. R. Acharya.** 1996. The refined crystal structure of toxic shock syndrome toxin-1 at 2.07 A resolution. *J. Mol. Biol.* **260**:553–569.

77. **Papageorgiou, A. C., C. M. Collins, D. M. Gutman, J. B. Kline, S. M. O'Brien, H. S. Tranter, and K. R. Acharya.** 1999. Structural basis for the recognition of superantigen streptococcal pyrogenic exotoxin A (SpeA1) by MHC class II molecules and T-cell receptors. *EMBO J.* **18**(1):9–21.

78. **Papageorgiou, A. C., C. P. Quinn, D. Beer, R. D. Brehm, H. S. Tranter, P. F. Bonventre, and K. R. Acharya.** 1996. Crystal structure of a biologically inactive mutant of toxic shock syndrome toxin-1 at 2.5 A resolution. *Protein Sci.* **5**:1737–1741.

79. **Papageorgiou, A. C., H. S. Tranter, and K. R. Acharya.** 1998. Crystal structure of microbial superantigen staphylococcal enterotoxin B at 1.5 A resolution: implications for superantigen recognition by MHC class II molecules and T-cell receptors. *J. Mol. Biol.* **277**:61–79.

80. **Peavy, D. L., W. H. Adler, and R. T. Smith.** 1970. The mitogenic effects of endotoxin and staphylococcal enterotoxin B on mouse spleen cells and human peripheral lymphocytes. *J. Immunol.* **105**(6):1453–1458.

81. **Petersson, K., G. Forsberg, and B. Walse.** 2004. Interplay between superantigens and immunoreceptors. *Scand. J. Immunol.* **59**(4):345–355.

82. **Petersson, K., M. Håkansson, H. Nilsson, G. Forsberg, L. A. Svensson, A. Liljas, and B. Walse.** 2001. Crystal structure of a superantigen bound to MHC class II displays zinc and peptide dependence. *EMBO J.* **20**(13):3306–3312.

83. **Petersson, K., H. Pettersson, N. J. Skartved, B. Walse, and G. Forsberg.** 2003. Staphylococcal enterotoxin H induces Valpha-specific expansion of T cells. *J. Immunol.* **170**(8):4148–4154.

84. **Petersson, K., M. Thunnissen, G. Forsberg, and B. Walse.** 2002. Crystal structure of a SEA variant in complex with MHC class II reveals the ability of SEA to crosslink MHC molecules. *Structure* **10**:1619–1626.

85. **Pless, D. D., G. Ruthel, E. K. Reinke, R. G. Ulrich, and S. Bavari.** 2005. Persistence of zinc-binding bacterial superantigens at the surface of antigen-presenting cells contributes to the extreme potency of these superantigens as T-cell activators. *Infect. Immun.* **73**(9):5358–5366.

86. **Pontzer, C. H., J. K. Russell, and H. M. Johnson.** 1991. Structural basis for differential binding of staphylococcal enterotoxin A and toxic shock syndrome toxin 1 to class II major histocompatibility molecules. *Proc. Natl. Acad. Sci. USA* **88**(1):125–128.

87. **Prasad, G. S., C. A. Earhart, D. L. Murray, R. P. Novick, P. M. Schlievert, and D. H. Ohlendorf.** 1993. Structure of toxic shock syndrome toxin 1. *Biochemistry* **32**(50):13761–13766.

88. **Prasad, G. S., R. Radhakrishnan, D. T. Mitchell, C. A. Earhart, M. M. Dinges, W. J. Cook, P. M. Schlievert, and D. H. Ohlendorf.** 1997. Refined structures of three crystal forms of toxic shock syndrome toxin-1 and of a tetramutant with reduced activity. *Protein Sci.* **6**:1220–1227.

89. **Proft, T., V. L. Arcus, V. Handley, E. N. Baker, and J. D. Fraser.** 2001. Immunological and biochemical characterization of streptococcal pyrogenic exotoxins I and J (SPE-I and SPE-J) from Streptococcus pyogenes. *J. Immunol.* **166**(11):6711–6719.

90. **Proft, T., S. L. Moffatt, C. J. Berkahn, and J. D. Fraser.** 1999. Identification and characterization of novel superantigens from Streptococcus pyogenes. *J. Exp. Med.* **189**(1):89–102.

91. **Proft, T., S. L. Moffatt, K. D. Weller, A. Paterson, D. Martin, and J. D. Fraser.** 2000. The streptococcal superantigen SMEZ exhibits wide allelic variation, mosaic structure, and significant antigenic variation. *J. Exp. Med.* **191**(10):1765–1776.

92. **Proft, T., P. D. Webb, V. Handley, and J. D. Fraser.** 2003. Two novel superantigens found in both group a and group C streptococcus. *Infect. Immun.* **71**(3):1361–1369.

93. **Roussel, A., B. F. Anderson, H. M. Baker, J. D. Fraser, and E. N. Baker.** 1997. Crystal structure of the streptococcal superantigen SPE-C: dimerization and zinc binding suggest a novel mode of interaction with MHC class II molecules. *Nat. Struct. Biol.* **4**(8):635–643.

94. **Russell, J. K., C. H. Pontzer, and H. M. Johnson.** 1990. The I-A beta b region (65-85) is a binding site for the superantigen, staphylococcal enterotoxin A. *Biochem. Biophys. Res. Commun.* **168**(2):696–701.

95. **Schad, E. M., A. C. Papageorgiou, L. A. Svensson, and K. R. Acharya.** 1997. A structural and functional comparison of staphylococcal enterotoxins A and C2 reveals remarkable similarity and dissimilarity. *J. Mol. Biol.* **269**(2):270–280.

96. **Schad, E. M., I. Zaitseva, V. N. Zaitsev, M. Dohlsten, T. Kalland, P. M. Schlievert, D. H. Ohlendorf, and L. A. Svensson.** 1995. Crystal structure of the superantigen staphylococcal enterotoxin type A. *EMBO J.* **14**:3292–301.

97. **Sundberg, E., and T. S. Jardetzky.** 1999. Structural basis for HLA-DQ binding by the streptococcal superantigen SSA. *Nat. Struct. Biol.* **6**(2):123–129.

98. **Sundberg, E. J., P. S. Andersen, P. M. Schlievert, K. Karjalainen, and R. A. Mariuzza.** 2003. Structural, energetic, and functional analysis of a protein-protein interface at distinct stages of affinity maturation. *Structure* **11**(9):1151–1161.

99. **Sundberg, E. J., H. Li, A. S. Llera, J. K. McCormick, J. Tormo, P. M. Schlievert, K. Karjalainen, and R. A. Mariuzza.** 2002. Structures of two streptococcal superantigens bound to TCR beta chains reveal diversity in the architecture of T cell signaling complexes. *Structure* **10**(5):687–699.

100. **Sundberg, E. J., Y. Li, and R. A.Mariuzza.** 2002. So many ways of getting in the way: diversity in the molecular architecture of superantigen-dependent T-cell signaling complexes. *Curr. Opin. Immunol.* **14**(1):36–44.

101. **Sundberg, E. J., M. W. Sawicki, S. Southwood, P. S. Andersen, A. Sette, and R. A. Mariuzza.** 2002. Minor structural changes in a mutated human melanoma antigen correspond to dramatically enhanced stimulation of a CD4+ tumor-infiltrating lymphocyte line. *J. Mol. Biol.* **319**(2):449–461.

102. **Sundstrom, M., L. Abrahmsen, P. Antonsson, K. Mehindate, W. Mourad, and M. Dohlsten.** 1996. The crystal structure of staphylococcal enterotoxin type D reveals Zn2+-mediated homodimerization. *EMBO J.* **15**(24):6832–6840.

103. **Sundstrom, M., D. Hallen, A. Svensson, E. Schad, M. Dohlsten, and L. Abrahmsen.** 1996. The co-crystal structure of staphylococcal enterotoxin type A with Zn^{2+} at 2.7 A resolution. Implications for major histocompatibility complex class II binding. *J. Biol. Chem.* **271**(50):32212–32216.

104. **Swaminathan, S., W. Furey, J. Pletcher, and M. Sax.** 1992. Crystal structure of staphylococcal enterotoxin B, a superantigen. *Nature* **359**(6398):801–806.

105. **Swaminathan, S., W. Furey, J. Pletcher, and M. Sax.** 1995. Residues defining V beta specificity in staphylococcal enterotoxins. *Nat. Struct. Biol.* **2**:680–686.

106. **Thompson, J. D., D. G. Higgins, and T. J. Gibson.** 1994. CLUSTAL W: improving the sensitivity of progressive multiple sequence alignment through sequence weighting, position-specific gap penalties and weight matrix choice. *Nucleic Acids Res.* **22**(22):4673–4680.

107. **Tiedemann, R. E., and J. D. Fraser.** 1996. Cross-linking of MHC class II molecules by staphylococcal enterotoxin A is essential for antigen-presenting cell and T cell activation. *J. Immunol.* **157**(9):3958–3966.

108. **Tiedemann, R. E., R. J. Urban, J. L. Strominger, and J. D. Fraser.** 1995. Isolation of HLA-DR1.(staphylococcal enterotoxin A)2 trimers in solution. *Proc. Natl. Acad. Sci. USA* **92**(26):12156–12159.

109. **Trowsdale, J.** 2005. HLA genomics in the third millennium. *Curr. Opin. Immunol.* **17**(5):498–504.

110. **Wen, R., D. R. Broussard, S. Surman, T. L. Hogg, M. A. Blackman, and D. L. Woodland.** 1997. Carboxy-terminal residues of major histocompatibility complex class II-associated peptides control the presentation of the bacterial superantigen toxic shock syndrome toxin-1 to T cells. *Eur. J. Immunol.* **27**(3):772–781.

111. **Wen, R., G. A. Cole, S. Surman, M. A. Blackman, and D. L. Woodland.** 1996. Major histocompatibility complex class II-associated peptides control the presentation of bacterial superantigens to T cells. *J. Exp. Med.* **183**(3):1083–1092.

112. **White, J., A. Herman, A. M. Pullen, R. Kubo, J. W. Kappler, and P. Marrack.** 1989. The V beta-specific superantigen staphylococcal enterotoxin B: stimulation of mature T cells and clonal deletion in neonatal mice. *Cell* **56**(1):27–35.

113. **Wikstrom, M., T. Drakenberg, S. Forsen, U. Sjobring, and L. Bjorck.** 1994. Three-dimensional solution structure of an immunoglobulin light chain-binding domain of protein L. Comparison with the IgG-binding domains of protein G. *Biochemistry* **33**(47):14011–14017.

114. **Woodland, D. L., R. Wen, and M. A. Blackman.** 1997. Why do superantigens care about peptides? *Immunol. Today* **18**(1):18–22.

115. **Zavala-Ruiz, Z., I. Strug, M. W. Anderson, J. Gorski, and L. J. Stern.** 2004. A polymorphic pocket at the P10 position contributes to peptide binding specificity in class II MHC proteins. *Chem. Biol.* **11**:1395–1402.

116. **Zavala-Ruiz, Z., I. Strug, B. D. Walker, P. J. Norris, and L. J. Stern.** 2004. A hairpin turn in a class II MHC-bound peptide orients residues outside the binding groove for T cell recognition. *Proc. Natl. Acad. Sci. USA* **101**:13279–13284.

117. **Zavala-Ruiz, Z., E. J. Sundberg, J. D. Stone, D. B. DeOliveira, I. C. Chan, J. Svendsen, R. A. Mariuzza, and L. J. Stern.** 2003. Exploration of the P6/P7 region of the peptide-binding site of the human class II major histocompatibility complex protein HLA-DR1 *J. Biol. Chem.* **278**:44904–44912.

118. **Zhao, Y., Z. Li, S. J. Drozd, Y. Guo, W. Mourad, and H. Li.** 2004. Crystal structure of Mycoplasma arthritidis mitogen complexed with HLA-DR1 reveals a novel superantigen fold and a dimerized superantigen-MHC complex. *Structure* **12**(2):277–288.

Superantigens: Molecular Basis for Their Role in Human Diseases
Edited by Malak Kotb and John D. Fraser
© 2007 ASM Press, Washington, D.C.

Chapter 8

Superantigens: Structure, Function, and Diversity

Matthew D. Baker and K. Ravi Acharya

In the years since the first three-dimensional structure of a bacterial superantigen was solved a wealth of structural information has been amassed that has greatly enhanced our understanding of these molecules and their interactions with the immune system (61). As the diversity of the family increases, structural information and the ability to assign specific functions to regions of the toxin, including assessing the roles of individual residues, provides a basis for a detailed comparison of this unique toxin family.

Bacterial superantigens (SAgs) are powerful T-cell stimulatory molecules produced primarily by *Staphylococcus aureus* and *Streptococcus pyogenes*. Unlike conventional antigens, SAgs are not processed internally by antigen-presenting cells (APCs), and so act as a fully intact native protein rather than a short antigenic peptide. Bacterial SAgs possess the unique ability to cross-link major histocompatibility complex (MHC) class II molecules and T-cell receptors, which in turn is responsible for their ability to illicit an immune response several orders of magnitude greater than that of conventional peptide antigens (45).

The number of known bacterial proteins with superantigenic properties and/or high homology with classical bacterial SAgs has grown considerably over the past decade. In addition, several other SAgs have been discovered with little or no homology to the family, both from bacterial and viral sources. Further, viral proteins with homology to bacterial SAgs have also been identified (44). The staphylococcal enterotoxins (SEs) A, B, C1–3, D, E, H, I, J, toxic shock syndrome toxin-1 (TSST-1); the streptococcal pyogenic exotoxins (Spes) A, C, H; streptococcal mitogenic exotoxin SME-Z_2 and streptococcal superantigen (SSA) are the most well studied of the bacterial superantigens (9, 10).

The division of staphylococcal and streptococcal SAgs into subfamilies based on amino acid sequence, structure, and physiological information has caused some disagreement in the scientific community. However, using purely sequence and structural information, the bacterial SAgs can be grouped into four subfamilies (63, 67). Group I comprises staphylococcal enterotoxins SEA, SED, SEE, SEH, SEI, and SEJ. Toxins from both *S. aureus* and

Matthew D. Baker and K. Ravi Acharya • Department of Biology and Biochemistry, University of Bath, Claverton Down, Bath BA2 7AY, United Kingdom.

S. pyogenes form group II, which is composed of SEB, SEC1–3, SpeA1-3, SSA, and SEG. Group III contains streptococcal pyogenic and mitogenic toxins: SpeC, SpeJ, SpeG, SpeH, SME-Z, SME-Z$_2$ and *Streptococcus dysgalactiae*-derived mitogen (SDM). The staphylo-coccal enterotoxin-like toxins (SSLs) and TSST-1 form group IV. Other pathogens, such as *Mycoplasma arthritidis* and *Yersinia pseudotuberculosis,* have also been shown to secrete superantigenic proteins and their crystal structures have recently been determined (14, 19, 69). *M. arthritidis* mitogen (MAM) and *Y. pseudotuberculosis* mitogen (YPM) have no se-quence or structure homology to the rest of the bacterial SAgs and therefore cannot be grouped with any of these subfamilies (14, 31).

The advent of genomics has enabled the discovery of putative SAgs based on se-quence alignment (21, 37). Such examples include SEQ (47) and SER (46) from *S. au-reus,* and several SAg-like motifs have been found in the genome of severe acute respira-tory syndrome (SARS)-associated coronavirus (44). Structural homology is also seen in the absence of sequence homology in other *S. aureus* proteins such as the chemotaxis-inhibitory protein of *S. aureus* (CHIPS), which has a striking homology to the super-antigen C-terminal domain (25).

The structural homology of the classical SAgs (groups I, II, III, and IV) allows their di-rect comparison and indicates a conserved three-dimensional architecture (9).

Bacterial SAgs consist of two domains: the N-terminal domain (also know as the B do-main or small domain) and the C-terminal domain (also known as the A domain or large do-main). Both domains are separated by a long, solvent-accessible α-helix, which runs across the center of the molecule (Color Plate 11). Notable features of the N-terminal domain are the presence of hydrophobic residues within solvent-exposed areas and a structural similar-ity to the oligosaccharide/oligonucleotide-binding fold (OB-fold). The C-terminal domain comprises a four-stranded β-sheet crowned by a central α-helix and resembles the β-grasp motif. Features common to most, but not all members of the bacterial superantigen family include a highly flexible disulfide loop, located in the N-terminal domain, and the presence of one or more zinc atoms (Color Plate 11, Table 1). Recently, several structures from the staphylococcal enterotoxin-like (SSL) toxin subfamily have been elucidated. These proteins show considerable sequence and structural homology to the classical SAgs yet have no su-perantigenic properties. SSL5 and SSL9 structures indicate that this common architecture is preserved among this related group of proteins (5, 8). The closest relative to SSL5 of the "true" superantigens is TSST-1. However, there are significant structural differences from other members of the SAg family. First, the β6- and β7-strands of the C-terminal domain are extended such that the β6–β7 loop protrudes significantly from the surface of the mole-cule. Second, there is a widespread positive charge over the surface of the protein, which is concentrated in particular around the area of the central α-helix and the outer face on the N-terminal domain. The biological importance of these features is as yet unclear, but as more studies are carried out on these intriguing additions to the family, the role of these proteins in pathogenesis and significance of their homology to superantigens will no doubt become clearer.

The topology of the family has been further extended by the crystal structures for MAM and *Y. pseudotuberculosis* mitogen a (YPMa) (19, 69). In this case, these two pro-teins show no sequence or structural similarities to the classical SAgs (Color Plate 11), yet both possess considerable superantigenicity. MAM (69) is composed of two α-helical domains arranged to form an L-shape (Color Plate 11). The N-terminal domain consists

Table 1. Role of zinc ion in superantigen function

Superantigen	M_r (kDa)	MHC-II generic site	Zinc usage	Dimer formation	Disulfide loop	PDB ID
S. aureus						
SEA	27.1	Yes	High-affinity site	Yes	Yes	1ESF
			Low-affinity site			
SEB	28.4	Yes	No		Yes	3SEB
SEC1–3	27.5	Yes		Yes	Yes	1STE (SEC2), 1CK1 (SEC3)
SED	26.3	Yes	High-affinity or dimer?	Yes	Yes	–
			Low-affinity site			
SEE	26.4	Yes	High or low		Yes	–
SEG	27		No		Yes	–
SEH	25.2	No generic site	Single		Yes	1ENF
SEI	24.9		No		No	–
TSST-1	22	Yes	No		No	2QIL
S. pyogenes						
SpeA	25.7	Yes	Single	Yes	Yes	1B1Z
SpeC	24.4	No generic site	Single	Yes	No	1AN8
SpeG	24.6	No generic site	Single[a]			
SpeH	23.6	No generic site	Single		Yes	1ET9
SpeJ	23.3	No generic site	Single	Yes	No	1TY0
SME-Z	24.3	No generic site	Single[a]		No	–
SME-Z2	24.2	No generic site	Single		No	1ET6
SSA	26.9	Yes	No		Yes	1BXT
S. dysgalactiae						
SDM	25		Single[a]		No	–
Y. pseudotuberculosis						
YPM	14.5				–	1PM4
M. arthritidis						
MAM	27		Yes		–	1R5I

[a]Proposed based on sequence alignment.

of a four α-helix bundle, which is wrapped by a 25-residue N-terminal loop, while the C-terminal domain contains six α-helices. YPMa is only 14 kDa and as such is much smaller than the classical staphylococcal and streptococcal SAgs. It consists of a jelly-roll fold comprising two β-sheets, each containing four antiparallel strands (19). Again, the structure is unlike that of any of the other known SAgs (including MAM) and is structurally comparable to viral capsid proteins and members of the tumor necrosis factor superfamily (Color Plate 11).

COMPLEX FORMATION BY THE SAgs

Conventional antigens are processed internally by APCs and displayed as discrete peptides on the cell surface by MHC class II molecules. These peptide antigens are then recognized by T-cell receptors (TCRs) specific to that peptide (Color Plate 12). To effect an immune response on the scale of a typical superantigen, the toxin must also interact with both an MHC class II molecule and a TCR as a whole intact toxin. Structural evidence shows SAgs bind to APCs on the outside of MHC class II molecule (32, 35, 43, 50) and to T cells via the external face of the TCR V_β element (22, 42) (Color Plate 12). The superantigen binds between the TCR and MHC class II molecule displacing the antigenic peptide away from the TCR-combining site. Thus, superantigenicity will occur irrespective of the TCR specificity for the antigenic peptide-MHC II complex (6). While the formation of this complex is comparable to conventional antigen recognition, there are considerable differences that allow SAgs their increased potency. To consider the nature of the trimolecular complex, we must first examine the interactions of these toxins with both MHC class II molecules and TCRs, separately. Complexes of SAgs with both MHC class II molecules (32, 35, 43, 50) and TCR molecules (22, 42), along with a considerable amount of mutagenesis studies, have revealed many similarities and differences in the way that this family of proteins interacts with its receptors.

BINDING TO MHC CLASS II MOLECULES

Structural data have revealed that there are two distinct modes in which staphylococcal and streptococcal SAgs can interact with MHC class II molecules. The first mode is via a low-affinity binding site (also known as the generic site) located on the α-chain of the MHC class II molecule while the second mode is via a high-affinity (~100 times higher affinity than the generic site) zinc-dependent site that is located on the β-chain of the MHC class I molecule (Color Plates 11 and 12). Crystal structures of SAgs in complex with MHC class II molecules via both the generic site (SEB and TSST-1 in complex with HLA-DR1) (32, 35) and the high-affinity site SpeC in complex with HLA-DR2 (43) and SEH in complex with HLA-DR1 (50) have allowed a detailed examination of these interactions. Individual SAgs bind to either one or both of the binding sites, providing diversity among the family. Further diversity is observed within the family as each SAg has been shown to bind differentially to distinct alleles of MHC class II molecules. Most of the SAgs such as TSST-1, SEB, and MAM bind preferentially to HLA-DR alleles, while SAgs SEC, SpeA, and SSA bind principally to HLA-DQ alleles (20, 58).

The complexes of SAgs bound to MHC class II molecules via the generic site (SEB–HLA-DR1 and TSST-1–HLA-DR1) indicate a binding mode similar to the DR1 α-chain with the solvent-exposed hydrophobic core of the SAg's N-terminal domain having a crucial role. Comparison of SEB and TSST-1 with other members of the classical SAg family shows similar hydrophobic core regions exist and thus would form the generic MHC class II binding site in these toxins. A notable difference between the SEB– and TSST-1–HLA-DR1 complexes is the presence of additional contacts with the peptide antigen in the

TSST-1–HLA-DR1 complex (35). Further, the composition of the peptide antigen present in the peptide-binding groove has been shown to affect the binding of TSST-1 to MHC class II molecules. This is highlighted by the fact that truncating the C-terminal end of the antigenic peptide dramatically affects TSST-1 binding to murine I-Ab (66). (For a more detailed view of the effects of peptide antigen on the activity of SAg, see reference 68 and references therein.)

THE ROLE OF THE ZINC ION IN SUPERANTIGEN FUNCTION

Many members of the superantigen family (except SEB, TSST-1, SSA, SSLs, and YPM) possess at least one zinc binding site (for details, see Table 1, Color Plates 11 and 12). For those SAgs that possess them, the zinc binding site represents an important, high-affinity alternative to the generic site for MHC class II recognition. This high-affinity zinc binding site has been identified at the C-terminal domain of SEA by a combination of mutational and structural analysis. This zinc site displays a K_d of 100 nM for MHC β-chain, and when compared to the zinc-independent generic site at the N-terminal domain of SEA (K_d of 10 μM), it highlights the importance of the zinc ion for MHC class II binding (23). In addition, it has been shown that the concurrent existence of these binding sites causes SEA to exhibit a K_d of 13 nM, and the mutation of residues in either of these sites abolishes toxin-induced cytokine expression in peripheral blood mononuclear cells (PBMCs) (2). The presence of two distinct MHC class II binding sites seems to enable SEA to form trimeric SEA-MHC-SEA complexes, as observed in solution experiments (64): SEE possesses zinc ligands identical with SEA, suggesting a similar mechanism for this toxin too. In SED and SpeC, the dimerization mechanism varies slightly (54, 60). SED can form zinc-dependent homodimers, while SpeC forms zinc-independent homodimers. Both SED and SpeC bind to the β-chain of the MHC class II molecule through a zinc-mediated mechanism similar to that of SEA, suggesting that formation of trimers and/or tetramers is possible. A similar binding mechanism has been proposed for SEH, which, importantly, lacks a generic MHC class II binding site and as such would rely entirely on the zinc binding site to interact with MHC class II molecules (26). A homologous high-affinity site to that of SEA is not present in either SEC or SpeA. However, a separate, lower-affinity zinc binding site with an estimated dissociation constant for the zinc ion of less than 1 μM (SEC) is present. This secondary zinc binding site is located within the N-terminal domain of these toxins and also appears to be important for MHC class II binding (Color Plate 11) (49).

A complete picture of the role of the zinc binding site is provided by the crystal structures of SpeC complexed with HLA-DR2 and SEH complexed with HLA-DR1 via the high-affinity zinc-dependent site (43, 50). The interactions between both SAgs and their MHC class II molecules are governed by a tetrahedrally coordinated bridging zinc ion. Three coordinating side chains (His 167, His 201, and Asp 203) provided by SpeC, and two (His 206 and Asp 208 plus a third provided by a water molecule) by SEH combine with His 81 from the MHC class II β1-helix. The stability of the SAg–MHC class II complex is maintained through interaction with the antigenic class II-associated peptide (approximately one third of the contact area between SpeC and MHC class II is taken up by antigenic peptide) and in both cases most of the interactions with the antigenic peptide are via its backbone atoms. Despite the composition of the peptides differing in each complex, similar interactions with the antigenic peptide are displayed by SEH and SpeC, demonstrating that, although the peptide plays an important role in the complex interaction, MHC class II binding is not entirely peptide specific.

A zinc ion also plays a critical role in the binding of SME-Z$_2$, SpeG, and SpeH to MHC class II molecules, as the binding of all three of these toxins to LG-2 cells is significantly reduced by chelating the zinc (53). The postulated zinc binding site of each of these SAgs is shown to be closest to that of SEA and SpeC, both of which have geometrically and spatially equivalent sites (53, 54). As the presence of zinc-binding ligands within the amino acid sequence of these toxins suggests, all three of these SAgs have been shown to bind to MHC class II molecules in a zinc-dependent fashion. To increase the complexity of the role of zinc further, a second zinc binding site was recently discovered in SEC2 (48). This distinct binding site, located close to the generic MHC class II binding site, is postulated to serve as a site of dimerization for SEC2. If this is the case, the generic MHC class II site would be blocked by the dimer interface, and binding to MHC class II molecules would have to be mediated by the SEC2 primary zinc binding site. This would result in SEC2 being able to bind a zinc-mediated dimer to MHC class II molecules. SpeA1 and SpeC are also able to form zinc-independent homodimers. SpeA1 is able to exist in a disulfide-linked dimeric form (11) via cysteine residues located within the flexible disulfide loop, while the SpeC dimer is formed by using the surface that is usually used as a generic MHC class II binding site (54).

The SSL proteins are unique among the superantigen family in that they do not bind to MHC class II molecules and do not appear to be superantigenic (8). Therefore, it is likely that the conserved amino acids appear to preserve the overall superantigen fold rather than play any role in interactions with MHC class II molecules. In addition, the number of non-conservative substitutions within the region homologous to the generic MHC class II binding site means MHC II binding is doubtful.

Despite the enormous structural and sequence differences between the classical SAgs and MAM, zinc was initially thought to play a role in MAM binding to MHC class II molecules and/or in its dimerization (20, 38). However, the crystal structure of dimeric MAM in complex with HLA-DR1 showed that zinc performs neither role, and the exact role of zinc in the action of this novel superantigen requires further investigation (69).

Although the structure of MAM complexed with HLA-DR1 bares no resemblance to the classical staphylococcal and streptococcal SAgs there are some general similarities in their binding mechanisms. Upon complex formation, there are no major structural changes at the interface between MAM and MHC class II molecule that are comparable with the complexes between classical SAgs and MHC class II. Further, substantial interaction occurs between the N-terminal loop of MAM and the antigenic peptide. The binding mode of each of the two MAM monomers with a single HLA-DR1 is identical. MAM is shown to be present as both monomer and homodimers in solution, indicating that it may be able to act on MHC class II molecules as both monomer and dimer. The interaction between the two molecules does not involve zinc ion and is formed by the C-terminal domain on one monomer sitting in the V-shaped cleft formed by both the N- and C-terminal domain of the second monomer (Color Plate 11).

The MAM–HLA-DR1 complex is formed through contacts between the N-terminal domain of MAM and the several regions of HLA-DR1, specifically the β1-β2 loop, the β3-β4 loop, and the α1-helix of the DR1 α-chain, the β1-helix of the DR1 β-chain, and the hemagglutinin (HA) antigenic peptide displayed by the HLA-DR1 molecule. The particular areas of the N-terminal domain of MAM that interact with HLA-DR1 are the α3- and α4-helices that bind to the α1-helix, the β1-β2 loop and the β3-β4 loop of the DR1 α-chain. The MAM binding site on HLA-DR1 appears to overlap with the generic binding site for classical staphylococcal and streptococcal SAgs. In support of this, SEB and TSST-1 have been shown to block MAM binding to MHC class II on THP-1 cells (12). Binding is also abolished by the presence of classical SAgs binding to the high-affinity zinc site, as the MAM binding site on MHC class II also encompasses a region on the MHC β-chain within which His 81 is located (69).

At present, very little is known about the interactions of YPM with MHC class II molecules. In the absence of structural evidence of the complex with MHC class II, and no homology to the rest of the superantigen family, mutagenesis studies provided the only real information (31). However, the crystal structure of YPM has revealed that most of the mutations that affected activity were buried within the toxin and therefore are unlikely to be involved in MHC binding. A probable explanation is that these mutations caused conformational changes and/or misfolding of the protein which resulted in inability to bind MHC class II molecules. As a result, it is essential that further work be carried out to fully characterize the functional regions of this toxin.

As the number and complexity of ways in which SAgs can mediate binding with MHC class II molecules increases, it has become apparent that these mechanisms play an integral role in the toxin's ability to regulate its own function. So far several mechanisms are apparent: zinc-mediated interaction or generic site interaction as a monomer, as a homodimer (which in turn can be either zinc or non-zinc mediated), or a combination of all three.

BINDING TO THE T-CELL RECEPTOR

At first glance, the interaction of SAgs with TCRs seems much less complex than their interactions with MHC class II molecules. Superantigens were thought to bind exclusively to TCR via the TCR V_β element via a generally similar mechanism mediated by interactions between the side chains of the SAg and the backbone atoms of the V_β element. As such, each superantigen is able to expand T cells bearing certain specific V_β elements, while excluding others (33).

The wealth of structural information available for SAgs has allowed extensive comparison of their TCR-binding regions. This analysis has revealed a similar framework of residues that would provide a common binding mechanism, with specific amino acid differences that may supply V_β specificity. The TCR binding site is located between the two domains of the molecule as a shallow cavity. In general this cavity is formed by the amino acid residues of the α2-helix, the β2-β3 loop, the β4-strand and β4-β5 loop, the β5-strand and the α5-helix (61) (Color Plate 11). This site, first characterized in SEB, has been shown to have equivalent regions in other SAgs based on structure-based sequence alignment. Conclusive details of the classical SAg TCR binding site have been provided by the crystal structures of several SAgs in complex with their TCR V_β elements (22, 42, 59). The structures of SEB, SEC2, and SEC3 support the idea of a simple binding mechanism; a majority of the contacts made involved interactions between the side chains of the SAg and backbone atoms of the TCR V_β element. In the cases of SEC2, SEC3, and SEB the main interactions are shown to be between their side-chain atoms and both complementarity-determining regions one and two (CDRs 1 and 2), and hypervariable region 4 (HV4) of the V_β-chain. Examination of the TCR binding sites of SEC2/3 and comparison with the corresponding regions of SEA and SEB shows an invariant asparagine residue (Asn 23 in SEB/SECs; Asn 25 in SEA) as being crucial for interaction with TCR. Mutational studies in SEB show that T-cell stimulation is lost upon mutation of this residue (34). Asn 23 is exposed to the solvent in SEA, SEB, and SEC, and sequence alignments suggest that it has similar interactions in all of the SEs. To further understand the role of individual residues in TCR binding, those residues in the crystal structure of the SEC3/V_β complex shown to be involved in complex stabilization were subjected to alanine-scanning mutagenesis (40). Asn 23, Tyr 90, and Gln 210 were seen to have the most influence on the binding of the TCR β-chain. Tyr 90 and Gln 210 are conserved among SEC1-3, SEB, and SpeA, and SSA has analogous residues Asn 49, Tyr 116, and Gln 223 (57, 61). It is likely therefore that these residues are among those that provide the common framework for binding to TCR V_β elements. The variation between different superantigens in terms of TCR affinity and specificity can be explained by the presence of those residues unique to each particular SAg, including any topological effect that each of these might have. For example, residue Tyr 26 of SEC2 confers specificity between SEC1 and SEC2 via its interaction with Gly 53 from the V_β-chain (18) and is not conserved in other SAgs. Val 91 of SEC2 is also implicated in TCR binding and is not conserved in SEA (Tyr 94) or SEB (Tyr 91) either (64), and it is possible that the exchange of Val 91 for a tyrosine residue in SEB may explain its decreased affinity for the Vβ8.2-chain (22). Those residues that govern the specificity of SEA for TCR are thought to include Ser 206, Asn 207, and Thr 21 (62). This is supported by the fact that exchanging residues 206 and 207 in SEA for their homologues in SEE causes the responding T cells to switch the profile of V_β elements to that of the profile normally seen for T cells stimulated by SEE (30): Ser 206 and Asn 207 in SEA correspond to Gln 210 and Ser 211, respectively, in both SEB and SEC2. The preceding evidence shows that the residues that define the specificity of a superantigen for particular V_β elements are relatively few. Moreover, it is these residues that make the greatest energetic contribution to the overall stability of the V_β superantigen complex (41).

Our simple mechanism of TCR binding for superantigens becomes a little more complicated with the inclusion of the evidence obtained from the crystal structures of SpeA1 in complex with mouse V_β 8.2 and SpeC in complex with human V_β 2.1 (36, 41). Examination of the SpeC complex shows that SpeC binds to significantly more V_β residues than either SEC2/3 or SEB and also includes areas of the CDR1 and CDR3 loops of the TCR β-chain. The enhanced number of contacts is most likely due to the differing topology of SpeC in and around the TCR binding site: SpeC has a deeper and broader cleft between its N- and C-terminal domains where the TCR binding site is located. Unlike SEB and SEC2/3, SpeC also forms numerous interactions with both main-chain and side-chain atoms of the TCR V_β-chain. The interaction of SpeA1 with the TCR V_β-chain is more similar to that of SEB, with the three hydrogen bonds observed between SEB and the TCR SpeA1 preserved in the SpeA1–TCR complex. However, SpeA1 also forms an additional five hydrogen bonds on top of those seen for SEB. Differences in the TCR binding sites of both of these SAgs and the interactions of amino acid side chains on both the superantigen and the TCR V_β-chain suggest that binding to TCR receptors is not merely one of simple conformational dependence as first thought (22, 41).

Given the wealth of structural information available on the toxin, it is somewhat surprising that the TCR binding site of TSST-1 is as yet not fully characterized. Its structural similarity to SpeC hints that it may share similar TCR binding characteristics. Again, because of the lack of a structure of TSST-1 in complex with TCR, we rely on mutagenesis data for information. The location of the TCR binding site of TSST-1 is thought to lie between the C-terminal domain on the long α2-helix, the β7-β8 and α2-β9 loops and part of the α1-helix. This would make its position unique among the SEs (3). The region encompassing residues 115 to 144 has been shown to be of great importance in TCR binding by TSST-1 due to the effect on mitogenicity observed upon mutation of residues within this area, in particular, residues Tyr 115, Glu 132, His 135, Ile 140, His 141, and Tyr 144 (3, 17). Mutation of these residues produces substantially fewer mitogenic toxins, but they can still be recognized by TSST-1-specific antibodies, indicating that the toxins produced are still fully folded (17).

The SSL family of proteins is unable to elicit a V_β-restricted T-cell response, which given the high degree of similarity with TSST-1 is perhaps a little surprising (8). However, upon closer examination of the structure of SSL5 it is apparent that amino acid conservation is restricted to those residues that would preserve the structural integrity of the protein. This is particularly so in and around the region joining N- and C-terminal domains of SSL5 where the TCR binding site is located in TSST-1. Further changes in specific surface residues also serve to change the nature of the protein more still, making it impossible for interaction with TCR molecules to occur.

Both MAM and YPM are known to bind to the TCR V_β-chain (1, 13, 65). However, no structural information is available for these toxins in complex with a TCR molecule. Although their individual crystal structures have allowed some speculative deduction as to how they may interact with TCRs, at present not enough data are available to produce a detailed model or fully characterize these interactions. It will be interesting to see if these novel SAgs add a further dimension to the interactions of SAgs with TCR molecules or if they bind in a similar fashion to the staphylococcal and streptococcal SAgs.

The available structural data have allowed detailed examination of the TCR V_β-chain binding sites of many SAgs. The sum of these data is that while interactions with TCR share a common core of residues among a majority of SAgs, specificity for particular V_β elements is supplied by amino acid residues unique to each toxin. This in turn demonstrates that, in parallel with their interactions with MHC class II molecules, SAgs are also able to interact with TCR molecules by multiple modes. In summary, a high-specificity binding mode involves several contacts by both backbone atoms and side-chain atoms over a large area, as adopted by SpeC. This mode has a high affinity for only a few TCR V_β elements. A second, moderate specificity mode with fewer interactions over a reduced contact area is also apparent. This mode has a reasonable affinity for an increased group of TCR V_β elements such as observed in SpeA1. The third mode, as displayed by SEB and SEC2, is a promiscuous binding mode allowing binding to TCR V_β-chains in a more simple conformation-dependent manner. The TCR binding modes of the SAgs do not end here, however; further complexities were discovered when it was revealed that SEH, in contrast to all other SAgs, stimulates T cells in a V_α-specific manner and completely lacks any V_β-restricted response (51). The possible reasons for SEH's unique TCR interaction are unclear, but it is proposed that SEH may bind to TCR because of its lack of a generic MHC class II binding site and its subsequent presentation by MHC class II molecules via a zinc atom. Whether other SAgs that are presented to TCR by MHC class II in the same way can bind to V_α in a similar fashion remains to be seen, but with the discovery of yet more SAgs from more diverse sources, it remains a distinct possibility.

FORMATION OF THE TRIMERIC COMPLEX FOR SIGNAL TRANSDUCTION

The precise mechanism leading to the formation of the MHC II–SAg–TCR complex is still not fully understood. The mechanism relies on the proximity of the APC and the T cell, and the favorable interaction of the TCR and MHC class II molecules at the cell surface. The existence of dimeric SAgs and SAgs with multiple MHC class II binding sites leading to the formation of complexes with more than one MHC class II molecule or TCR adds further complexity to the mechanism.

In addition, while considering the formation of a complex, the character of membrane-bound receptors must be taken into account (16). If a complex is to form, cell membranes need to be brought close enough together to interact, and receptors must diffuse to this site of interaction. For superantigenic T-cell activation to occur less than 0.3% of the MHC class II molecules must be occupied by SAg (39); higher concentrations of bound toxin result in an aborted T-cell response after a few cell divisions. Thus, a low local concentration of MHC class II molecules on the cell interface is preferable for optimum superantigenicity. The binding of a SAg to TCR induces clustering of the TCRs on the cell surface and the assembly of the intracellular components required for signal transduction (24). It is thought that this occurs in a manner that mimics the way peptide antigens induce receptor clustering either through direct clustering events as proposed by the TCR oligomerization model, or by the binding of superantigen homodimers to multiple MHC class II molecules, which in turn induces T-cell clustering (64, 68). Molecular modeling suggests that signal transduction stimulated by SEA through large-scale assembly is limited to four or five TCR–(DR1β–SEA–DR1α) tetramers and requires the dimerization of MHC class II molecules. While TCRs would be clustered together in this model, TCR dimerization is thought unlikely (15). SEA is not unique in its ability to form zinc-mediated dimers (64). SED (60) and SEC2 (48) can form zinc-dependent homodimers, while SpeA1 forms a non-zinc-mediated, disulfide-linked dimer (11), and a SpeC dimer can also be formed in the absence of zinc (54). MAM has also been shown to be able to form zinc-dependent and zinc-independent dimers (38, 69); YPM is thought to be able to form zinc-independent trimers (19). This clearly demonstrates that SAgs have evolved slightly different ways of inducing receptor clustering. SAgs that act as monomers and possess only a single MHC class II binding site appear to rely on the interactions of the TCR V_{β} with MHC class II-β1, which increases the stability of the ternary complex to within the range seen for conventional antigen. A stable MHC–SAg–TCR complex with an extended half-life would therefore assist receptor clustering. The differences in mechanism between those SAgs that utilize zinc and those that do not are further highlighted by the persistence of zinc-binding SAgs at the surface of APCs (52). Zinc-binding SAgs persist at the cell surface, binding MHC class II molecules in an essentially irreversible manner. The mechanism by which they do this is unclear, but it is postulated that the zinc binding sites allow SAgs to cross-link multiple MHC class II molecules forming MHC II oligomers. In turn, the stability of the oligomers' surface location is enhanced enabling the prolonged stimulation of T cells.

OTHER STRUCTURAL FEATURES AND IDIOSYNCRASIES

SAgs possess several other features implicated in their activity; these include a disulfide loop, a possible cell binding site, and a novel region distinct from the MHC II and TCR sites that is directly involved in lethality (7).

Common symptoms of superantigen-mediated diseases are vomiting and diarrhea, but the exact relationship between SAg structure and the symptoms emesis and diarrhea is unclear. In addition, the association between these activities and superantigenicity is also vague. It is thought that the flexible disulfide loop is, in part, responsible for these properties; exchange of the two cysteine residues that form this disulfide loop for alanine is shown to eliminate the emetic activity in SEC1 (29). It has been shown that the disulfide bond itself is not an absolute requirement for emetic activity but the conformation within or adjacent to the loop is important for emesis. The corresponding cysteine residues in SpeA have also been implicated in T-cell stimulation, and their mutation significantly reduces the ability of the toxin to stimulate certain populations of T cells (36). This suggests that there is some correlation between superantigenicity and emesis, but recent work indicates that emesis may not be wholly linked with superantigenicity in all toxins (27). His 225 of SEA has been demonstrated to be important for both superantigenic and emetic activity, while His 61 appears to be important only for emetic activity (28). Further, regions of the N-terminal fragment of SEA that are important for both emetic and superantigenic functions have also been identified (27). The emetic activity of SEB can be eliminated by carboxymethylation of its histidine residues, yet the modified toxin is still able to induce peripheral blood cell proliferation in monkeys (4). Further, the C-terminal fragment of SEC1 induces diarrhea but not emesis in primates (56). In combination, this evidence would suggest that the two activities are separable in the staphylococcal enterotoxins at least. But to fully to assess the contribution of particular amino acids to these symptoms, further research will be required.

Residues 150 to 160 of SEB and homologous residues in other SAgs have been identified as a novel domain within the classical superantigen family (7). A synthetic peptide containing this sequence was able to prevent Sag-induced lethality from a wide range of SAgs. It has been proposed that the peptide blocks the costimulatory signals required for T-cell activation and thus the corresponding region of the toxins themselves encompasses a novel binding domain for costimulatory molecules.

The ability of TSST-1 to cause systemic or localized symptoms in a site-dependent manner has led to the suggestion that, unlike other staphylococcal enterotoxins, TSST-1 must be able to cross the epithelial barrier and enter the cell (55). The mechanism by which TSST-1 is able to cross membranes could involve either passive diffusion or the use of specific cellular receptors. If a cellular receptor is utilized, then TSST-1 must possess an equivalent binding site. Structurally, evidence can be provided by the differences between TSST-1 and the other SAgs. These include the lack of a α-helix in the C-terminal domain, an extension to the N-terminal domain and the absence of a disulfide loop. TSST-1 also has unique patches of hydrophobic and neutral residues on the front and rear of the β-barrel at the N-terminal domain. In combination, these features could produce a receptor-specific binding site such that TSST-1 is able traverse epithelial cells and allow systemic shock.

Further support is provided by the SSL group of proteins (5, 8). SSL7 and SSL9 have been shown to interact selectively with monocytes via specific saturable binding sites leading to their uptake. Therefore, both SSL7 and SSL9 must possess cell binding domains. It is unclear if this is also the case with SSL5, but its structure reveals a widespread positive charge over its surface, suggesting a likely binding site for a negatively charged binding partner (5).

Modeling exercises with SSL5 and the amino acid sequences of several of the SSL proteins show that the general surface features change throughout the group, indicating that the classical superantigen fold may have been evolved to produce a group of similar proteins, each with differing function(s), although the exact nature of the functions of these molecules is yet to be established.

REFERENCES

1. **Abe, J., T. Takeda, Y. Watanabe, H. Nakao, N. Kobayashi, D. Y. Leung, and T. Kohsaka.** 1993. Evidence for superantigen production by *Yersinia pseudotuberculosis. J. Immunol.* **151:**4183–4188.

2. **Abrahmsen, L., M. Dohlsten, S. Segren, P. Bjork, E. Jonsson, and T. Kalland.** 1995. Characterization of two distinct MHC class II binding sites in the superantigen Staphylococcal enterotoxin A. *EMBO J.* **14:**2978–2986.

3. **Acharya, K. R., E. F. Passalacqua, E. Y. Jones, K. Harlos, D. I. Stuart, R. D. Brehm, and H. S. Tranter.** 1994. Structural basis of superantigen action inferred from crystal structure of toxic-shock syndrome toxin-1. *Nature* **367:**94–97.

4. **Alber, G., D. K. Hammer, and B. Fleischer.** 1990. Relationship between enterotoxic- and T lymphocyte-stimulating activity of Staphylococcal enterotoxin B. *J. Immunol.* **144:**4501–4506.

5. **Al-Shangiti, A. M., C. E. Naylor, S. P. Nair, D. C. Briggs, B. Henderson, and B. M. Chain.** 2004. Structural relationships and cellular tropism of Staphylococcal superantigen-like proteins. *Infect. Immun.***72:**4261–4270.

6. **Anderson, P. S., P. M. Lavoie, R. P. Sekaly, H. Churchill, and D. M. Kranz.** 1999. Role of the T cell receptor α-chain in stabilising TCR-Superantigen-MHC class II complexes. *Immunity* **10:**473–483.

7. **Arad, G., R. Levy, D. Hillman, and R. Kaempfer.** 2000. Superantigen antagonist protects against lethal shock and defines a new domain for T-cell activation. *Nat. Med.* **6:**414–421.

8. **Arcus, V. L., R. Langley, T. Proft, J. D. Fraser, and E. N. Baker.** 2002. The three-dimensional structure of a superantigen-like protein, SET3, from a pathogenicity island of the Staphylococcus aureus genome. *J. Biol. Chem.* **277:**32274–32281.

9. **Baker, M. D., and K. R. Acharya.** 2003 Superantigens. Structure, function, and diversity. *Methods. Mol. Biol.* **214:**1–31.

10. **Baker, M. D., and K. R. Acharya.** 2004. Superantigens: structure-function relationships. *Int. J. Med. Microbiol.* **293:**529–537.

11. **Baker, M. D., I. Gendlina, C. M. Collins, and K. R. Acharya.** 2004. Crystal structure of a dimeric form of Streptococcal pyrogenic exotoxin A (SpeA1). *Protein. Sci.* **13:**2285–2290.

12. **Bernatchez, C., R. Al-Daccak, P. E. Mayer, K. Mehindate, L. Rink, S. Mecheri, and W. Mourad.** 1997. Functional analysis of Mycoplasma arthritidis-derived mitogen interactions with class II molecules. *Infect. Immun.* **65:**2000–2005.

13. **Cole, B. C.** 1991. The immunobiology of *Mycoplasma arthritidis* and its superantigen MAM. *Curr. Top. Microbiol. Immunol.* **174:**107–119.

14. **Cole, B. C., K. L. Knudtson, A. Oliphant, A. D. Sawitzke, A. Pole, M. Manohar, L. S. Benson, E. Ahmed, and C. L. Atkin.** 1996. The sequence of the *Mycoplasma arthritidis* superantigen, MAM: identification of functional domains and comparison with microbial superantigens and plant lectin mitogens. *J. Exp. Med.* **183:**1105–1110.

15. **Cuff, L., R. G. Ulrich, and M. A. Olson.** 2003. Prediction of the multimeric assembly of Staphylococcal enterotoxin A with cell-surface protein receptors. *J. Mol. Graph. Model.* **21:**473–486.

16. **Davis, S. J., S. Ikemizu, E. J. Evans, L. Fugger, T. R. Bakker, and P. A. van der Merwe.** 2003. The nature of molecular recognition by T cells. *Nat. Immunol.* **4:**217–224.

17. **Deresiewicz, R. L., J. Woo, M. Chan, R. W. Finberg, and D. L. Kasper.** 1994. Mutations affecting the activity of toxic shock syndrome toxin-1. *Biochemistry* **33:**12844–12851.

18. **Deringer, J. R., R. J. Ely, C. V. Stauffacher, and G. A. Bohach.** 1996. Subtype-specific interactions of type C Staphylococcal enterotoxins with the T-cell receptor. *Mol. Microbiol.* **22:**523–534.

19. **Donadini, R., C. W. Liew, A. H. Kwan, J. P. Mackay, and B. A. Fields.** 2004. Crystal and solution structures of a superantigen from *Yersinia pseudotuberculosis* reveal a jelly-roll fold. *Structure* **12:**145–156.

20. **Etongue-Mayer, P., M. A. Langlois, M. Ouellette, H. Li, S. Younes, R. Al-Daccak, and W. Mourad.** 2002. Involvement of zinc in the binding of Mycoplasma arthritidis-derived mitogen to the proximity of the HLA-DR binding groove regardless of histidine 81 of the β chain. *Eur. J. Immunol.* **32:**50–58.

21. **Ferretti, J. J., W. M. McShan, D. Ajdic, D. J. Savic, G. Savic, K. Lyon, C. Primeaux, S. Sezate, A. N. Suvorov, S. Kenton, H. S. Lai, S. P. Lin, Y. Qian, H. G. Jia, F. Z. Najar, Q. Ren, H. Zhu, L. Song, J. White, X. Yuan, S. W. Clifton, B. A. Roe, and R. McLaughlin.** 2001. Complete genome sequence of an M1 strain of *Streptococcus pyogenes*. *Proc. Natl. Acad. Sci. USA* **98:**4658–4663.

22. **Fields, B. A., E. L. Malchiodi, H. Li, X. Ysern, C. V. Stauffacher, P. M. Schlievert, K. Karjalainen, and R. A. Mariuzza.** 1996. Crystal structure of a T-cell receptor β-chain complexed with a superantigen. *Nature* **384:**188–192.

23. **Fraser, J. D., R. G. Urban, J. L. Strominger, and H. Robinson.** 1992. Zinc regulates the function of two superantigens. *Proc. Natl. Acad. Sci USA* **89:**5507–5511.

24. **Germain, R. N.** 1997. T-cell signalling: the importance of receptor clustering. *Curr. Biol.* **7:**640–644.

25. **Haas, P. J., C. J. C. de Haas, M. J. J. C. Poppelier, K. P. M. van Kessel, J. A. G. van Strijp, K. Dijkstra, R. M. Scheek, H. Fan, J. A. W. Kruijtzer, R. M. J. Liskamp, and J. Kemmink.** 2005. The Structure of C5a receptor-blocking domain of chemotaxis inhibitory protein of *Staphylococcus aureus* is related to a group of immune evasive molecules. *J. Mol. Biol.* **353:**859–872.

26. **Hakansson, M., K. Petersson, H. Nilsson, G. Forsberg, P. Bjork, P. Antonsson, and L. A. Svensson.** 2000. The crystal structure of Staphylococcal enterotoxin H: implications for binding properties to MHC class II and TcR molecules. *J. Mol. Biol.* **302:**527–537.

27. **Harris, T. O., and M. J. Betley.** 1995. Biological activities of Staphylococcal enterotoxin type A mutants with N-terminal substitutions. *Infect. Immun.* **63:**2133–2140.

28. **Hoffman, M., M. Tremaine, J. Mansfield, and M. Betley.** 1996. Biochemical and mutational analysis of the histidine residues of Staphylococcal enterotoxin A. *Infect. Immun.* **64:**885–890.

29. **Hovde, C. J., J. C. Marr, M. L. Hoffmann, S. P. Hackett, Y. I. Chi, K. K. Crum, D. L. Stevens, C. V. Stauffacher, and G. A. Bohach.** 1994. Investigation of the role of the disulphide bond in the activity and structure of Staphylococcal enterotoxin C1. *Mol. Microbiol.* **13:**897–909.

30. **Hudson, K. R., H. Robinson, and J. D. Fraser.** 1993. Two adjacent residues in Staphylococcal enterotoxins A and E determine T cell receptor Vβ specificity. *J. Exp. Med.* **177:**175–184.

31. **Ito, Y., G. Seprenyi, J. Abe, and T. Kohsaka.** 1999. Analysis of functional regions of YPM, a superantigen derived from gram-negative bacteria. *Eur. J. Biochem.* **263:**326–337.

32. **Jardetzky, T. S., J. H. Brown, J. C. Gorga, L. J. Stern, R. G. Urban, Y. I. Chi, C. Stauffacher, J. L. Strominger, and D. C. Wiley.** 1994. Three-dimensional structure of a human class II histocompatibility molecule complexed with superantigen. *Nature* **368:**711–718.

33. **Kappler, J., B. Kotzin, L. Herron, E. W. Gelfand, R. D. Bigler, A. Boylston, S. Carrel, D. N. Posnett, Y. Choi, and P. Marrack.** 1989. V$_\beta$ specific stimulation of human T cells by Staphylococcal toxins. *Science* **244:**811–813.

34. **Kappler, J. W., A. Herman, J. Clements, and P. Marrack.** 1992. Mutations defining functional regions of the superantigen staphylococcal enterotoxin B. *J. Exp. Med.* **175:**387–396.

35. **Kim, J., R. G. Urban, J. L. Strominger, and D. C. Wiley.** 1994. Toxic shock syndrome toxin-1 complexed with a class II major histocompatibility molecule HLA-DR1. *Science* **266:**1870–1874.

36. **Kline, J. B., and C. M. Collins.** 1997. Analysis of the interaction between the bacterial superantigen Streptococcal pyrogenic exotoxin A (SpeA) and the human T-cell receptor. *Mol. Microbiol.* **24:**191–202.

37. **Kuroda, M., T. Ohta, I. Uchiyama, T. Baba, H. Yuzawa, I. Kobayashi, L. Cui, A. Oguchi, K. Aoki, Y. Nagai, J. Lian, T. Ito, M. Kanamori, H. Matsumaru, A. Maruyama, H. Murakami, A. Hosoyama, Y. Mizutani-Ui, N. K. Takahashi, T. Sawano, R. Inoue, C. Kaito, K. Sekimizu, H. Hirakawa, S. Kuhara, S. Goto, J. Yabuzaki, M. Kanehisa, A. Yamashita, K. Oshima, K. Furuya, C. Yoshino, T. Shiba, M. Hattori, N. Ogasawara, H. Hayashi, and K. Hiramatsu.** 2001. Whole genome sequencing of methicillin-resistant *Staphylococcus aureus*. *Lancet* **357:**1225–1240.

38. **Langlois, M. A., Y. El Fakhry, and W. Mourad.** 2003. Zinc-binding sites in the N terminus of Mycoplasma arthritidis-derived mitogen permit the dimer formation required for high affinity binding to HLA-DR and for T cell activation. *J. Biol. Chem.* **278:**22309–22315.

39. **Lavoie, P. M., H. McGrath, N. H. Shoukry, P. A. Cazenave, R. P. Sekaly, and J. Thibodeau.** 2001. Quantitative relationship between MHC class II-superantigen complexes and the balance of T cell activation versus death. *J. Immunol* **166:**7229–7237.

40. **Leder, L., A. Llera, P. M. Lavoie, M. I. Lebedeva, H. Li, R. P. Sekaly, G. A. Bohach, P. J. Gahr, P. M. Schlievert, K. Karjalainen, and R. A. Mariuzza.** 1998. A mutational analysis of the binding of Staphylococcal enterotoxins B and C3 to the T cell receptor β-chain and major histocompatibility complex class II. *J. Exp. Med.* **187:**823–833.

41. **Li, H., A. Llera, and R. A. Mariuzza.** 1998. Structure-function studies of T-cell receptor-superantigen interactions. *Immunol. Rev.* **163:**177–186.

42. **Li, H., A. Llera, D. Tsuchiya, L. Leder, X. Ysern, P. M. Schlievert, K. Karjalainen, and R. A. Mariuzza.** 1998. Three-dimensional structure of the complex between a T cell receptor β-chain and the superantigen Staphylococcal enterotoxin B. *Immunity* **9:**807–816.

43. **Li, Y., H. Li, N. Dimasi, J. K. McCormick, R. Martin, P. Schuck, P. M. Schlievert, and R. A. Mariuzza.** 2001. Crystal structure of a superantigen bound to the high-affinity, zinc- dependent site on MHC class II. *Immunity* **14:**93–104.

44. **Li, Y., C. Luo, W. Lei, Z. Xu, C. Zeng, S. Bi, J. Yu, J. Wu, and H. Yang.** 2004. Structure-based preliminary analysis of immunity and virulence of SARS Coronavirus. *Viral. Immun.* **17:**528–534.

45. **Marrack, P., and J. Kappler.** 1990. The staphylococcal enterotoxins and their relatives. *Science* **248:**1066.

46. **Omoe, K., D. L. Hu, H. Takahashi-Omoe, A. Nakane, and K. Shinagawa.** 2003. Identification and characterization of a new Staphylococcal enterotoxin-related putative toxin encoded by two kinds of plasmids. *Infect. Immun.* **71:**6088–6094.

47. **Orwin, P. M., D. Y. Leung, T. J. Tripp, G. A. Bohach, C. A. Earhart, D. H. Ohlendorf, and P. M. Schlievert.** 2002. Characterization of a novel Staphylococcal enterotoxin-like superantigen, a member of the group V subfamily of pyrogenic toxins. *Biochemistry* **41:**14033–14040.

48. **Papageorgiou, A. C., M. D. Baker, J. D. McLeod, S. K. Goda, C. N. Manzotti, D. M. Sansom, H. S. Tranter, and K. R. Acharya.** 2004. Identification of a secondary zinc-binding site in Staphylococcal enterotoxin C2. Implications for superantigen recognition. *J. Biol. Chem.* **279:**1297–1303.

49. **Papageorgiou, A. C., C. M. Collins, D. M. Gutman, J. B. Kline, S. M. O'Brien, H. S. Tranter, and K. R. Acharya.** 1999. Structural basis for the recognition of superantigen streptococcal pyrogenic exotoxin A (SpeA1) by MHC class II molecules and T-cell receptors. *EMBO J.* **18:**9–21.

50. **Petersson, K., M. Hakansson, H. Nilsson, G. Forsberg, L. A. Svensson, A. Liljas, and B. Walse.** 2001. Crystal structure of a superantigen bound to MHC class II displays zinc and peptide dependence. *EMBO J.* **20:**3306–3312.

51. **Petersson, K., H. Pettersson, N. J. Skartved, B. Walse, and G. Forsberg.** 2003. Staphylococcal enterotoxin H induces V_α specific expansion of T cells. *J. Immunol.* **170:**4148–4154.

52. **Pless, D. D., G. Ruthel, E. K. Reinke, R. G. Ulrich, and S. Bavari.** 2005. Persistence of zinc-binding bacterial superantigens at the cell surface of antigen-presenting cells contributes to the extreme potency of these superantigens as T-cell activators. *Infect. Immun.* **73:**5358–5366.

53. **Proft, T., S. L. Moffatt, C. J. Berkahn, and J. D. Fraser.** 1999. Identification and characterization of novel superantigens from *Streptococcus pyogenes*. *J. Exp. Med.* **189:**89–102.

54. **Roussel, A., B. F. Anderson, H. M. Baker, J. D. Fraser, and E. N. Baker.** 1997. Crystal structure of the Streptococcal superantigen SPE-C: dimerization and zinc binding suggest a novel mode of interaction with MHC class II molecules. *Nat. Struct. Biol.* **4:**635–643.

55. **Schlievert, P. M., L. M. Jablonski, M. Roggiani, I. Sadler, S. Callantine, D. T. Mitchell, D. H. Ohlendorf, and G. A. Bohach.** 2000. Pyrogenic toxin superantigen site specificity in toxic shock syndrome and food poisoning in animals. *Infect. Immun.* **68:**3630–3634.

56. **Spero, L., and B. A. Morlock.** 1978. Biological activities of the peptides of Staphylococcal enterotoxin C formed by limited tryptic hydrolysis. *J. Biol. Chem.* **253:**8787–8791.

57. **Stevens, K. R., M. Van, J. G. Lamphear, and R. R. Rich.** 1996. Altered orientation of Streptococcal superantigen (SSA) on HLA-DR1 allows unconventional regions to contribute to SSA V_β specificity. *J. Immunol.* **157:**4970–4978.

58. **Sundberg, E., and T. S. Jardetzky.** 1999. Structural basis for HLA-DQ binding by the Streptococcal superantigen SSA. *Nat. Struct. Biol.* **6:**123–129.

59. **Sundberg, E. J., H. Li, A. S. Llera, J. K. McCormick, J. Tormo, P. M. Schlievert, K. Karjalainen, and R. A. Mariuzza.** 2002. Structures of two Streptococcal superantigens bound to TCR β chains reveal diversity in the architecture of T cell signalling complexes. *Structure* **10:**687–699.

60. **Sundstrom, M., L. Abrahmsen, P. Antonsson, K. Mehindate, W. Mourad, and M. Dohlsten.** 1996. The crystal structure of Staphylococcal enterotoxin type D reveals Zn^{2+}-mediated homodimerization. *EMBO J.* **15:**6832–6840.

61. **Swaminathan, S., W. Furey, J. Pletcher, and M. Sax.** 1992. Crystal structure of Staphylococcal enterotoxin B, a superantigen. *Nature* **359:**801–806.

62. **Swaminathan, S., W. Furey, J. Pletcher, and M. Sax.** 1995. Residues defining V_β specificity in staphylococcal enterotoxins. *Nature. Struct. Biol.* **2:**680–686.

63. **Thomas, P., P. D. Webb, V. Handley, and J. D. Fraser.** 2004. Identification & characterisation of the two novel Streptococcal pyrogenic exotoxins SPE-L & SPE-M. *Indian J. Med. Res.* **119**(Suppl.):37–43.

64. **Tiedemann, R. E., R. J. Urban, J. L. Strominger, and J. D. Fraser.** 1995. Isolation of HLA-DR1.(Staphylococcal enterotoxin A)2 trimers in solution. *Proc. Natl. Acad. Sci. USA* **92:**12156–12159.

65. **Uchiyama, T., T. Miyoshi-Akiyama, H. Kato, W. Fujimaki, K. Imanishi, and X. J. Yan.** 1993. Superantigenic properties of a novel mitogenic substance produced by Yersinia pseudotuberculosis isolated from patients manifesting acute and systemic symptoms. *J. Immunol.* **151:**4407–4413.

66. **Wen, R., D. R. Broussard, S. Surman, T. L. Hogg, M. A. Blackman, and D. L. Woodland.** 1997. Carboxy-terminal residues of major histocompatibility complex class II- associated peptides control the presentation of the bacterial superantigen toxic shock syndrome toxin-1 to T cells. *Eur. J. Immunol.* **27:**772–781.

67. **Williams, R. J., J. M. Ward, B. Henderson, S. Poole, B. P. O'Hara, M. Wilson, and S. P. Nair.** 2000. Identification of a novel gene cluster encoding Staphylococcal exotoxin-like proteins: characterization of the prototypic gene and its protein product, SET1. *Infect. Immun.* **68:**4407–4415.

68. **Woodland, D. L., R. Wen, and M. A. Blackman.** 1997. Why do superantigens care about peptides? *Immunol. Today* **18:**18–22.

69. **Zhao, Y., Z. Li, S. J. Drozd, Y. Guo, W. Mourad, and H. Li.** 2004. Crystal structure of Mycoplasma arthritidis mitogen complexed with HLA-DR1 reveals a novel superantigen fold and a dimerized superantigen-MHC complex. *Structure* **12:**277–288.

Section III

SUPERANTIGENS AND HUMAN DISEASES

Superantigens: Molecular Basis for Their Role in Human Diseases
Edited by Malak Kotb and John D. Fraser
© 2007 ASM Press, Washington, D.C.

Chapter 9

Role of Superantigens in Skin Disease

Sang-Hyun Cho and Donald Y. M. Leung

The skin is an important target for microbial infection. One key strategy by which microbes exacerbate skin disease is via the production of microbial toxins. This has been most clearly demonstrated for staphylococcal and streptococcal superantigens which exacerbate and sustain skin inflammation in skin diseases such as atopic dermatitis (AD) and guttate psoriasis (50). In the current chapter, we will therefore primarily focus on the role of staphylococcal and streptococcal superantigens in human skin diseases, beginning with a review of the properties of superantigens and the mechanisms by which they cause cutaneous immunologic responses.

PATHOPHYSIOLOGY OF SUPERANTIGENS ON THE SKIN

The reader is referred to chapter 2 of this book for a detailed discussion of the biologic and immunologic properties of superantigens as this chapter will focus on the effects that superantigens have on the skin and immunologic events that contribute to superantigen-induced skin inflammatory disease. Direct exposure of normal human skin to staphylococcal and streptococcal superantigens has been demonstrated to induce an acute skin inflammatory response or dermatitis within a 24- to 48-h period (85). In certain individuals this dermatitis, induced by transient exposure to superantigens, persists for over one month, which is interesting in light of previous reports that following superantigen-mediated diseases such as toxic shock syndrome some patients develop chronic eczema (66).

The mechanisms by which superantigens induce skin inflammation have been studied extensively (summarized in Table 1). To determine whether superantigen-induced dermatitis is primarily due to superantigen-induced T-cell activation or represents nonspecific inflammation due to the release of proinflammatory cytokines from HLA-DR+ skin cells, we have studied the effects of microgram quantities of SEB, vehicle or sodium lauryl sulfate (SLS) for 24 h on normal skin and atopic subjects. Skin biopsies

Sang-Hyun Cho • Department of Dermatology, The Catholic University of Korea, Seoul, Korea 403-720.
Donald Y. M. Leung • Department of Pediatrics, National Jewish Medical and Research Center, Denver, CO 80206, and University of Colorado Health Sciences Center, Denver, CO 80262.

Table 1. Immunologic features of superantigen-mediated disease

- T cell and macrophage activation
- Correlation between exacerbation of illness and expansion or deletion of Vβ-specific T cells
- Isolation of a microorganism that produces a superantigen capable of inducing the relevant Vβ-specific T-cell expansion
- In vivo exposure to the superantigen induces the disease
- Treatment of offending superantigen eliminates the disease

were then taken from all treated areas after 48 h (83). From all subjects, skin biopsies of SEB-treated areas demonstrated selective accumulation of T cells expressing the SEB-reactive T-cell receptors (TCR) Vβ12 and 17, but not other TCR Vβs. This selective upregulation was not found in the SLS-treated areas. These data support the concept that superantigen-induced T-cell activation is involved in the dermatitis seen following experimental application of superantigen on intact skin and thus may contribute to skin inflammation when superantigen-producing *Staphylococcus aureus* colonizes or infects the skin.

Although microgram quantities of superantigens may occur in acute exudative AD skin lesions where 10^6 *S. aureus* cells exist per mm^2 of skin, it is unlikely that these concentrations of toxin are reached in chronic AD or psoriasis where there are only several hundred thousand *S. aureus* per mm^2. Therefore we also examined the ability of nanogram quantities of topically applied purified TSST-1, SEB, and streptococcal pyrogenic enterotoxin (SPE) types A and C to induce inflammatory reactions in clinically uninvolved skin of subjects with psoriasis, AD, lichen planus, and normal controls (89). Nanogram quantities of superantigen were unable to induce a clinical skin reaction on intact normal human skin. Employing a protocol of epidermal modification by tape stripping (used to simulate the scratching known to elicit eczema in AD or the Koebner reaction in psoriasis) followed by 48 h of closed patch testing of superantigens, we found that superantigens triggered a significantly greater inflammatory skin response in psoriatics than healthy subjects or patients with AD or lichen planus. Surprisingly, skin biopsies from superantigen-induced skin reactions were not associated with the predicted TCR Vβ stimulatory properties of the superantigen. Skin biopsies obtained 6 and 24 h after patch testing with superantigens, however, demonstrated increased tumor necrosis factor alpha (TNF-α) mRNA in the epidermis, but not the dermis, of skin biopsies from psoriatics compared with healthy subjects. Immunohistochemical studies revealed significantly higher levels of HLA-DR expression in keratinocytes of skin biopsies from psoriatic than from control subjects. However, a mutant TSST-1 protein (G31S/S32P), unable to bind HLA-DR, did not elicit an inflammatory skin reaction. These findings indicate that HLA-DR expression on activated keratinocytes results in direct inflammatory skin responses to superantigens with no selective expansion of T cells. This is an important observation as it demonstrates a T-cell-independent mechanism by which superantigens contribute to the pathogenesis of inflammatory skin diseases associated with HLA-DR expression on their keratinocytes such as chronic AD and psoriasis.

Effects on Skin Antigen-Presenting Cells

In addition to activated keratinocytes, several other skin cell types constitutively express HLA-DR on their cell surface and are therefore targets for superantigen action. These include epidermal Langerhans cells and dermal macrophages that release a variety of proinflammatory cytokines, such as interleukin-1 (IL-1) and TNF-α, upon stimulation with superantigens (55). Superantigen-mediated stimulation of monocytes is a consequence of binding and transducing a positive signal through major histocompatibility complex (MHC) class II molecules (4, 45). This process can be blocked by anti-MHC class II antibodies, and gamma interferon (IFN-γ)-induced upregulation of MHC class II enhances responsiveness. Superantigens also inhibit monocyte/macrophage apoptosis and may thereby perpetuate chronic skin inflammation (12, 13).

The type of antigen-presenting cell (APC) used to present superantigen may influence T-cell development. T cells stimulated by SEB in the presence of dermal dendrocytes produced a T-helper type 1 (Th1) pattern of IL-2 and IFN-γ, while T cells stimulated in the presence of MHC class II$^+$ keratinocytes produced only IL-4 (32). This difference is related to defective IL-12 production by keratinocytes during the activation. This fact suggests that the nature of the primary T-cell response is determined by the accessory cell used for antigen presentation. This may have important implications for the mechanisms by which cutaneous T-helper type 2 (Th2) cell responses evolve in AD or Th1 cell-mediated skin reactions develop in the challenge phase of allergic contact dermatitis.

The ability of Langerhans cells and/or keratinocytes to function as accessory cells in T-cell responses to staphylococcal superantigens has been studied. Epidermal Langerhans cells or IFN-γ-treated epidermal cells can act as accessory cells in presenting SEB to murine splenic T cells (34). Similarly, MHC class II$^+$ human keratinocytes treated in vitro with IFN-γ acquire the ability to activate T cells in the presence of superantigen (70). This interaction can be blocked by antibodies to MHC (HLA-DR, HLA-DQ), to intercellular adhesion molecule-1 (ICAM-1), or to lymphocyte function-associated antigen-1 (LFA-1). Thus, cell adhesion and MHC class II molecules are necessary for superantigen-induced activation. In contrast, MHC class II$^+$ keratinocytes are not able to present nominal peptide antigens to naive T cells, presumably because keratinocytes can not process antigen for presentation in the antigen-binding groove of the MHC class II molecule, and because they lack costimulatory molecules to deliver the second signal in T-cell activation (69, 70).

Effects on T Cells

Superantigens activate cytokine production and proliferation of T cells expressing specific TCR Vβ regions and these T cells can migrate into tissues to orchestrate inflammation. Such T cells may include autoreactive T cells that migrate to skin containing the autoantigen recognized by that T cell and mediate damage via cytotoxic mechanisms or the secretion of proinflammatory cytokines. Different superantigens cause the expansion of diverse portions of the T-cell repertoire (2, 64), so superantigens differ in their capacity to expand autoreactive T cells with varying specificities. Also note that under certain conditions T-cell expansion by superantigens may be followed in time by anergy and/or deletion of the stimulated T cells (92).

Superantigenic stimulation of T cells promotes skin homing by upregulation of the skin-homing receptor, cutaneous lymphoid antigen (CLA), which promotes localization of T cells to the skin (52, 78). The heterogeneous expression of lymphocyte-homing receptors on memory T-cell population is thought to define lymphocytes with tissue-selective recirculatory potential. Skin T cells, as compared with peripheral blood T cells, are highly enriched for the CLA^+ subset of cells (78). Leung and colleagues (16) have shown that in vitro stimulation of peripheral blood mononuclear cells (PBMCs) with SEB, TSST-1, SPEA, and SPEC induces a significant increase in the numbers of CLA^+ T-cell blasts, but not blasts bearing the mucosa-associated adhesion molecule, $\alpha e \beta 7$-integrin, compared with T cells stimulated with phytohemagglutinin (PHA). Induction of superantigen-induced CLA expression was blocked by anti-IL-12, and the addition of IL-12 to PHA-stimulated T cells induced CLA, but not $\alpha e \beta 7$-integrin, expression. These data suggest that bacterial toxins induce the expansion of skin-homing CLA^+ T cells in an IL-12-dependent manner (52). This characteristic of superantigens would greatly favor the development of skin rashes in superantigen-mediated diseases.

Studies by Laouini et al. (48) have demonstrated that epicutaneous application of superantigens to BALB/c mouse skin results in a local inflammatory skin response characterized by dermal infiltration of mononuclear cells and eosinophils and increased expression of Th2 cytokines, i.e., increased IL-4 but not IFN-γ. Naturally occurring $CD4^+CD25^+$ regulatory T cells (nTreg) have important suppressive effects on T-effector cells. Loss of nTreg cell suppressive function has been implicated in the pathogenesis of autoimmune and allergic inflammatory conditions (20). Superantigens have been found to cause potent abrogation of nTreg activity, thereby suggesting a novel mechanism by which superantigens could augment T-cell-activated responses in human autoimmune and inflammatory diseases. Recently, it has been shown that inhibition of the nTreg proliferation status by superantigens occurs due to induction of glucocorticoid-induced TNF receptor-related protein ligand (GITR-L) on APCs followed by engagement of GITR on effector T cells (16, 76).

Staphylococcal superantigens have also been shown to induce human T-cell resistance to corticosteroids and may thereby complicate the treatment of AD and other inflammatory diseases treated with corticosteroids (35, 36). Recently, we found that peripheral blood T cells stimulated with superantigens, but not anti-CD3, induced corticosteroid-resistant T cells suggesting that costimulatory signals must act in concert with the T-cell receptor to cause steroid resistance (60). Blockade of CD40-CD40L interaction had no effect on superantigen-induced corticosteroid resistance. However, CD28 costimulation with T-cell receptor activation induced corticosteroid resistance of human T cells in a dose-dependent manner. Treatment with MEK/ERK inhibitors, but not a p38 inhibitor or a JNK inhibitor, restored the response to steroids as indicated by proliferation assays. Of note, superantigen-induced corticosteroid resistance was associated with abrogation of glucocorticoid receptor nuclear translocation (60). This effect could be reversed by treatment with MEK/ERK pathway inhibitors. Thus, superantigen-induced corticosteroid resistance involves the Raf-MEK-ERK1/2 pathway of T-cell receptor signaling which leads to glucocorticoid receptor phosphorylation and inhibition of dexamethasone-induced glucocorticoid receptor nuclear translocation. These are important observations because they provide a clear therapeutic target, i.e., inhibition of the MEK/ERK pathway, for reversal of superantigen-induced steroid resistance.

Effects on B Cells

Superantigens have also been found to activate B cells and could thus lead to increased synthesis of immunoglobulin E (IgE) or autoantibodies (41, 42). Studies have suggested that staphylococcal superantigens can stimulate autoantibody or IgE production by crosslinking the MHC class II molecule on B cells with the TCR on T cells (37). This form of B-cell activation likely depends on the release of local cytokines in the vicinity of B cells previously primed by autoantigen or allergen. Stimulation as opposed to inhibition of immunoglobulin synthesis depends on the concentration of bacterial superantigen present in the local milieu; picogram or femtogram concentrations of superantigen induce polyclonal B-cell activation. In contrast, nanogram or greater concentrations of staphylococcal superantigen inhibit B-cell activation by inducing B-cell apoptosis.

Overall these observations indicate that superantigens can act on various cell types to influence the skin immune or inflammatory response. The particular response of skin cells to superantigens likely depends on a combination of factors including their stage of development and activation, cytokine milieu, avidity for specific superantigens, as well as costimulatory signals provided by the superantigen-presenting cell. These marked immunomodulatory effects of superantigens on T cells, APCs, and other immune effector cells have led to widespread speculation that these molecules provide the basis by which microbes may mediate a variety of diseases associated with autoimmune and inflammatory skin diseases.

ROLE OF STAPHYLOCOCCAL SUPERANTIGENS IN SKIN DISEASES

S. aureus is a common cause of cutaneous bacterial infections. The potential role that superantigens may play in contributing to the evolution of skin rashes is supported by the observation that systemic illnesses known to be caused by superantigens such as staphylococcal toxic shock syndrome are often accompanied by skin rashes (27). Furthermore following toxic shock syndrome and Kawasaki Disease, which is also thought to be caused by superantigens, patients have been reported to develop persistent eczema (14, 66). In the next section of this chapter, we will focus in particular on atopic dermatitis where substantial data suggests a role for superantigens in the pathogenesis of this common skin disease.

Atopic Dermatitis

Atopic dermatitis (AD) is a chronic, relapsing, highly pruritic inflammatory skin disease affecting more than 10% of children and characterized by infiltration of T cells, monocyte/macrophages, and eosinophilia into skin lesions (51). The majority of patients with AD have a personal or family history of respiratory allergy. Serum IgE levels are elevated in approximately 80% of patients with AD. Many factors can trigger the AD skin inflammation cascade including irritants, foods, aeroallergens, emotional stress, and infectious agents including *S. aureus*.

Substantial evidence supports a role for staphylococcal superantigens in the pathophysiology of AD. First, *S. aureus* is found on the skin of most patients with AD (32). In contrast, only 5% of healthy subjects harbor this bacterium on their skin. The density of *S. aureus* on acutely inflamed AD lesions is frequently more than 1,000 times higher than on nonlesional atopic skin. These patients often have an exacerbation of their skin disease and respond rapidly to antibiotic therapy (58). The propensity of AD skin toward skin infection appears to be due to a combination of factors including reduced skin innate immune responses, augmented Th2 responses, and reduced skin-barrier function (71, 74).

Second, several studies have demonstrated that the majority of *S. aureus* isolated from AD skin produces superantigens, such as SEB or TSST-1 (15, 53). Skin biopsies of AD patients have identified staphylococcal superantigens by immunofluorescence as deeply into the skin as on the inflammatory cells infiltrating into the dermis.

Third, direct evidence for in vivo superantigen effects in AD have been demonstrated by comparing the superantigen profiles of *S. aureus* cultured from the skin of chronic AD subjects to the TCR Vβ repertoire of their skin-homing (CLA$^+$) T cells in peripheral blood and skin biopsies. In one study, superantigen-secreting *S. aureus* strains were identified in half of AD patients, and all of these subjects manifested significant TCR Vβ skewing within the CLA$^+$, but not the CLA$^-$ subsets of both their CD4$^+$ and CD8$^+$ T cells that reflected the superantigens found on their skin (86). TCR Vβ skewing was not present within the CLA$^+$ T-cell subset of patients with plaque psoriasis and normal controls. TCR BV genes from the presumptively superantigen-expanded populations of skin-homing T-cells were cloned and sequenced from three subjects and, consistent with a superantigen-driven effect, were found to be polyclonal. These data support the concept that staphylococcal superantigens can contribute to AD pathogenesis by increasing the frequency of memory T cells able to migrate to and be activated within AD lesions. This is consistent with data from skin biopsies of AD patients demonstrating that TCR Vβ expression in skin T-cell infiltrates relates to the superantigen-producing *S. aureus* found on their skin (15).

Finally, most AD patients make specific IgE antibodies directed against the staphylococcal superantigens found on their skin (53). Basophils from patients with IgE to superantigens release histamine on exposure to the relevant superantigen, but not in response to superantigens to which they make no specific IgE. These findings raise the intriguing possibility that superantigens induce specific IgE in AD patients and chronic mast cell degranulation in vivo when the superantigens penetrate their disrupted epidermal barrier. This promotes the itch-scratch cycle and skin rashes in AD. Indeed, a correlation has been found between the presence of IgE to superantigens and severity of AD. Furthermore, colonization with superantigen-producing *S. aureus* is at greatest density in patients with IgE to staphylococcal superantigens. Of note, in one study there was no difference in skin severity between patients with or without superantigen-producing *S. aureus* unless patients made an IgE response to the superantigen present on their skin (72).

Patients with superantigens on their skin in general have increased IgE levels to specific allergens. This is consistent with in vitro studies demonstrating that superantigens augment allergen-specific IgE synthesis by binding to HLA-DR on B cells (41, 42). Utilizing a humanized murine model of skin inflammation, *S. aureus* superantigen plus allergen was found to have an additive effect in inducing cutaneous inflammation (40). Skin-homing CLA$^+$ T cells have also been shown to respond to superantigen and contribute to eosinophilia and IgE production in AD (1). Thus superantigens contribute to skin disease in AD via a combination of actions on the local and systemic immune system.

Staphylococcal Scalded Skin Syndrome (SSSS)/Bullous Impetigo/Staphylococcal Scarlatiniform Eruption

Three types of skin lesions have been reported to be produced by phage group II *S. aureus*, particularly strains 77 and 55: (i) bullous impetigo, (ii) exfoliative disease (SSSS), and (iii) nonstreptococcal scarlatiniform eruption (staphylococcal scarlet fever). All three represent varying cutaneous responses to extracellular ETA or ETB produced by these staphylococci. ETA acts as a serine protease of desmoglein 1 (Dsg-1), the desmosomal cadherin that is also the target of autoantibodies in *Pemphigus foliaceus* (3).

SSSS is a generalized exanthematous disorder with cutaneous tenderness, widespread blistering, and superficial denudation/desquamation. SSSS represents the severe end of a spectrum of blistering skin diseases that includes localized bullous impetigo. These disorders are caused by ETs A or B, produced by certain strains of *S. aureus*, usually belonging to phage group 2 (46). Initial studies suggested that phage lytic group II *S. aureus* (types 71 and 55) were mainly responsible for ET production, but it is now known that all phage groups are able to produce ET and cause SSSS (25). About 5% of all *S. aureus* produce ET and two different serotypes affecting humans (ETA and ETB) have been identified (47). Although they possess some physicochemical differences, ETA and ETB have 40% sequence homology and produce identical dermatological effects (7).

A controversy exists concerning whether the ETs possess superantigenic activity. Initial work suggesting that the toxins were able to stimulate human Vβ2 and murine Vβ3 T cells (68) were refuted by studies suggesting that recombinant ET cloned into either non-toxin-producing *S. aureus* (31) or *Escherichia coli* (79) did not possess any superantigenic activity, despite the recombinant toxin retaining its exfoliative activity. The authors suggested that the superantigenic activity in previous studies was probably due to contamination by other staphylococcal superantigens, such as TSST-1 or the enterotoxins. Vath et al. (91), however, showed that cloning ETA into a nonsuperantigenic strain of *S. aureus* resulted in superantigenic activity, and that recombinant ETA with a mutated active site (Ser195Cys) lost its exfoliative activity, but retained its mitogenic activity, suggesting that the mitogenic activity of the ET was separate from its exfoliative activity. ETA is also able to activate murine macrophages to release high levels of TNF-α, IL-6, and nitric oxide and cause contact-dependent cytotoxicity in transformed embryo fibroblast cells. More recent work suggests that the ETs may possess a unique and very specific superantigenic activity. Using highly purified recombinant ETs, Monday's group showed that, in the presence of APCs, both ETA and ETB were able to induce selective polyclonal expansion of several human Vβ-bearing T cells (but not Vβ2), and only those murine Vβ T cells that were highly homologous to the human forms (67).

Evidence is accumulating that these toxins may act as atypical glutamate-specific serine proteases as follows: (i) incubating ETA with neonatal mouse epidermis or A431 epidermal cells results in caseinolytic activity in the supernatant (87); (ii) the toxins have significant sequence homology to V8 protease, another staphylococcal protein with homology to the trypsinlike serine proteases (26); (iii) modifying residue serine 195 of the predicted serine protease active site of ETA results in loss of exfoliating activity in newborn mice (80, 81); (iv) three-dimensional computer modeling of the toxins shows that their structure can be modeled on other glutamate-specific trypsinlike serine proteases, such as α-thrombin, chymotrypsin, *Streptomyces griseus* protease, and *Achromobacter* protease (9); and (v) recent three-dimensional crystallographic images of both ETA and ETB show that the toxins consist of two domains, each made up of six antiparallel β-strands that form a β-barrel common to all members of the trypsin family, along with a serine protease catalytic triad of serine, histidine, and aspartic acid. In addition, the toxins possess Thr190 and His213 in the N-terminal pocket that is conserved in all glutamate-specific serine proteases. However, ETA differs from other serine proteases in that it possesses a large amphipathic N-terminal portion that covers the active site. This region may bind a specific epidermal receptor and cause a conformational change that opens the active site to induce serine protease activity. A similar mechanism has been proposed for other proteases, including thrombin and hepatitis C virus NS3 protease (17). The structure of ETB is similar to ETA except that the oxyanion hole, which forms part of the catalytic site, is in the closed or inactive conformation for ETA, but in the open or active conformation for ETB (77). Laboratory studies suggest that ETB may be more pyrogenic than ETA and enhances susceptibility to lethal shock in rabbits (67), while clinical studies have shown that, although both serotypes were equally responsible for localized SSSS, ETB was isolated more frequently from children with generalized SSSS (80% versus 8% of 24 cases each) and may also be able to cause generalized exfoliation in apparently healthy adults (75).

ETA cleaves Dsg-1 in both murine and human skin. Dsg-1 is a desmosomal cadherin involved in intercellular adhesion and is found only in the superficial epidermis (3). Disruption of this structure results in loss of cell-to-cell adhesion and separation at the level of the zona granulosa. ETA cleaves the extracellular domain of mouse and human Dsg-1 in a dose-dependent manner. ETA acts as an atypical glutamate-specific serine protease that binds and cleaves Dsg-1 in the region of amino acid number 170, where there are several glutamic acid residues. This could explain several aspects of SSSS, including the specific site of action in the superficial epidermis and why the mucous membranes are not affected in SSSS, since Dsg-1 is only found in the epidermis. Minor variations in the sequence or structure of Dsg-1 may also explain the species specificity of SSSS (47).

In a study of bullous impetigo, 51% of patients had concurrent *S. aureus* cultured from the nose or throat; 79% of cultures grew the same strain from both sites (49). Bullous impetigo occurs most commonly in the newborn and in older infants, and is characterized by the rapid progression of vesicles to flaccid bullae. Bullae usually arise on areas of grossly normal skin. The Nikolsky's sign is not present.

Staphylococcal scarlatiniform eruption is identical with the generalized scarlatiniform rash with skin tenderness observed in the initial stage of SSSS. Staphylococci belonging to phage group II are recovered from sites of staphylococcal infection (conjunctivitis, abscesses, bacteremia, and external otitis). In general, these strains produce SEs similar to toxins responsible for TSS. Thus, staphylococcal scarlet fever may be a milder form of TSS.

Recurrent Toxin-Mediated Perineal Erythema

This was described by Manders et al. (62) in 1996 as a recurrent, toxin-mediated disease sharing some of the clinical characteristics of Kawasaki Syndrome but occurring in young adults, rather than small children. Clinical features include macular erythema of the perineum within 24 to 48 h of a bacterial pharyngitis, strawberry tongue, and extremity changes including erythema, edema, and convalescent desquamation. No fever or hypotension is noted and recurrences are frequent. Culture of the pharynx during the acute pharyngitis identified a TSST-1-producing *S. aureus* or a SPEA- and B-producing group A *Streptococcus* (61).

Cutaneous T-Cell Lymphomas

Cutaneous T-cell lymphomas (CTCL) are T-cell lympho-infiltrative malignancies that follow an indolent, chronic course. Since T cells can show morphological changes similar to those of Sézary tumor cells after mitogenic stimulation and in vivo in benign inflammatory cutaneous disorders, the idea that sustained stimulation might drive the initial phase of the course of mycosis fungoides and/or Sézary syndrome has been raised by several authors, and the malignant nature of the initial phase of mycosis fungoides has even been questioned (6).

Despite much effort to identify a unique antigen in this disease, the etiology remains unknown. Microbial involvement has been suggested based on a decrease in erythema and tumor size in CTCL with systemic as well as topical antibiotic therapy in some cases (44). Moreover, 90% of $V\beta2.1^+$ Sézary cells in the peripheral blood of patients could be activated in vitro by TSST-1, but not SEB, which showed specificity for both the $V\beta$ sequence and the toxin. In a large prospective cohort of CTCL patients, 32 of 42 showed *S. aureus* in either skin or blood samples and 78.6% of patients investigated had superantigen-producing *S. aureus*. Instead of a monoclonal expansion of a certain $V\beta$ subset, an oligoclonal expansion was found, although patients with TSST-1-producing strains revealed the expected expansion of the $V\beta2$ gene (43). This study suggested that *S. aureus* superantigen enterotoxins could provide or potentiate lymphocytic infiltration and chronic antigenic stimulation leading to T-cell clonal expansion in CTCL.

ROLE OF STREPTOCOCCAL SUPERANTIGENS IN SKIN DISEASE

As in *S. aureus*, several group A streptococcal superantigens have been identified. These include SPE (or erythrogenic exotoxin) A to C, F, and G to J, streptococcal superantigen, and streptococcal mitogenic exotoxin Z. Systemic streptococcal diseases associated with superantigen involvement including toxic shock syndrome and rheumatic fever are often associated with skin disease as a manifestation of their illness, suggesting a role for superantigens in skin disease (23). The role of these superantigens in skin disease has been demonstrated most clearly in psoriasis, particularly guttate psoriasis.

Psoriasis is a chronic relapsing disease of the skin with diverse clinical presentations and polygenic inheritance (21, 73). This skin disease is thought to be immune mediated because of the presence of a significant number of activated T cells within the altered hyperproliferating epidermis and dermis, by macrophages, and by the proven beneficial effects of immunosuppressive or immunomodulating therapy. Second, the increased, persistent keratinocyte proliferation found in skin lesions occurs in conjunction with a characteristic skin inflammatory pattern. Further, the genetic predisposition represents a hallmark of psoriasis; the inheritance is polygenic with a genetic risk ratio of nearly 10 for first-degree relatives of patients with early-onset psoriasis (30).

T-lymphocyte activation is believed to play a central role in the pathogenesis of psoriasis. Histologic examination of early skin lesions of psoriasis indicates that infiltration of T cells and macrophages into the skin precedes the characteristic epidermal proliferation that is found in psoriasis (5). T-cell clones isolated from psoriatic plaques release growth factors that stimulate keratinocyte proliferation (84). The T-cell cytokine pattern in lesional psoriatic skin is Th1-like, characterized by IL-1, IFN-γ, and TNF-α expression (90). The strongest evidence linking T-cell activation to psoriasis is the observation that immunosuppressive drugs inhibiting T-cell activation and cytokine release, such as anti-CD3, corticosteroids, and cyclosporine A, are effective treatments for psoriasis (94). Furthermore, administration of a fusion protein combining fragments of diphtheria toxin and human IL-2 toxin eliminated activated T cells expressing IL-2 receptors (CD25) and caused significant clinical resolution of psoriasis (33).

To establish a direct cause-and-effect relationship between immune activation and the development of psoriasis, animal models have been used in which full-thickness clinically uninvolved skin from psoriasis patients was grafted onto SCID mice. Boehncke and colleagues (11) found that intradermal injection of a bacterial superantigen, ET, induced development of histologic features of psoriasis. Furthermore, when patients' superantigen-stimulated PBMCs were administered intraperitoneally, homing of T cells to the graft epidermis was observed.

Using a SCID mouse-human skin chimeric model, Wrone-Smith and Nickoloff (93) stimulated autologous PBMCs from psoriasis patients with IL-2 and SEB. Intradermal injection of these superantigen-stimulated PBMCs into uninvolved skin induced the development of plaques with scaling of the skin and histologic features suggestive of psoriasis. Immunoperoxidase staining demonstrated the presence of CD4$^+$ and CD8$^+$ T cells in the epidermis and dermis. These studies, combined with the previous isolation of T cells from psoriatic lesions that produced cytokines capable of inducing psoriatic changes, suggest that superantigen-stimulated T cells play a role in the development of psoriasis.

Infections have long been recognized as a trigger for the onset or exacerbation of psoriasis. The frequency with which infections trigger psoriasis varies and up to 54% of children are reported to have exacerbation of existing psoriasis during the 2- to 3-week interval after an upper respiratory tract infection (10, 72). Acute guttate psoriasis frequently follows an acute streptococcal infection by 1-2 weeks. Among patients with acute guttate psoriasis, 56 to 85% have immediately preceding streptococcal disease. Streptococcal infections may play a role in exacerbating other forms of psoriasis. *Streptococcus pyogenes* (β-hemolytic streptococci, group A) was isolated in 26% of patients with acute guttate psoriasis, 14% of patients with guttate flare of plaque psoriasis, and 16% of patients with chronic psoriasis, while in 7% of the control population (88).

Guttate Psoriasis

Several reports support the concept that bacterial infection is an important trigger of acute guttate psoriasis (38, 56, 63). In this illness, acute guttate psoriasis lesions are preceded by streptococcal pharyngitis and are accompanied by rises in serum antistreptococcal titers (38). Patients with guttate psoriasis frequently show improvement of their skin disease after treatment with antistreptococcal antibiotics.

The first experimental support for these clinical observations was provided by Cole and Wuepper (22), who found that alcohol precipitates of cell-free culture filtrates from *S. pyogenes* (strain NY-5) induced increased keratinocyte proliferation following intradermal injection into rabbit skin. These culture filtrates also had marked mitogenic activity on human lymphocytes and contained high levels of superantigens, that is, SPEA,

SPEB, and SPEC. Intradermal injections of small amounts of streptococcal extracts into normal skin of psoriatic patients also induced lesions with histologic characteristics of psoriasis (82). Furthermore, T lymphocytes isolated from guttate and chronic plaque psoriasis proliferate in response to group A streptococcal antigens (8).

These studies have led to the hypothesis that bacterial superantigenic toxins induce psoriasis in some patients by activating epidermal keratinocytes, infiltrating T lymphocytes, and monocytes (56). To confirm that superantigens played a role in the acute induction of guttate psoriasis, it was important to determine whether expansion of particular Vβ populations of T cells was observed in the peripheral blood or skin of patients with guttate psoriasis, to identify pathogenic bacteria and their superantigens, to determine whether the TCR Vβ pattern in tissue was what would be predicted based on the superantigens isolated from these patients, and to induce new lesions with superantigen challenge.

Lewis and colleagues (59) studied the T-cell repertoire in the peripheral blood and skin lesions of patients with guttate psoriasis and chronic plaque psoriasis, using a panel of nine monoclonal TCR Vβ antibodies. Both types of psoriasis showed a selective expansion of Vβ2$^+$ T lymphocytes in the skin lesions compared with peripheral blood. The marked expansion of Vβ2 was consistent with activation by a superantigen secreted during streptococcal pharyngitis. However, the observation of a local expansion of Vβ-specific T cells did not exclude the possibility of clonotypic T-cell expansion via an immunodominant peptide.

Leung and colleagues (54) subsequently demonstrated the accumulation of Vβ2$^+$ T cells infiltrating into the perilesional and lesional skin of patients with guttate psoriasis. Vβ2$^+$ T cells accounted for over 50% of the T-cell infiltrate in some lesions. This increased Vβ2$^+$ T cell expansion was not seen in perilesional or lesional skin from AD patients, or inflammatory irritant skin lesions induced by SLS in healthy subjects. Note, no increases in Vβ2$^+$ T cells have been observed in normal skin (28). Thus, the observed increase in Vβ2$^+$ T cells appeared to be specific for guttate psoriasis skin lesions rather than resulting from nonspecific skin inflammation.

These investigators also provided further support for the concept that the Vβ2$^+$ T-cell expansion in guttate psoriasis is the result of superantigen activation by demonstrating a selective expansion of Vβ2$^+$ cells in both the CD4 and the CD8$^+$ subsets of infiltrating T cells in guttate psoriasis skin lesions. More importantly, sequence analysis of TCR β-chain genes of Vβ2-expressing T cells in the skin from patients with guttate psoriasis showed extensive junctional region diversity consistent with superantigen stimulation.

To identify the superantigen that might be involved in Vβ2$^+$ T-cell activation in guttate psoriasis, streptococcal isolates from these patients were analyzed by M typing and secretion of SPEA, SPEB, and SPEC. Similar to previous studies on guttate psoriasis, streptococci from their patients did not express any consistent M protein type (88). Some of the isolates secreted SPEA or SPEB, which could explain the expansion of Vβ8 seen in some patients. However, all streptococci secreted SPEC, a superantigen known to stimulate the marked expansion of Vβ2$^+$ T cells. This consistent expression of SPEC by streptococci from guttate psoriasis patients suggests that it may have an important role in this skin disease. When PBMCs of healthy donors and psoriasis patients were stimulated with aqueous extracts of normal facial and plantar stratum corneum, there was a potent stimulation of PBMCs of both healthy donors and patients with autologous and allogenic extracts. The response was T cell driven and the activity was inhibited by an anti-HLA-DR monoclonal antibody, indicating the presence of antigen or superantigen. Taken together with studies demonstrating that superantigens activate the expression of CLA in T cells (52), these findings support the hypothesis that T-lymphocyte activation by streptococcal superantigens following streptococcal pharyngitis induces cutaneous localization and expansion of $V\beta2^+$ T cells, which initiates the lymphocyte-driven inflammation leading to clinical psoriasis.

Chronic Plaque Psoriasis

In patients with chronic plaque psoriasis, local exacerbation of skin disease is commonly seen in the intergluteal cleft, in the inframammary region, in the groin, and in the scalp. All of these areas are potential reservoirs of bacteria or fungi that might trigger local plaque formation. It had been demonstrated that a subset of patients with plaque psoriasis harbor *S. aureus* on their skin. Leung and colleagues (56) first reported that the $V\beta$ pattern of T lymphocytes in psoriatic plaques corresponded to the same $V\beta$s expanded by superantigen-secreting microbes cultured from the plaques. Unfortunately, in plaque psoriasis there is not the same type of hard evidence as there is in guttate psoriasis that superantigens selectively expand particular T-cell populations bearing the appropriate TCR $V\beta$. The expression of $V\beta3$ and/or $V\beta13.1$ mRNA in the $CD8^+$, but not $CD4^+$, T cells is increased in the lesions of most patients, and the persistence of $V\beta3$- and/or $V\beta13.1$-bearing $CD8^+$ T cells in lesions that did not undergo resolution suggests their role as effector cells (19). The consistent clonal expansion of $CD8^+$ lymphocytes of limited $V\beta$ specificity strongly suggests an antigen-driven response, potentially from an infectious agent that cross-reacts with a normal epidermal protein (71). Other T-cell populations, such as $V\beta19$, $V\beta22^+$ (74), or $V\beta2^+$ T cells, also have been reported to be involved in psoriasis.

The host factors and immunologic triggers likely differ among patients who develop chronic psoriasis. Nearly 70% of patients with guttate psoriasis develop chronic plaque psoriasis. In such patients, superantigens may activate skin-infiltrating autoreactive T cells that remain persistently activated due to the abnormal recognition of specific skin antigens. Other factors that determine whether patients have self-limited guttate psoriasis or develop chronic plaque psoriasis are unknown. These conditions may depend on host genetic factors that are involved in antigen binding, such as MHC molecules, as well as the actual antigen triggering T-cell activation. Potential candidate skin autoantigens include keratins (65), which have cross-reactive determinants with bacterial antigens. Alternatively, superantigens may activate either cutaneous professional or nonprofessional APCs to locally stimulate the T cells to induce keratinocyte proliferation. Since the perilesional skin of patients with guttate psoriasis, which has increased $V\beta2^+$ T cells, does not necessarily become a chronic lesion, a second event in the skin is probably needed for complete evolution of the chronic psoriatic skin lesion.

Travers and colleagues (89) have further demonstrated that application of SEB, SPEC, and TSST-1 on tape-abraded skin of psoriatic patients induces an inflammatory lesion with a mononuclear cell infiltrate and epidermal thickening. Patch skin testing with the same superantigens in healthy subjects or on unaffected skin of patients with AD did not produce the same degree of inflammation. The T cells in the dermis and epidermis of these positive patch tests to superantigens do not show preferential TCR $V\beta$ skewing corresponding to the superantigen applied. These results are most consistent with the hypothesis that epicutaneous superantigens may activate local proinflammatory cytokine release by $HLA\text{-}DR^+$ keratinocytes and cause the influx of inflammatory cells, including autoimmune T cells that may recognize local skin antigens. In this situation, induction of skin inflammation does not require superantigenic expansion of T lymphocytes, thus adding to the complexity of mechanisms by which bacteria contribute to skin inflammation.

Potential Role of Superantigens in Psoriasis

These studies suggest several distinct pathways by which bacterial superantigens can act to induce or maintain psoriasis. Acute guttate psoriasis is triggered by pharyngeal infection with superantigen-secreting streptococci, but it is rarely associated with the presence of streptococci on local skin lesions. Since these patients do not develop TSS and there is no evidence for Vβ expansion of circulating T cells, it is possible that following streptococcal pharyngitis, Vβ2$^+$ T cells expressing the CLA skin-homing receptor are induced in lymph nodes draining the pharynx, that is, at a site distant from the skin. Following activation, these T cells home to the skin, where the secretion of Th1 cell-derived cytokines contributes to the development of psoriasis. This is consistent with our observation that the percentage of Vβ2$^+$ T cells in perilesional skin is much higher than that found in the actual guttate psoriasis lesion. In those patients who subsequently develop chronic plaque psoriasis, there may be further local activation by a "skin specific antigen" that is recognized by Vβ2$^+$ T cells in a host genetically predisposed to the development of this autoimmune skin disease.

The situation is probably more complex in patients with chronic plaque psoriasis, in which superantigens are likely to be only one of a number of factors. Nevertheless, the data using SCID mouse-human skin chimeric models demonstrating the ability of superantigens to induce psoriatic changes in uninvolved skin, the isolation of superantigen-producing *S. aureus* from nearly 50% of psoriasis patients, the induction of CLA on T cells by bacterial superantigens via IL-12 production, and the development of plaque psoriasis in the majority of patients with guttate psoriasis support the concept that superantigens can play a role in this form of psoriasis. Induction of psoriatic lesions is likely to involve professional APCs in the dermis or the epidermis, presenting either circulating superantigen, or epicutaneous superantigen delivered through injured skin. The APCs for superantigens in the skin include MHC class II-bearing Langerhans cells in the epidermis and dermal dendritic cells (18, 29), or epidermal macrophages entering the epidermis (24).

Taken together, superantigen-driven T-cell activation might contribute to the heterogeneity in psoriasis in several different ways. First, reactions to different superantigens can produce lesions with different TCR Vβ patterns and therefore the recruitment of T cells that recognize different skin antigens. Second, reactions to particular superantigens may differ. Although most MHC class II haplotypes are able to present superantigens, different alleles vary in their ability to present particular superantigens (39). Hence, the development of particular types of psoriasis may be favored by MHC class II haplotypes associated with preferential presentation of particular superantigens, as well as autoimmune epidermal peptide antigens. The pattern of T-cell activation would therefore vary among different patients, resulting in clinical heterogeneity of psoriasis.

CONCLUSIONS

Superantigens have received a great deal of attention since the discovery of their mechanisms in 1989. Since then, a wealth of knowledge about their structure and molecular mechanisms as well as the immunobiology and the different strategies they use to cause diseases has been presented. This chapter has reviewed the importance of bacterial superantigens in

Table 2. Evidence of role of straphylococcal superantigens in atopic dermatitis

- Epicutaneous application of superantigens induces eczematoid dermatitis
- AD severity correlates with presence of IgE antibodies to superantigens
- Superantigens augment allergen-induced skin inflammation by activating infiltrating mononuclear cells and inducing mast cell degranulation
- Patients recovering from toxic shock syndrome develop chronic eczema
- Superantigens induce the skin-homing receptor on T cells
- Peripheral blood mononuclear cells from AD, as compared with healthy controls, have higher proliferation responses to superantigens

the pathogenesis of inflammatory skin diseases (Table 2). Evidence that bacterial superantigens may have the potential to influence the pathogenesis of chronic skin diseases, including AD and psoriasis, has been increasing.

Both *S. aureus* and *S. pyogenes* are commensal organisms in humans, so the fact that they have the potential to activate the immune response in such a dramatic fashion means that their expression must be tightly controlled and that the immune system must deal with their continuous presence. Superantigen production from the bacterium in AD and psoriasis affects T-cell activation, T-cell CLA expression, keratinocyte proliferation, and IgE production. Nevertheless, the detailed reactions involving superantigens in the inflammatory process are still not fully understood. Numerous host and environmental factors influence the expression and effect of secreted superantigens and thereby their influence on pathology. More basic studies and properly controlled clinical trials are clearly required to elucidate the role of bacterial superantigens in the etiology of superantigen-mediated diseases.

In the future, identification of the antigens or superantigens that trigger particular diseases is likely to provide physicians with more effective and objective methods to diagnose and treat superantigen-mediated diseases. Certain of these diseases in the future may become more amenable to early treatment with antimicrobial agents, antibodies directed against superantigens including those present in intravenous gamma globulin, or the development of vaccines for prevention of superantigen-mediated diseases. Considering the emergence of multi-drug-resistant bacteria and the ability of superantigens to alter response to steroid therapy, new synthetic antibiotics, MAPK inhibitors, cytokine inhibitors, and superantigen peptide antagonists targeting the steps of the immune activation cascade offer the most potential for future therapeutic efficacy. In this regard, synthetic cationic steroid antibiotics, which share similar structural and antibacterial properties to antimicrobial peptides, such as cathelicidins, are promising.

REFERENCES

1. **Akdis, M., C. A. Akdis, L. Weigl, R. Disch, and K. Blaser.** 1997. Skin-homing, CLA+ memory T cells are activated in atopic dermatitis and regulate IgE by an IL-13-dominated cytokine pattern: IgG4 counter-regulation by CLA- memory T cells. *J. Immunol.* **159:**4611–4619.
2. **Alouf, J. E., and H. Muller-Alouf.** 2003. Staphylococcal and streptococcal superantigens: molecular, biological and clinical aspects. *Int. J. Med. Microbiol.* **292:**429–440.
3. **Amagai, M., N. Matsuyoshi, Z. H. Wang, C. Andl, and J. R. Stanley.** 2000. Toxin in bullous impetigo and staphylococcal scalded-skin syndrome targets desmoglein 1. *Nat. Med.* **6:**1275–1277.

4. **Baadsgaard, O., K. D. Cooper, S. Lisby, H. C. Wulf, and G. L. Wantzin.** 1987. Dose response and time course for induction of T6- DR+ human epidermal antigen-presenting cells by *in vivo* ultraviolet A, B, and C irradiation. *J. Am. Acad. Dermatol.* **17:**792–800.

5. **Baadsgaard, O., G. Fisher, J. J. Voorhees, and K. D. Cooper.** 1990. The role of the immune system in the pathogenesis of psoriasis. *J. Invest. Dermatol.* **95:**32S–34S.

6. **Bachelez, H.** 2001. Is there a role for epigenetic factors in the pathogenesis of epidermotropic cutaneous T-cell lymphomas (mycosis fungoides and Sézary syndrome)? *Hematol. J.* **2:**286–289.

7. **Bailey, C. J., J. de Azavedo, and J. P. Arbuthnott.** 1980. A comparative study of two serotypes of epidermolytic toxin from *Staphylococcus aureus. Biochim. Biophys. Acta.* **624:**111–120.

8. **Baker, B. S., S. Bokth, A. Powles, J. J. Garioch, H. Lewis, H. Valdimarsson, and L. Fry.** 1993. Group A streptococcal antigen-specific T lymphocytes in guttate psoriatic lesions. *Br. J. Dermatol.* **128:**493–499.

9. **Barbosa, J. A., J. W. Saldanha, and R. C. Garratt.** 1996. Novel features of serine protease active sites and specificity pockets: sequence analysis and modelling studies of glutamate-specific endopeptidases and epidermolytic toxins. *Protein Eng.* **9:**591–601.

10. **Boehncke, W. H., D. Dressel, T. M. Zollner, and R. Kaufmann.** 1996. Pulling the trigger on psoriasis. *Nature* **379:**777.

11. **Boehncke, W. H., C. Kuenzlen, T. M. Zollner, V. Mielke, and W. Sterry.** 1994. Predominant usage of distinct T-cell receptor V beta regions by epidermotropic T cells in psoriasis. *Exp. Dermatol.* **3:**161–163.

12. **Bratton, D. L., Q. Hamid, M. Boguniewicz, D. E. Doherty, J. M. Kailey, and D. Y. Leung.** 1995. Granulocyte macrophage colony-stimulating factor contributes to enhanced monocyte survival in chronic atopic dermatitis. *J. Clin. Invest.* **95:**211–218.

13. **Bratton, D. L., K. R. May, J. M. Kailey, D. E. Doherty, and D. Y. Leung.** 1999. Staphylococcal toxic shock syndrome toxin-1 inhibits monocyte apoptosis. *J. Allergy Clin. Immunol.* **103:**895–900.

14. **Brosius, C. L., J. W. Newburger, J. C. Burns, P. Hojnowski-Diaz, S. Zierler, and D. Y. Leung.** 1988. Increased prevalence of atopic dermatitis in Kawasaki disease. *Pediatr. Infect. Dis. J.* **7:**863–866.

15. **Bunikowski, R., M. Mielke, H. Skarabis, U. Herz, R. L. Bergmann, U. Wahn, and H. Renz.** 1999. Prevalence and role of serum IgE antibodies to the *Staphylococcus aureus*-derived superantigens SEA and SEB in children with atopic dermatitis. *J. Allergy Clin. Immunol.* **103:**119–124.

16. **Cardona, I. D., L.-S. Ou, E. Goleva, and D. Y. M. Leung.** 2006. Staphylococcal enterotoxin B inhibits regulatory T cells by inducing GITR-L on monocytes. *J. Allergy Clin. Immunol.* **117:**688–695.

17. **Cavarelli, J., G. Prevost, W. Bourguet, L. Moulinier, B. Chevrier, B. Delagoutte, A. Bilwes, L. Mourey, S. Rifai, Y. Piemont, and D. Moras.** 1997. The structure of *Staphylococcus aureus* epidermolytic toxin A, an atypic serine protease, at 1.7 A resolution. *Structure* **5:**813–824.

18. **Cerio, R., C. E. Griffiths, K. D. Cooper, B. J. Nickoloff, and J. T. Headington.** 1989. Characterization of factor XIIIa positive dermal dendritic cells in normal and inflamed skin. *Br. J. Dermatol.* **121:**421–431.

19. **Chang, J. C., L. R. Smith, K. J. Froning, B. J. Schwabe, J. A. Laxer, L. L. Caralli, H. H. Kurland, M. A. Karasek, D. I. Wilkinson, D. J. Carlo, et al.** 1994. CD8+ T cells in psoriatic lesions preferentially use T-cell receptor V beta 3 and/or V beta 13.1 genes. *Proc. Natl. Acad. Sci. USA* **91:**9282–9286.

20. **Chatila, T. A.** 2005. Role of regulatory T cells in human diseases. *J. Allergy Clin. Immunol.* **116:**949–959.

21. **Christophers, E., and T. Henseler.** 1987. Contrasting disease patterns in psoriasis and atopic dermatitis. *Arch. Dermatol. Res.* **279**(Suppl.):S48–S51.

22. **Cole, G. W., and K. D. Wuepper.** 1978. Isolation and partial characterization of a keratinocyte proliferative factor produced by *Streptococcus pyogenes* (strain NY-5). *J. Invest. Dermatol.* **71:**219–223.

23. **Cone, L. A., D. R. Woodard, P. M. Schlievert, and G. S. Tomory.** 1987. Clinical and bacteriologic observations of a toxic shock-like syndrome due to *Streptococcus pyogenes. N. Engl. J. Med.* **317:**146–149.

24. **Cooper, K. D., G. R. Neises, and S. I. Katz.** 1986. Antigen-presenting OKM5+ melanophages appear in human epidermis after ultraviolet radiation. *J. Invest. Dermatol.* **86:**363–370.

25. **Dajani, A. S.** 1972. The scalded-skin syndrome: relation to phage-group II staphylococci. *J. Infect. Dis.* **125:**548–551.

26. **Dancer, S. J., R. Garratt, J. Saldanha, H. Jhoti, and R. Evans.** 1990. The epidermolytic toxins are serine proteases. *FEBS Lett.* **268:**129–132.

27. **Deresewicz, R.** 1997. Staphylococcal toxic shock syndrome, p. 435–480. *In* D. Y. M. Leung, B. Huber, and P. M. Schlievert (ed.), *Superantigens: Molecular Biology, Immunology and Relevance to Human Disease.* Marcel Dekker, New York, N.Y.

28. **Dunn, D. A., A. S. Gadenne, S. Simha, E. A. Lerner, M. Bigby, and P. A. Bleicher.** 1993. T-cell receptor V beta expression in normal human skin. *Proc. Natl. Acad. Sci. USA* **90:**1267–1271.

29. **Duraiswamy, N., Y. Tse, C. Hammerberg, S. Kang, and K. D. Cooper.** 1994. Distinction of class II MHC+ Langerhans cell-like interstitial dendritic antigen-presenting cells in murine dermis from dermal macrophages. *J. Invest. Dermatol.* **103:**678–683.

30. **Elder, J. T., R. P. Nair, T. Henseler, S. Jenisch, P. Stuart, N. Chia, E. Christophers, and J. J. Voorhees.** 2001. The genetics of psoriasis 2001: the odyssey continues. *Arch. Dermatol.* **137:**1447–1454

31. **Fleischer, B., and C. J. Bailey.** 1992. Recombinant epidermolytic (exfoliative) toxin A of *Staphylococcus aureus* is not a superantigen. *Med. Microbiol. Immunol. (Berl).* **180:**273–278.

32. **Goodman, R. E., F. Nestle, Y. M. Naidu, J. M. Green, C. B. Thompson, B. J. Nickoloff, and L. A. Turka.** 1994. Keratinocyte-derived T cell costimulation induces preferential production of IL-2 and IL-4 but not IFN-gamma. *J. Immunol.* **152:**5189–5198.

33. **Gottlieb, S. L., P. Gilleaudeau, R. Johnson, L. Estes, T. G. Woodworth, A. B. Gottlieb, and J. G. Krueger.** 1995. Response of psoriasis to a lymphocyte-selective toxin (DAB389IL-2) suggests a primary immune, but not keratinocyte, pathogenic basis. *Nat. Med.* **1:**442–447.

34. **Grossman, D., R. G. Cook, J. T. Sparrow, J. A. Mollick, and R. R. Rich.** 1990. Dissociation of the stimulatory activities of staphylococcal enterotoxins for T cells and monocytes. *J. Exp. Med.* **172:**1831–1841.

35. **Hauk, P. J., Q. A. Hamid, G. P. Chrousos, and D. Y. Leung.** 2000. Induction of corticosteroid insensitivity in human PBMCs by microbial superantigens. *J. Allergy Clin. Immunol.* **105:**782–787.

36. **Hauk, P. J., and D. Y. Leung.** 2001. Tacrolimus (FK506): new treatment approach in superantigen-associated diseases like atopic dermatitis? *J. Allergy Clin. Immunol.* **107:**391–392.

37. **He, X. W., J. Goronzy, and C. Weyand.** 1992. Selective induction of rheumatoid factors by superantigens and human helper T cells. *J. Clin. Invest.* **89:**673–680.

38. **Henderson, C. A., and A. S. Highet.** 1988. Acute psoriasis associated with Lancefield Group C and Group G cutaneous streptococcal infections. *Br. J. Dermatol.* **118:**559–561.

39. **Herman, A., G. Croteau, R. P. Sekaly, J. Kappler, and P. Marrack.** 1990. HLA-DR alleles differ in their ability to present staphylococcal enterotoxins to T cells. *J. Exp. Med.* **172:**709–717.

40. **Herz, U., N. Schnoy, S. Borelli, L. Weigl, U. Kasbohrer, A. Daser, U. Wahn, E. Kottgen, and H. Renz.** 1998. A human-SCID mouse model for allergic immune response bacterial superantigen enhances skin inflammation and suppresses IgE production. *J. Invest. Dermatol.* **110:**224–231.

41. **Hofer, M. F., R. J. Harbeck, P. M. Schlievert, and D. Y. Leung.** 1999. Staphylococcal toxins augment specific IgE responses by atopic patients exposed to allergen. *J. Invest. Dermatol.* **112:**171–176.

42. **Hofer, M. F., M. R. Lester, P. M. Schlievert, and D. Y. Leung.** 1995. Upregulation of IgE synthesis by staphylococcal toxic shock syndrome toxin-1 in peripheral blood mononuclear cells from patients with atopic dermatitis. *Clin. Exp. Allergy* **25:**1218–1227.

43. **Jackow, C. M., J. C. Cather, V. Hearne, A. T. Asano, J. M. Musser, and M. Duvic.** 1997. Association of erythrodermic cutaneous T-cell lymphoma, superantigen-positive *Staphylococcus aureus*, and oligoclonal T-cell receptor V beta gene expansion. *Blood* **89:**32–40.

44. **Jappe, U.** 2000. Superantigens and their association with dermatological inflammatory diseases: facts and hypotheses. *Acta Derm. Venereol.* **80:**321–328.

45. **Kotzin, B. L., D. Y. Leung, J. Kappler, and P. Marrack.** 1993. Superantigens and their potential role in human disease. *Adv. Immunol.* **54:**99–166.

46. **Ladhani, S.** 2001. Recent developments in staphylococcal scalded skin syndrome. *Clin. Microbiol. Infect.* **7:**301–307.

47. **Ladhani, S., C. L. Joannou, D. P. Lochrie, R. W. Evans, and S. M. Poston.** 1999. Clinical, microbial, and biochemical aspects of the exfoliative toxins causing staphylococcal scalded-skin syndrome. *Clin. Microbiol. Rev.* **12:**224–242.

48. **Laouini, D., S. Kawamoto, A. Yalcindag, P. Bryce, E. Mizoguchi, H. Oettgen, and R. S. Geha.** 2003. Epicutaneous sensitization with superantigen induces allergic skin inflammation. *J. Allergy Clin. Immunol.* **112:**981–987.

49. **Lee, P. K., M. T. Zipoli, A. N. Weinberg, M. N. Swartz, and R. A. Johnson.** 2003. Pyodermas: *Staphylococcus aureus*, streptococcus, and other gram-positive bacteria, p. 1856–1878. *In* I. M. Freeberg, A. Z. Eisen, K. Wolff, K. F. Austen, L. A. Goldsmith, and S. I. Katz (ed.), *Fitzpatrick's Dermatology in General Medicine*, 6th ed. McGraw-Hill, New York, N.Y.

50. **Leung, D. Y.** 2003. Infection in atopic dermatitis. *Curr. Opin. Pediatr.* **15:**399–404.

51. **Leung, D. Y., M. Boguniewicz, M. D. Howell, I. Nomura, and Q. A. Hamid.** 2004. New insights into atopic dermatitis. *J. Clin. Invest.* **113:**651–657.

52. **Leung, D. Y., M. Gately, A. Trumble, B. Ferguson-Darnell, P. M. Schlievert, and L. J. Picker.** 1995. Bacterial superantigens induce T cell expression of the skin-selective homing receptor, the cutaneous lymphocyte-associated antigen, via stimulation of interleukin 12 production. *J. Exp. Med.* **181:**747–753.

53. **Leung, D. Y., R. Harbeck, P. Bina, R. F. Reiser, E. Yang, D. A. Norris, J. M. Hanifin, and H. A. Sampson.** 1993. Presence of IgE antibodies to staphylococcal exotoxins on the skin of patients with atopic dermatitis. Evidence for a new group of allergens. *J. Clin. Invest.* **92:**1374–1380.

54. **Leung, D. Y., J. B. Travers, R. Giorno, D. A. Norris, R. Skinner, J. Aelion, L. V. Kazemi, M. H. Kim, A. E. Trumble, M. Kotb, et al.** 1995. Evidence for a streptococcal superantigen-driven process in acute guttate psoriasis. *J. Clin. Invest.* **96:**2106–2112.

55. **Leung, D. Y., J. B. Travers, and D. A. Norris.** 1995. The role of superantigens in skin disease. *J. Invest. Dermatol.* **105:**37S–42S.

56. **Leung, D. Y., P. Walsh, R. Giorno, and D. A. Norris.** 1993. A potential role for superantigens in the pathogenesis of psoriasis. *J. Invest. Dermatol.* **100:**225–228.

57. Reference deleted.

58. **Lever, R., K. Hadley, D. Downey, and R. Mackie.** 1988. Staphylococcal colonization in atopic dermatitis and the effect of topical mupirocin therapy. *Br. J. Dermatol.* **119:**189–198.

59. **Lewis, H. M., B. S. Baker, S. Bokth, A. V. Powles, J. J. Garioch, H. Valdimarsson, and L. Fry.** 1993. Restricted T-cell receptor V beta gene usage in the skin of patients with guttate and chronic plaque psoriasis. *Br. J. Dermatol.* **129:**514–520.

60. **Li, L. B., E. Goleva, C. F. Hall, L. S. Ou, and D. Y. Leung.** 2004. Superantigen-induced corticosteroid resistance of human T cells occurs through activation of the mitogen-activated protein kinase kinase/extracellular signal-regulated kinase (MEK-ERK) pathway. *J. Allergy Clin. Immunol.* **114:**1059–1069.

61. **Manders, S. M.** 1998. Toxin-mediated streptococcal and staphylococcal disease. *J. Am. Acad. Dermatol.* **39:**383–400.

62. **Manders, S. M., W. R. Heymann, E. Atillasoy, J. Kleeman, and P. M. Schlievert.** 1996. Recurrent toxin-mediated perineal erythema. *Arch. Dermatol.* **132:**57–60.

63. **Marples, R. R., C. L. Heaton, and A. M. Kligman.** 1973. *Staphylococcus aureus* in psoriasis. *Arch. Dermatol.* **107:**568–570.

64. **Marrack, P., and J. Kappler.** 1990. The staphylococcal enterotoxins and their relatives. *Science* **248:**705–711.

65. **McFadden, J., H. Valdimarsson, and L. Fry.** 1991. Cross-reactivity between streptococcal M surface antigen and human skin. *Br. J. Dermatol.* **125:**443–447.

66. **Michie, C. A., and T. Davis.** 1996. Atopic dermatitis and staphylococcal superantigens. *Lancet* **347:**324.

67. **Monday, S. R., G. M. Vath, W. A. Ferens, C. Deobald, J. V. Rago, P. J. Gahr, D. D. Monie, J. J. Iandolo, S. K. Chapes, W. C. Davis, D. H. Ohlendorf, P. M. Schlievert, and G. A. Bohach.** 1999. Unique superantigen activity of staphylococcal exfoliative toxins. *J. Immunol.* **162:**4550–4559.

68. **Morlock, B. A., L. Spero, and A. D. Johnson.** 1980. Mitogenic activity of staphylococcal exfoliative toxin. *Infect. Immun.* **30:**381–384.

69. **Nickoloff, B. J., R. S. Mitra, J. Green, Y. Shimizu, C. Thompson, and L. A. Turka.** 1993. Activated keratinocytes present bacterial-derived superantigens to T lymphocytes: relevance to psoriasis. *J. Dermatol. Sci.* **6:**127–133.

70. **Nickoloff, B. J., R. S. Mitra, J. Green, X. G. Zheng, Y. Shimizu, C. Thompson, and L. A. Turka.** 1993. Accessory cell function of keratinocytes for superantigens. Dependence on lymphocyte function-associated antigen-1/intercellular adhesion molecule-1 interaction. *J. Immunol.* **150:**2148–2159.

71. **Nomura, I., E. Goleva, M. D. Howell, Q. A. Hamid, P. Y. Ong, C. F. Hall, M. A. Darst, B. Gao, M. Boguniewicz, J. B. Travers, and D. Y. Leung.** 2003. Cytokine milieu of atopic dermatitis, as compared to psoriasis, skin prevents induction of innate immune response genes. *J. Immunol.* **171:**3262–3269.

72. **Nomura, I., K. Tanaka, H. Tomita, T. Katsunuma, Y. Ohya, N. Ikeda, et al.** 1999. Evaluation of the staphylococcal exotoxins and their specific IgE in childhood atopic dermatitis. *J. Allergy Clin. Immunol.* **104:**441–446.

73. **Nyfors, A., and K. Lemholt.** 1975. Psoriasis in children. A short review and a survey of 245 cases. *Br. J. Dermatol.* **92:**437–442.

74. **Ong, P. Y., T. Ohtake, C. Brandt, I. Strickland, M. Boguniewicz, T. Ganz, R. L. Gallo, and D. Y. Leung.** 2002. Endogenous antimicrobial peptides and skin infections in atopic dermatitis. *N. Engl. J. Med.* **347:**1151–1160.

75. **Opal, S. M., A. D. Johnson-Winegar, and A. S. Cross.** 1988. Staphylococcal scalded skin syndrome in two immunocompetent adults caused by exfoliatin B-producing *Staphylococcus aureus. J. Clin. Microbiol.* **26:**1283–1286.

76. **Ou, L. S., E. Goleva, C. Hall, and D. Y. Leung.** 2004. T regulatory cells in atopic dermatitis and subversion of their activity by superantigens. *J. Allergy Clin. Immunol.* **113:**756–763.

77. **Papageorgiou, A. C., L. R. Plano, C. M. Collins, and K. R. Acharya.** 2000. Structural similarities and differences in *Staphylococcus aureus* exfoliative toxins A and B as revealed by their crystal structures. *Protein Sci.* **9:**610–618.

78. **Picker, L. J., R. J. Martin, A. Trumble, L. S. Newman, P. A. Collins, P. R. Bergstresser, and D. Y. Leung.** 1994. Differential expression of lymphocyte homing receptors by human memory/effector T cells in pulmonary versus cutaneous immune effector sites. *Eur. J. Immunol.* **24:**1269–1277.

79. **Plano, L. R., D. M. Gutman, M. Woischnik, and C. M. Collins.** 2000. Recombinant *Staphylococcus aureus* exfoliative toxins are not bacterial superantigens. *Infect. Immun.* **68:**3048–3052.

80. **Prevost, G., S. Rifai, M. L. Chaix, and Y. Piemont.** 1991. Functional evidence that the Ser-195 residue of staphylococcal exfoliative toxin A is essential for biological activity. *Infect. Immun.* **59:**3337–3339.

81. **Redpath, M. B., T. J. Foster, and C. J. Bailey.** 1991. The role of the serine protease active site in the mode of action of epidermolytic toxin of *Staphylococcus aureus. FEMS Microbiol. Lett.* **65:**151–155.

82. **Rosenberg, E. W., and P. W. Noah.** 1988. The Koebner phenomenon and the microbial basis of psoriasis. *J. Am. Acad. Dermatol.* **18:**151–158.

83. **Skov, L., J. V. Olsen, R. Giorno, P. M. Schlievert, O. Baadsgaard, and D. Y. Leung.** 2000. Application of Staphylococcal enterotoxin B on normal and atopic skin induces up-regulation of T cells by a superantigen-mediated mechanism. *J. Allergy Clin. Immunol.* **105:**820–826.

84. **Strange, P., L. Skov, and O. Baadsgaard.** 1994. Interferon gamma-treated keratinocytes activate T cells in the presence of superantigens: involvement of major histocompatibility complex class II molecules. *J. Invest. Dermatol.* **102:**150–154.

85. **Strange, P., L. Skov, S. Lisby, P. L. Nielsen, and O. Baadsgaard.** 1996. Staphylococcal enterotoxin B applied on intact normal and intact atopic skin induces dermatitis. *Arch. Dermatol.* **132:**27–33.

86. **Strickland, I., P. J. Hauk, A. E. Trumble, L. J. Picker, and D. Y. Leung.** 1999. Evidence for superantigen involvement in skin homing of T cells in atopic dermatitis. *J. Invest. Dermatol.* **112:**249–253.

87. **Takiuchi, I., M. Kawamura, T. Teramoto, and D. Higuchi.** 1987. Staphylococcal exfoliative toxin induces caseinolytic activity. *J. Infect. Dis.* **156:**508–509.

88. **Telfer, N. R., R. J. Chalmers, K. Whale, and G. Colman.** 1992. The role of streptococcal infection in the initiation of guttate psoriasis. *Arch. Dermatol.* **128:**39–42.

89. **Travers, J. B., Q. A. Hamid, D. A. Norris, C. Kuhn, R. C. Giorno, P. M. Schlievert, E. R. Farmer, and D. Y. Leung.** 1999. Epidermal HLA-DR and the enhancement of cutaneous reactivity to superantigenic toxins in psoriasis. *J. Clin. Invest.* **104:**1181–1189.

90. **Valdimarsson, H., B. S. Baker, I. Jonsdottir, A. Powles, and L. Fry.** 1995. Psoriasis: a T-cell-mediated autoimmune disease induced by streptococcal superantigens? *Immunol. Today* **16:**145–149.

91. **Vath, G. M., C. A. Earhart, J. V. Rago, M. H. Kim, G. A. Bohach, P. M. Schlievert, and D. H. Ohlendorf.** 1997. The structure of the superantigen exfoliative toxin A suggests a novel regulation as a serine protease. *Biochemistry (Mosc.)* **36:**1559–1566.

92. **White, J., A. Herman, A. M. Pullen, R. Kubo, J. W. Kappler, and P. Marrack.** 1989. The V beta-specific superantigen staphylococcal enterotoxin B: stimulation of mature T cells and clonal deletion in neonatal mice. *Cell* **56:**27–35.

93. **Wrone-Smith, T., and B. J. Nickoloff.** 1996. Dermal injection of immunocytes induces psoriasis. *J. Clin. Invest.* **98:**1878–1887.

94. **Yamauchi, P. S., and N. J. Lowe.** 2006. Cessation of cyclosporine therapy by treatment with etanercept in patients with severe psoriasis. *J. Am. Acad. Dermatol.* **54**(3 Suppl. 2)**:**S135–S5138.

EXPERIMENTAL MODELS
FOR SUPERANTIGEN-MEDIATED DISEASES

Superantigens: Molecular Basis for Their Role in Human Diseases
Edited by Malak Kotb and John D. Fraser
© 2007 ASM Press, Washington, D.C.

Chapter 10

Pathogenetic Mechanisms and Therapeutic Approaches in Superantigen-Induced Experimental Autoimmune Diseases

Andrej Tarkowski

INTRODUCTION

In the past decade, attention has focused on the contribution of environment to the pathogenesis of autoimmune diseases. In this context, microbial superantigens are highly suspected as causative agents in both the inductive phase and in chronic stages of autoimmune diseases. Superantigens represent a group of molecules that are able to cause massive activation of the host immune system irrespective of the antigenic specificity of the T or B cell. The fact that superantigens potently activate the immune system led to the hypothesis that they might also affect the course of autoimmune diseases either by initiating the autoimmune process and/or by inducing relapse of an already established autoimmune condition. Importantly, the knowledge about how superantigens mediate their detrimental action will help designing efficient treatment remedies.

In principle, three distinct mechanisms mediate superantigenic impact on the onset/relapse of autoimmune disease. First, superantigens may, following presentation on antigen-presenting cells, directly activate autoreactive T and B cells, which will migrate to the appropriate organ and once there contribute to tissue destruction by production of chemokines, proinflammatory cytokines, and tissue destructive proteinases. Excessive autoantibody synthesis, being an outcome of exposure of the immune system to superantigen-producing bacteria (3, 13), will lead to immune complex formation with ensuing activation of the complement cascade leading to tissue damage. Second, innocent (i.e., nonautoreactive) bystander lymphocytes will be activated, thereby triggering nonspecific inflammatory response that might lead to disease relapse in the chronic phase

Andrej Tarkowski • Department of Rheumatology and Inflammation Research, Göteborg University, Guldhedsgatan 10, S-413 46 Göteborg, Sweden.

of autoimmune disease. Finally, superantigens are able to activate the antigen-presenting cells, such as macrophages. Such an activation will not only lead to aberrantly high production of cytokines, chemokines, prostaglandins, and superoxides, but might also give rise to an altered antigen processing, resulting in presentation of cryptic epitopes as well as posttranslational alteration of endogenous molecules including citrullination and oxidation, both known to be of importance in induction of arthritis (17, 24).

CHARACTERISTICS OF MICROBIAL SUPERANTIGENS

Microbial superantigens encompass viral and bacterial proteins that share the ability to interact with major histocompatibility complex (MHC) class II and the T-cell receptor, thereby bypassing the conventional antigen-processing pathway. Indeed, whereas conventional antigens are loaded into the peptide-binding groove of the MHC molecule, the superantigen typically binds to either the α- or β-chain, or even the C-terminal domain of MHC class II, without any requirement for intracellular processing. Furthermore, superantigens interact with particular T-cell receptor (TCR) Vβ-chains, irrespective of the antigenic specificity of the given TCR. Indeed, certain superantigens are able to displace the antigenic peptide from its receptor (4). The mitogenic capacity of the superantigen seems to correlate with the binding affinity of a given TCR for the superantigen. Since the TCR repertoire comprises only a limited number of different Vβ-chains and each superantigen may interact with one or several Vβ members, low amounts of each superantigen may trigger the activation of up to 30% of the whole T-cell population.

The best characterized group of superantigens belongs to the pyrogenic family, and includes the staphylococcal enterotoxins A, B, C, D, E, G, I, toxic shock syndrome toxin-1 (TSST-1), streptococcal superantigen, and the streptococcal pyrogenic toxins A, B, C, G, H, I, J, SMEZ, and SSA. All of these pyrogenic toxins share a three-dimensional structure (25). Nonetheless, these toxins show important differences, not only with regard to their Vβ TCR specificities, but also with regard to the clinical symptoms they produce. Bacterial superantigens that do not belong to the pyrogenic family include the staphylococcal exfoliative toxins A and B, *Mycoplasma arthritidis* mitogen, and *Yersinia pseudotuberculosis* mitogen. Superantigens also occur outside the world of bacteria. Indeed, one of the best characterized superantigens is the mouse mammary tumor virus (MMTV)-encoded superantigens. These virus-encoded superantigens demonstrate a link between endogenous superantigens and infectious agents.

Staphylococcal protein A was first characterized as a molecule having the ability to interact with human immunoglobulin G (IgG) heavy chain in a nonimmune manner. The B-cell-activating property of protein A is attributed to its recognition of Fab-domains of V_HIII-encoded B-cell receptor immunoglobulins. In mice, Fab-mediated protein A-binding interactions are commonly displayed by 5 to 10% of mature B cells. Because of its V_HIII-restricted recognition of supraclonal B cells, protein A merits the designation B-cell superantigen.

The specificity of interaction of superantigens with TCR Vβ families and BCR V_H families provides a tool for the analysis of the impact of superantigens on different lymphocyte populations. The results indicate that responding lymphocytes may proliferate, become anergized, or undergo deletion as a consequence of these interactions.

IMPACT OF SUPERANTIGENS ON EXPERIMENTAL AUTOIMMUNE DISEASES

There is a body of indirect support indicating that superantigens may be of importance in human autoimmune diseases. This support is predominantly based on skewed usage of Vβ TCR families at the site of inflammatory insult. Such a predominance would indicate superantigen-driven T-cell expansion. Superantigens have been implicated in several inflammatory diseases with and without autoimmune background. With these conditions one can include Kawasaki syndrome, psoriasis, rheumatoid arthritis, autoimmune myositis, and diabetes mellitus. However, direct, i.e., causal, evidence proving the role of superantigens in human autoimmunity is still missing. Superantigenic manipulations in experimental models of autoimmune diseases have shed a light on how these molecules may corrupt immune responses by either increasing severity of tissue damage or alternatively protecting the host against autoimmune attack. The following chapter will highlight some experimental autoimmune and immune mediated diseases where the role of superantigens has been analyzed.

Experimental Allergic Encephalomyelitis (EAE)

Experimental allergic encephalomyelitis is an animal model of human multiple sclerosis. The ability of staphylococcal superantigen to aggravate the course of disease was documented in several well-performed studies (14, 35). The aggravation was documented both as exacerbation of preexisting disease being in a quiescent stage as well as amplification of the subclinical course of EAE giving rise to overt disease manifestations. The data generated suggest that the aggravation of disease was not due to VβTCR-specific (i.e., Vβ8 being of importance as a driving force in EAE) activation since superantigens lacking specificity for this TCR epitope also displayed similar capacity (35). Thus, the innocent-bystander-activating properties of staphylococcal superantigens are most probably of importance in generating (i) a cytokine storm and (ii) intramolecular epitope spreading (38), which in concert will ultimately end up in a bout of disease.

Experimental Arthritis

Superantigens are able to interact with synoviocytes thereby triggering their production of chemokines (RANTES, monocyte chemoattractant protein-1 [MCP-1], and interleukin-8 [IL-8]). More importantly, type A synoviocytes (i.e., macrophage-like cells) are able to present superantigens to cognate $CD4^+T$ cells residing in inflamed tissue of both rodents having chronic experimental arthritis and human beings with rheumatoid arthritis (RA). For these reasons it is not astonishing that superantigens contribute to the disease course in several rodent models of chronic rheumatic diseases. Indeed, in collagen II-induced arthritis, probably the most widespread model of human RA, exposure to *M. arthritidis* superantigen exacerbates the course of the disease (15). Also, use of TSST-1 in the same arthritis model led to upregulation of mRNA expression of proinflammatory molecules combined with aggravation of the course of arthritis (19). Just as in a case of EAE, even here the subclinical course of collagen II arthritis may be turned to an overt one by challenge with a superantigen (28). By the same token, TSST-1 is able to reactivate peptidoglycan-triggered arthritis (37).

Experimental Psoriasis

The impact of staphylococcal superantigens has also been studied in the model of human psoriasis, an inflammatory disorder characterized by cutaneous skin lesions containing activated keratinocytes and a plethora of inflammatory cells including T cells, macrophages, and neutrophils. To mimic human psoriasis, it is possible to transplant clinically uninvolved human skin from psoriasis patients to SCID mice. Such a xenogeneic tranplantation model will result in overt psoriatic lesions providing repetitive intradermal injections with bacterial superantigens combined with simultaneous intraperitoneal injections with superantigen-stimulated lymphocytes (12). Such a procedure will result in epidermal hyperproliferation, papillomatosis, focal expression of intercellular adhesion molecule-1 (ICAM-1), and infiltration of T cells characterized by expression of cutaneous lymphocyte-associated antigen. A similar model of psoriasis was employed by Yamamoto et al. (42). This group showed that to maintain human overtly psoriasiform epidermis transplanted to SCID mice for a long time, it was necessary to repeatedly provide superantigen (SEB)-stimulated peripheral blood mononuclear cells. In the transplanted epidermis of these mice one could detect occurrence of the mRNA encoding proinflammatory cytokines gamma interferon and IL-1β.

Infectious Diseases with Autoimmune Manifestations

An infectious disease that is commonly mediated by staphylococci and streptococci is septic arthritis. It is called "septic" since the bacteria that invade the human joints are almost invariably blood-borne. This disease is characterized both in humans and in murine models by a very fast joint destruction and significant mortality (40). Serologically, there is an overwhelming polyclonal B cell activation resulting in production of auto-antibodies including rheumatoid factors, antibodies specific for DNA and collagen type II (3). In the case of septic arthritis, it has been shown that mice inoculated intravenously with a superantigen-producing *Staphylococcus aureus* strain show more severe joint disease than the control mice infected with the same dose of an isogeneic, non-superantigen-producing strain (2). The reason for this outcome is the in situ expansion of a certain Vβ-specific CD4 T-cell family. Indeed, deletion of this relatively minute T-cell population leads to decreased severity of both septic arthritis and sepsis-mediated mortality (1).

Bacterial cell wall-expressed protein A triggers supraclonal B-cell responses both in vitro and in an in vivo model of staphylococcal infection (30). Protein A itself is a virulence determinant in arthritis, since specific inactivation of this molecule will downregulate the severity of septic arthritis (29).

To summarize, two scenarios can be suggested for the contribution of superantigens to the development of autoimmune disease (35). In a subject with preexisting disease, exposure to superantigens (e.g., in case of infection with superantigen-producing bacteria) may lead to an acute flare of the condition. In healthy subjects, exposure to superantigen may under certain conditions (e.g., "autoimmune-prone" MHC) lead to a non-antigen-specific expansion of autoreactive T cells, followed by amplification of these autoreactive clones of the lymphocyte-expressing, superantigen-specific VβTCR family.

HOW TO PREVENT SUPERANTIGEN-MEDIATED DISEASES?

Since the exact role of superantigens in human autoimmune disease remains speculative, the presentation below will merely focus on approaches of how to counteract either superantigen production or the superantigenic action of already secreted toxins on their target cells, or those that influence the downstream activation of the immune system by superantigens. These approaches are summarized below.

Downregulation of Superantigen Production

The seemingly simplest, but probably not the easiest way to stop the action of superantigens is to switch off their production in vivo. Many ways to achieve this goal may be envisaged. One of these would be the treatment of infected patients with either specific antisense DNA or siRNA. In both cases one might achieve specific silencing of the gene(s) that are responsible for superantigen production. However, there are several obstacles to these methods, including problems with passage of these molecules through the bacterial cell wall. An alternative, albeit less-specific way, is to interact with the bacterial quorum-sensing mechanism using the RNAIII molecule, which is encoded by the *agr* locus of staphylococci (27). This can be achieved by administering either RNAIII-inhibiting peptide or by injecting antibodies to the constitutively produced RNAIII-activating protein (8). Yet another means to downregulate the production of superantigens in a nonspecific way is to use antibiotics with protein-synthesis inhibitor properties, such as clindamycin (43).

Superantigen Neutralization

Once produced and secreted, the superantigens may be neutralized by interactions with either blocking peptides or specific antibodies. A very interesting approach to achieve neutralization was undertaken by Arad et al. (6, 7). This group proved that a peptide with similarity to SEB toxin residues 150 to 161, and also to SEA and TSST-1, displayed potent inhibition of superantigen-mediated cytokine production. Preformed antibodies to this peptide were also efficient in this respect, indicating interference between these antibodies and superantigen binding to either the TCR or MHC class II molecule. Most impressively, all of the mice that were administered the peptide intravenously survived lethal superantigenic challenge. In addition, upon rechallenge with superantigen a few weeks later, the mice continued to be protected. This persistent protection may have been mediated by endogenous specific antibody responses, despite the fact that the peptide itself was not involved in binding to either MHC class II or the Vβ-chain of the TCR. Yet another group (41) identified a peptide with antagonistic properties with respect to superantigen-triggered host responses. SEB, SEC, SED, and TSST-1 were antagonized by the peptide, which indicates that the peptide interacts either with conserved residues of the superantigens or the MHC class II molecule.

A more classical approach to neutralize superantigens is to use toxin-specific antibodies. Such antibodies occur naturally in normal human sera, indicating certain ongoing exposure to at least staphylococcal superantigens. Indirect support for therapeutic properties of these antibodies was the successful treatment of both streptococcal and staphylococcal diseases by the infusion of human IgG that contained superantigen-specific antibodies. However, to optimize the impact of antibodies one needs to increase their in vivo concentration, and more importantly, enhance the possibility that the host immune system will produce these molecules upon exposure to superantigens. The best way to achieve these goals may be to immunize the patient with superantigens themselves. However, since wild-type superantigens display toxic properties, one needs to use attenuated variants that retain antigenicity but have lowered toxicity. The attenuated superantigens (which lack the ability to bind to MHC class II) have proven to be highly immunogenic in the mouse, and to provide 100% protection against rechallenge with the wild-type toxin (9), which makes vaccination an interesting option at least with respect to toxic shock syndrome and superantigen-producing bacterial infections (26).

Downregulation of Superantigen-Triggered Inflammation

Bearing in mind the plethora of microorganisms that produce superantigenic molecules, and thus the necessity for multiple immunizations, the in vivo neutralization of superantigens may prove difficult. Therefore, many researchers have assessed the possibility of interacting with the inflammatory circuits that are triggered by superantigenic exposure to downregulate inflammation that per se leads to deleterious sequels in the host. The most straightforward possibility is to neutralize the proinflammatory molecules that are readily induced by infection with superantigen-producing bacteria, such as inflammatory cytokines (tumor necrosis factor [TNF], IL-1, IL-6, IL-8, and high-mobility group B-1 [HMGB-1]), reactive oxygen metabolites (such as H_2O_2), complement cascade components (e.g., C5a), platelet-activating factor (PAF), certain coagulation factors, and migration inhibition factor (MIF) (reviewed in reference 32). It has been convincingly shown that interaction with each of these molecules leads to downregulation of inflammation in experimental animal models. However, many of these molecules are important for the defense against microbial invasion itself. That is why some attempts to downregulate inflammation in human sepsis, by, e.g., the neutralization of TNF, have not been efficacious (31). Other approaches have been somewhat more successful in the human setting, e.g., the administration of activated protein C (11). This finding is of great interest, given the multiple interactions between the coagulation and inflammatory/immune systems. Yet another reasonably new approach is the usage of antagonists to HMGB-1, which exerts an important proinflammatory role in RA, for example (21).

An alternative approach to the neutralization of inflammatory molecules is to provide anti-inflammatory treatment. Early efforts included the use of corticosteroids. Such studies met with success both in experimental animal models of sepsis caused by superantigen-producing staphylococci (34), as well as in human sepsis (5). However, since glucocorticosteroids have many undesired effects on the immune system (e.g., downregulation of peripheral blood mononuclear cell activities) the dose and timing of the treatment seems to be of major importance.

Some newer treatment modalities, which are possibly less toxic than glucocorticosteroids, employ the administration of anti-inflammatory cytokines, primarily IL-10 alone or together with IL-4. These two Th2-type cytokines potently downregulate inflammation that is mediated by macrophages and Th1-type T cells, both of which are activated by superantigens (10).

Interaction with the Apoptotic Mechanisms of the Host

During superantigen exposure, ample evidence exists that T cells undergo rapid apoptosis. In experimental models of sepsis and inflammation, the overexpression of antiapoptotic proteins, such as Bcl-2 (18), and the inhibition of caspases result in the prolongation of the lymphocyte life span and increase the survival rate of experimental animals.

Blocking of MHC Class II, the TCR, and Costimulatory Molecules To Prevent Interaction with Superantigens

Several strategies have been developed to design soluble molecules that mimic MHC class II and the TCR, either as individual entities or as a fusion protein. A fusion protein of MHC class II and TCR inhibited the in vitro release of IL-2 upon stimulation of lymphocytes with superantigen (22). Alternatively, certain costimulatory molecules may be blocked, thereby interrupting T-cell activation by superantigens. Indeed, the in vivo use of soluble CTLA4Ig to block superantigen-induced signaling resulted in significantly increased survival of mice that were exposed concomitantly to superantigen and this chimeric protein as compared with control mice that were administered superantigen alone (33).

Induction of Superantigen-Specific Tolerance

Immunological tolerance may be induced by either central or peripheral deletion of specific lymphocyte clones, or alternatively by silencing of the lymphocytes that have the ability to respond to a given signal. Systemic administration of many superantigens readily induces T-cell activation followed by VβTCR-specific deletion of superantigen-recognizing T cells. This approach to inducing superantigen-specific tolerance would be highly undesirable from the therapeutic point of view, since the prerequisite for the state of tolerance would be systemic administration of the superantigen, which would give rise to life-threatening shock. An alternative approach is to use the nasal rather than the systemic route, thereby bypassing the induction of systemic T-cell activation. This approach has recently been assessed (16), whereby it was shown that (i) intranasal preexposure of the host to the superantigen protected against rapid death upon systemic challenge with the same (but not heterologous) superantigen, (ii) the protection provided was not due to deletion of responsive lymphocytes, nor was it due to triggering of neutralizing antibodies, (iii) protection was mediated by increased production of IL-10, since IL-10-deficient mice were unable to raise protective immunity, and (iv) to achieve protection one needed to provide the wild-type superantigen, since even modest modification of its structure led to failure in tolerance induction.

HOW CAN WE EMPLOY SUPERANTIGENS FOR THE BENEFIT OF THE HOST?

Although superantigens are powerful weapons in the armamentarium of microorganisms, their properties may, in certain situations, be used for the benefit of human beings. Because of their binding properties and their selective lymphocyte-killing properties, superantigens, alone or potentially engineered as conjugates with other proteins, are being used experimentally to interact with severe autoimmune diseases. For example, one could inject relatively low doses of superantigens, which would permit clonal deletion of T cells without inducing a state of hyperactivity in the host. Indeed, this approach has proven to be successful for the prophylaxis/treatment in experimental models of lupus (20) and in EAE (39). The prerequisite for success is the efficient targeting of the relevant T-cell populations (i.e., those that are autoreactive and simultaneously express the superantigen-specific VβTCR epitope (reviewed in reference 23).

FUTURE DIRECTIONS

It has been clear for a decade that microbial superantigens have a significant impact on the expression of autoimmune and immune-mediated diseases. Indeed, depending on the timing and dose of superantigen, injecting of superantigen may affect the incidence and course of an autoimmune disease as outlined above. Further studies on the therapeutic uses of superantigens as well as specific silencing of superantigen-mediated aberrant immune responses are definitely merited.

REFERENCES

1. **Abdelnour, A., T. Bremell, R. Holmdahl, and A. Tarkowski.** 1994. Clonal expansion of T lymphocytes causes arthritis and mortality in mice infected with toxic shock syndrome toxin-1-producing staphylococci. *Eur. J. Immunol.* **24:**1161–1166.
2. **Abdelnour, A., T. Bremell, and A. Tarkowski.** 1994. Toxic shock syndrome toxin 1 contributes to the arthritogenicity of Staphylococcus aureus. *J. Infect. Dis.* **170:**94–99.
3. **Abdelnour, A., and A. Tarkowski.** 1993. Polyclonal B-cell activation by an arthritogenic *Staphylococcus aureus* strain: contribution of T-cells and monokines. *Cell. Immunol.* **147:**279–293.
4. **Andersen, P. S., P. M. Lavoie, R. P. Sekaly, H. Churchill, D. M. Kranz, P. M. Schlievert, K. Karjalainen, and R. A. Mariuzza.** 1999. Role of the T cell receptor alpha chain in stabilizing TCR-superantigen-MHC class II complexes. *Immunity* **10:**473–483.
5. **Annane, D., V. Sebille, C. Charpentier, P. E. Bollaert, B. Francois, J. M. Korach, G. Capellier, Y. Cohen, E. Azoulay, G. Troche, P. Chaumet-Riffaut, and E. Bellissant.** 2002. Effect of treatment with low doses of hydrocortisone and fludrocortisone on mortality in patients with septic shock. *JAMA* **288:**862–871.
6. **Arad, G., D. Hillman, R. Levy, and R. Kaempfer.** 2001. Superantigen antagonist blocks Th1 cytokine gene induction and lethal shock. *J. Leukoc. Biol.* **69:**921–927.
7. **Arad, G., R. Levy, D. Hillman, and R. Kaempfer.** 2000. Superantigen antagonist protects against lethal shock and defines a new domain for T-cell activation. *Nat. Med.* **6:**414–421.
8. **Balaban, N., L. V. Collins, J. S. Cullor, E. B. Hume, E. Medina-Acosta, O. Vieira da Motta, R. O'Callaghan, P. V. Rossitto, M. E. Shirtliff, L. Serafim da Silveira, A. Tarkowski, and J. V. Torres.** 2001. Prevention of diseases caused by *Staphylococcus aureus* using the peptide RIP. *Peptides* **21:**1301–1311.
9. **Bavari, S., B. Dyas, and R. G. Ulrich.** 1996. Superantigen vaccines: a comparative study of genetically attenuated receptor-binding mutants of staphylococcal enterotoxin A. *J. Infect. Dis.* **174:**338–345.
10. **Bean, A. G., R. A. Freiberg, S. Andrade, S. Menon, and A. Zlotnik.** 1993. Interleukin 10 protects mice against staphylococcal enterotoxin B-induced lethal shock. *Infect. Immun.* **61:**4937–4939.
11. **Bernard, G. R., J. L. Vincent, P. F. Laterre, S. P. LaRosa, J. F. Dhainaut, A. Lopez-Rodriguez, J. S. Steingrub, G. E. Garber, J. D. Helterbrand, E. W. Ely, and C. J. Fisher, Jr.** 2001. Efficacy and safety of recombinant human activated protein C for severe sepsis. *N. Engl. J. Med.* **344:**699–709.
12. **Boehncke, W. H., T. M. Zollner, D. Dressel, and R. Kaufmann.** 1997. Induction of psoriasiform inflammation by a bacterial superantigen in the SCID-hu xenogeneic transplantation model. *J. Cutan. Pathol.* **24:**1–7.
13. **Bremell, T., A. Abdelnour, and A. Tarkowski.** 1992. Histopathological and serological progression of experimental *Staphylococcus aureus* arthritis. *Infect. Immun.* **60:**2976–2985.
14. **Brocke, S., A. Gaur, C. Piercy, A. Gautam, K. Gijbels, C. G. Fathman, and L. Steinman.** 1993. Induction of relapsing paralysis in experimental autoimmune encephalomyelitis by bacterial superantigen. *Nature* **365:**642–644.
15. **Cole, B. C., and M. M. Griffiths.** 1993. Triggering and exacerbation of autoimmune arthritis by the Mycoplasma arthritidis superantigen MAM. *Arthritis Rheum.* **36:**994–1002.
16. **Collins, L. V., K. Eriksson, R. G. Ulrich, and A. Tarkowski.** 2002. Mucosal tolerance to a bacterial superantigen indicates a novel pathway to prevent toxic shock. *Infect. Immun.* **70:**2282–2287.

17. **Collins, L. V., S. Hajizadeh, E. Holme, I. M. Jonsson, and A. Tarkowski.** 2004. Endogenously oxidized mitochondrial DNA induces in vivo and in vitro inflammatory responses. *J. Leukoc. Biol.* **75:**995–1000.

18. **Hotchkiss, R. S., P. E. Swanson, C. M. Knudson, K. C. Chang, J. P. Cobb, D. F. Osborne, K. M. Zollner, T. G. Buchman, S. J. Korsmeyer, and I. E. Karl.** 1999. Overexpression of Bcl-2 in transgenic mice decreases apoptosis and improves survival in sepsis. *J. Immunol.* **162:**4148–4156.

19. **Kageyama, Y., Y. Koide, T. Nagata, M. Uchijama, A. Yoshida, T. Arai, T. Miura, C. Miyamoto, and A. Nagano.** 2001. Toxic shock syndrome toxin-1 accelerated collagen-induced arthritis in mice. *J. Autoimmun.* **16:**125–131.

20. **Kim, C., K. A. Siminovitch, and A. Ochi.** 1991. Reduction of lupus nephritis in MRL/lpr mice by a bacterial superantigen treatment. *J. Exp. Med.* **174:**1431–1437.

21. **Kokkola, R., E. Sundberg, A. C. Avebrger, K. Palmblad, H. Yang, K. J. Tracey, U. Andersson, and H. E. Harris.** 2003. Successful treatment of collagen-induced arthritis in mice and rats by targeting extracellular high mobility group box chromosomal protein 1 activity. *Arthritis Rheum.* **48:**2052–2058.

22. **Lehnert, N. M., D. L. Allen, B. L. Allen, P. Catasti, P. R. Shiflett, M. Chen, B. E. Lehnert, and G. Gupta.** 2001. Structure-based design of a bispecific receptor mimic that inhibits T cell responses to a superantigen. *Biochemistry* **40:**4222–4228.

23. **Li, H., A. Llera, E. L. Malchiodi, and R. A. Mariuzza.** 1999. The structural basis of T cell activation by superantigens. *Annu. Rev. Immunol.* **17:**435–466.

24. **Lundberg, K., S. Nijenhuis, E. R. Vossenaar, K. Palmblad, W. J. van Venrooij, L. Klareskog, A. J. Zendman, and H. E. Harris.** 2005.Citrullinated proteins have increased immunogenicity and arthritogenicity and their presence in arthritic joints correlates with disease severity. *Arthritis Res. Ther.* **7:**R458–R467.

25. **McCormick, J. K., J. M. Yarwood, and P. M. Schlievert.** 2001. Toxic shock syndrome and bacterial superantigens: an update. *Annu. Rev. Microbiol.* **55:**77–104.

26. **Nilsson, I. M., M. Verdrengh, R. G. Ulrich, S. Bavari, and A. Tarkowski.** 1999. Protection against *Staphylococcus aureus* sepsis by vaccination with recombinant staphylococcal enterotoxin A devoid of superantigenicity. *J. Infect. Dis.* **180:**1370–1373.

27. **Novick, R. P., H. F. Ross, S. J. Projan, J. Kornblum, B. Kreiswirth, and S. Moghazeh.** 1993. Synthesis of staphylococcal virulence factors is controlled by regulatory RNA molecule. *EMBO J.* **12:**3967–3975.

28. **Omata, S., T. Sasaki, K. Kakimoto, and U. Yamashita.** 1997. Staphylococcal enterotoxin B induces arthritis in female DBA/1 mice but fails to induce activation of type II collagen-reactive lymphocytes. *Cell. Immunol.* **179:**138–145.

29. **Palmqvist, N., T. J. Foster, A. Tarkowski, and E. Josefsson.** 2002. Protein A is a virulence factor in Staphylococcus aureus arthritis and septic death. *Microb. Pathog.* **33:**239–249.

30. **Palmqvist, N., G. J. Silverman, E. Josefsson, and A. Tarkowski.** 2005. Bacterial cell wall-expressed protein A triggers supraclonal B-cell responses upon in vivo infection with Staphylococcus aureus. *Microbes Infect.* **7:**1501–1511.

31. **Reinhart, K., and W. Karzai.** 2001. Anti-tumor necrosis factor therapy in sepsis: update on clinical trials and lessons learned. *Crit. Care Med.* **29:**S121–S125.

32. **Riedemann, N. C., R. F. Guo, and P. A. Ward.** 2003. Novel strategies for the treatment of sepsis. *Nat. Med.* **9:**517–524.

33. **Saha, B., B. Jaklic, D. M. Harlan, G. S. Gray, C. H. June, and R. Abe.** 1996. Toxic shock syndrome toxin-1-induced death is prevented by CTLA4Ig. *J. Immunol.* **157:**3869–3875.

34. **Sakiniene, E., T. Bremell, and A. Tarkowski.** 1996. Addition of corticosteroids to antibiotic treatment ameliorates the course of experimental Staphylococcus aureus arthritis. *Arthritis Rheum.* **39:**1596–1605.

35. **Schiffenbauer, J., H. M. Johnson, E. J. Butfiloski, L. Wegrzyn, and J. M. Soos.** 1993. Staphylococcal enterotoxins can reactivate experimental allergic encephalomyelitis. *Proc. Natl. Acad. Sci. USA* **90:**8543–8546.

36. **Schiffenbauer, J., J. M. Soos, and H. M. Johnson.** 1998. The possible role of bacterial superantigens in the pathogenesis of autoimmune disorders. *Immunol. Today* **19:**117–120.

37. **Schwab, J. H., R. R. Brown, S. K. Anderle, and P. M. Schlievert.** 1993. Superantigen can reactivate bacterial cell wall-induced arthritis. *J. Immunol.* **150:**4151–4159.

38. **Soos, J. M., M. G. Mujtaba, J. Schiffenbauer, B. A. Torres, and H. M. Johnson.** 2002. Intramolecular epitope spreading induced by staphylococcal enterotoxin superantigen reactivation of experimental allergic encephalomyelitis. *J. Neuroimmunol.* **123:**30–34.

39. **Soos, J. M., J. Schiffenbauer, and H. M. Johnson.** 1993. Treatment of PL/J mice with the superantigen, staphylococcal enterotoxin B, prevents development of experimental allergic encephalomyelitis. *J. Neuroimmunol.* **43:**39–43.

40. Tarkowski, A., M. Bokarewa, L. V. Collins, I. Gjertsson, O. H. Hultgren, T. Jin, I. M. Jonsson, E. Josefsson, E. Sakiniene, and M. Verdrengh. 2002. Current status of pathogenetic mechanisms in staphylococcal arthritis. *FEMS Microbiol. Lett.* **217:**125–132.

41. Visvanathan, K., A. Charles, J. Bannan, P. Pugach, K. Kashfi, and J. B. Zabriskie. 2001. Inhibition of bacterial superantigens by peptides and antibodies. *Infect. Immun.* **69:**875–884.

42. Yamamoto, T., M. Matsuuchi, I. Katayama, and K. Nishioka. 1998. Repeated subcutaneous injection of staphylococcal enterotoxin B-stimulated lymphocytes retains epidermal thickness of psoriatic skin-graft onto severe combined immunodeficient mice. *J. Dermatol. Sci.* **17:**8–14.

43. Zimbelman, J., A. Palmer, and J. Todd. 1999. Improved outcome of clindamycin compared with beta-lactam antibiotic treatment for invasive Streptococcus pyogenes infection. *Pediatr. Infect. Dis. J.* **18:**1096–1100.

Chapter 11

Experimental Models of Superantigen-Mediated Neuropathology

Malte E. Kornhuber, Alexander Emmer, Kristina Gerlach,
and M. S. Staege

INTRODUCTION

Inflammatory diseases of the nervous system are frequent and often result in permanent disability. In some of these diseases etiology and pathogenesis have been largely established, as in herpes encephalitis. In contrast, the so-called autoimmune diseases of the central nervous system are less well understood. Superantigens have been suggested to play a role, in particular, in multiple sclerosis (MS) (21, 27, 31).

There have been different attempts with superantigen to modify experimental allergic encephalomyelitis (EAE), which is taken as an animal modal for MS. Relapses of EAE can be either attenuated (26, 30, 35) or precipitated by superantigen (4, 28). The contradictory results depend at least in part on whether encephalitogenic T cells are stimulated directly in a Vβ-specific manner and become anergic afterward, or if these T cells become activated or disinhibited indirectly after superantigenic stimulation (7). These observations are of therapeutic importance, since effects of superantigens in the more complex human immune system may be unforeseeable.

MS is not simply an inflammatory disease like EAE. It is well established that in MS chronic degeneration runs in parallel to outbreaks of inflammation. The portions of inflammation and degeneration may vary so that different types of disease course can be distinguished. Contrary to what might be expected, recent studies indicate that the degenerative process is not always secondary to but may also precede neuroinflammation. Weeks or months before cerebral inflammatory plaques became manifest by contrast enhancement on nuclear magnetic resonance imaging (NMRI), subtle changes developed in their place (11). Histological investigation of the newly forming plaque showed degeneration of myelin-forming oligodendrocytes without signs of inflammation (2). Therefore

Malte E. Kornhuber, Alexander Emmer, and Kristina Gerlach • Neurology Hospital, Martin Luther University, D-06097 Halle-Wittenberg, Germany. *M. S. Staege* • Children's Cancer Research Center, Division of Pediatric Hematology and Oncology, Martin Luther University, D-06097 Halle-Wittenberg, Germany.

plaques presumably display a peculiar evolution from pure degenerative lesions to a mixed inflammatory-degenerative state. Accordingly, different types of plaques with or without inflammation have been identified previously by histological techniques (20). In the earliest clinical phase of relapsing-remitting MS, when there were only very few plaques seen on NMRI, widespread axonal loss was already present (8, 9), which could not be attributed to the effects of focal lesions. This interpretation is supported by the fact that plaques vanish in parallel with interferon beta treatment, while accumulation of disability (24) or of diffuse axonal damage goes on (22).

Most if not all pieces of the pathogenetic puzzle of MS thus fit to a diffuse primary degenerative disease with secondary temporary and focal outbreaks of inflammation. Results of migration studies are in agreement with acquisition of MS early in life (5). There have been many attempts to search for such an infectious etiology in MS. Up to now no pathogen has been unequivocally established to be the cause of MS. Nevertheless, there are promising candidates such as MS-associated retrovirus (MSRV) (23). Actually, in parallel to EAE viral disease models for MS have been developed in laboratory animals, e.g., encephalomyelitis following infection with Theiler's virus or canine distemper virus (3, 32). In EAE and in the virus models inflammatory tissue damage is usually observed. However, silent progression as in MS is better reflected by the viral models. As viruses may encode for superantigens, these are candidates to connect viral degeneration with inflammation in central nervous system (CNS) tissue.

The following experiments demonstrate that superantigen expressed in the brain or spinal cord is capable of inducing neuroinflammation as in MS. Part of the data has previously been published (15).

EFFECTS OF INTRACEREBRAL T-CELL SUPERANTIGEN

Staphylococcal enterotoxin (SE) superantigens were purchased from Toxin Technology (Sarasota, Fla.). Forty-microliter aliquots of superantigen or saline were slowly injected intracerebrally through a small burr hole in isoflurane-anesthetized male 300-g Lewis rats 2.5 mm lateral from the midline at the bregma at a depth of 3.5 mm. Histological analysis was performed after fixing the brain with 4% buffered paraformaldehyde. Horizontal sections of the cerebral hemispheres at the corpus callosum and at the level of the lateral ventricles were stained with hematoxylin/eosin. In a pilot trial two animals were injected with 1 mg/ml SEA. The brains were removed 5 days later in deep anesthesia. Cuffings of perivascular round cells were identified scattered around the injection canal in both animals. When the initial experiments with SEA were repeated several times with different intervals from 1 to 32 days between injection and sacrification ($n = 36$), the results were disappointing in that the reproducibility of focal perivascular round cell cuffings was low. In the first 3 days, more or less, few perivascular round cells could be observed in both hemispheres with a preponderance in the corpus callosum and the periventricular white matter. Thereafter perivascular round cells were detected around the injection canal in several animals up to 12 days after SEA injection. Maximum response in the injected hemisphere was seen up to 8 days after injection (Fig. 1). On average 6.7 ± 6.1 reactive vessels were detected between days 4 and 8 ($n = 12$). The effect of SEE, SEB, toxic shock syndrome toxin (TSST) 1 or saline was investigated 5 days after intracerebral injection (two animals in each group). Reactive blood vessels were identified after injection of SEE or TSST1 but not with SEB or saline (Fig. 1).

The cerebral perivascular inflammatory reaction demonstrated that superantigen expressed in the brain can induce round cells to invade the CNS and persist around blood vessels in the vicinity of the injection site. Thus, superantigens were presumably bound by constitutively major histocompatibility complex (MHC)-positive perivascular cells, presumably microglial cells. Round cells surveilling the brain came in contact with superantigen-presenting cells. A relatively short-lived inflammatory reaction was initiated lasting for 1 to 2 weeks. As no similar response was seen with saline or SEB, the effect could not be attributed to nonspecific effects of the injection procedure, but was considered as superantigen specific. The lack of stimulatory potency of SEB in Lewis rats is in accord with previous results (26).

We wondered why the response to superantigen was so variable and disappointingly low. Relatively good results had been obtained in the two pilot animals. While experiments were performed at least 2 weeks after shipment of the animals, in the pilot trial the two animals had been treated on the day after receipt from the breeder. Therefore, the stress of transportation might have somehow influenced the results. We argued also that relapses in multiple sclerosis are often precipitated by some nonspecific immune stress-like infection. Furthermore, it was known that only activated immune cells were capable of invading the CNS (33). For these reasons we tried to imitate the stress response by loading the blood with activated lymphocytes.

ACTIVATED SPLENOCYTES AMPLIFY SUPERANTIGEN ENCEPHALITIS

The experimental procedure was as described above. Activated syngeneic splenocytes were injected in volumes of 0.5 ml through the tail vein or penis vein on the third day after intracerebral injection of superantigen. Activation of splenocytes was achieved in the following way (all steps were performed under sterile conditions): A spleen was removed from a male 300-g Lewis rat under deep isoflurane anesthesia. The spleen was cut and the content passaged through a sieve into isotonic NaCl. Cells were washed three times and the pellet finally resuspended in Click's RPMI (Seromed, Berlin, Germany) with 5% heat-inactivated fetal calf serum (Vitromex, Selters, Germany) and with a final concentration of 2 μg/ml concanavalin A (ConA) (Pharmacia, Uppsala, Sweden). Cells were harvested and washed three times after 3 days in culture when they were maximally stimulated. They were kept in NaCl on ice for injection purposes. Usually 10^7 cells were injected intravenously under brief general anesthesia with isoflurane. The time course of the tissue reaction to 1 mg/ml SEA was investigated with 24 animals. In general, perivascular round cell infiltrates were more numerous and more reproducible than without adding activated splenocytes. In the first 3 days after splenocyte injection, reactive vessels were seen in the corpus callosum and around the ventricles in both hemispheres. Thereafter, inflamed blood vessels were confined to the injected hemisphere. The response was most intense 4 to 8 days after intravenous injection and vanished up to the 12th day. Thereafter, no reactive vessel could be identified. On days 4 through 8 after intravenous injection, on average 18.5 ± 11.4 (7 through 39) vessels with round cell cuffs were observed ($n = 14$ animals). When compared to the corresponding numbers obtained without activated splenocytes, the difference was statistically significant ($P < 0.05$;

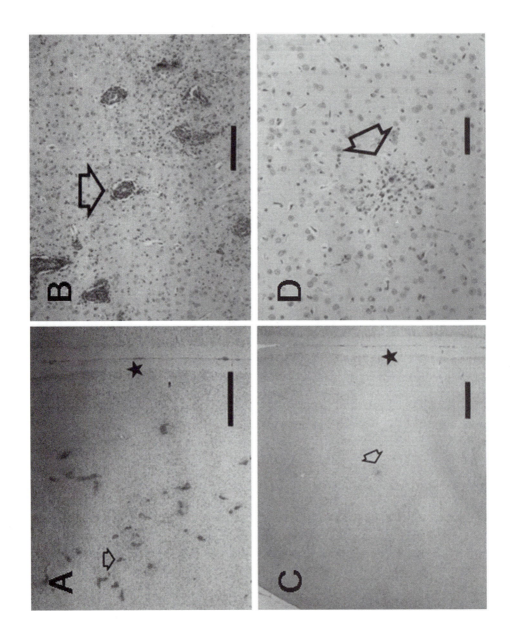

two-sided U test). Similarly high numbers of reactive blood vessels were obtained with intracerebral SEE or TSST1 5 days after intravenous loading of 10^7 activated splenocytes per animal, but not with saline or SEB (two animals in each group).

In further experiments the influence of the superantigen concentration or of the number of activated splenocytes on the tissue reaction was investigated. When the amount of activated splenocytes was kept constant at 10^7 per animal, the number of reactive blood vessels increased linearly with the concentration of SEA ($n = 10$; Fig. 2a). When the injected SEA was kept constant at 1 mg/ml, the number of reactive blood vessels increased linearly with the number of activated splenocytes injected intravenously ($n = 6$; Fig. 2b).

In four rats SEA was injected into the lateral ventricle followed by intravenous injection of 10^7 ConA-activated splenocytes 3 days later. All these animals developed a prominent inflammatory reaction within the meninges. Meningitis has not been our main interest and was not further studied. Nevertheless, the results are in accord with the view that T-cell superantigen is capable of inducing or at least enhancing viral or bacterial meningitis.

The results obtained with activated splenocytes confirm the conclusions drawn above. Actually, the amplification of an inflammatory response in the brain by antigen-naive splenocytes comes close to the situation in MS where relapses are precipitated by various nonspecific challenges of the immune system.

In the Lewis rat SEA does not stimulate T cells specific for myelin basic protein (MBP) (26). Although a role for myelin-specific T cells cannot be completely ruled out in superantigen encephalitis, these cells are not necessary to explain the presented results.

We wondered whether superantigen encephalitis shared further similarities with neuroinflammation as seen in MS. For this purpose, the inflammatory response to SEA was investigated by immunocytochemistry or by gene expression profiles. Results from these experiments have not been published previously.

CD8(+) SUPPRESSOR T-CELLS PREVAIL
IN SUPERANTIGEN ENCEPHALITIS

Experiments were performed as described above with minor modifications. Animals were perfused through the aorta ascendens with 0.9% NaCl prior to sacrifice. After removal from the skull, brains were immediately frozen at $-80°C$ in isohexan on dry ice for 1 min. Cryocut (4°C) tissue sections of 4-μm thickness were fixed with acetone for 10 min and washed in Tris buffer between every working step. Nonspecific binding was blocked with 5% heat-inactivated goat serum (Intrastat) for 20 min. All antibodies were used in a dilution of 1:50 in 0.9% sodium phosphate buffer (BD Biosciences Pharmingen). Slices were incubated at room temperature for 60 min with the primary antibody, for 30 min with the secondary antibody coupled with streptavidin. After light-brown color was seen with diaminobenzidine

Figure 1. The figure illustrates the effects of intracerebral superantigen alone. Frontal sections of the rat brain at the level of the corpus callosum (cc), hematoxylin and eosin stain. The interhemispheric cleft has been marked by a star. (A) Five days after intracerebral SEA (bar, 1 mm). (B) Part of A at higher magnification. (C, D) Seven days after intracerebral SEB injection (SEB does not activate T cells in rats) and 4 days after intravenous ConA-blast injection; no reactive vessels are observed. The injection canal is surrounded by a few brownish macrophages, presumably containing blood degeneration products.

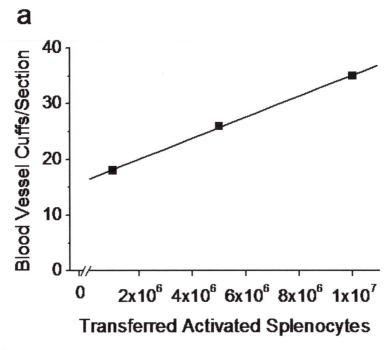

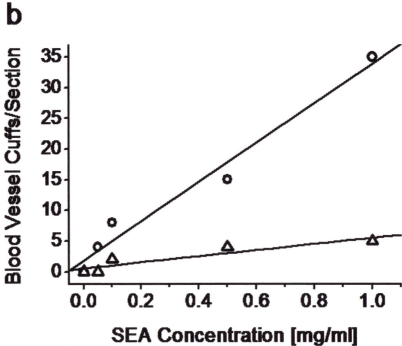

Figure 2. Each data point represents the mean value obtained from at least two animals. All data sets were supplied with a linear fit. (a) The number of reactive blood vessels per tissue section rises linearly with the number of activated splenocytes injected intravenously. (b) The number of vessel cuffs on representative brain sections is displayed over the SEA concentration. SEA per se, open upward triangles; SEA plus ConA blasts, open circles (see text).

(DAB), slices were washed with tap water and incubated for 1 minute with Mayer's Hämalaun. Sections were fixed in alcohol and saved with Rotihistokitt. Monoclonal primary antibodies were used to detect CD3 (T cells), CD4 (T-helper cells), CD8 (T-suppressor cells), CD45 (primarily staining B cells in rats), and CD68 (microglia).

The superantigen encephalitis consisted almost completely of CD3+ T cells. These were mainly CD8+ suppressor/cytotoxic T cells, while less than 10% were CD4+ helper T cells. Few CD45+ B cells were identified (less than 1%). Beside the perivascular distribution, cells could also be seen scattered in the parenchyma. During the following days, the numbers of T cells decreased as seen previously. A strong activation of microglial elements (CD68+) was identified in the inflamed area with a perivascular and a periventricular distribution.

EAE is commonly mediated by CD4+ helper T cells. By way of contrast, a preponderance of CD8+ T cells is common to superantigen encephalitis and to the inflammatory MS plaque (1, 29). In the MS plaque, part of the CD8+ suppressor/cytotoxic T cells belong to few clones that have in common certain Vβ subtypes of the T-cell receptor (1, 17, 29), features that can be expected when a superantigen is involved in the pathogenesis.

GENE EXPRESSION PROFILE OF SUPERANTIGEN ENCEPHALITIS

Because superantigen encephalitis shares striking similarities with neuroinflammation in MS, we became interested whether this was also true for gene expression. Male Lewis rats weighing 300 g were treated as described above. Three rats received SEA intracerebrally and activated splenocytes intravenously. Another three rats were injected with saline intracerebrally and with activated splenocytes intravenously. Brains were removed 5 days after intravenous injection and after perfusing the animals through the ascending aorta with 0.9% NaCl in deep anesthesia. Immediately afterward coronary 1.5-mm slices were taken from both hemispheres separately at the injection site from each animal. The slices were shock frozen in isohexan on dry ice for 1 min and stored at −80°C until analysis. Total RNA was prepared in TRIzol (Invitrogen) and purified with RNeasy kit (Quiagen). cDNA was prepared using Superscript-Choice-System (Invitrogen). Rat Genome U34A microarrays were used to study gene expression profiles. SAM 2.0 was used for statistical purposes. In addition to the required statistical significance, acceptance of differential gene expression demanded a minimum cut-off of two times above or below the control level.

In the SEA group 276 of 8,800 genes showed a significantly higher gene expression level than controls, whereas expression of 380 genes was significantly lower. Table 1 shows part of the results for genes that showed elevated expression levels in the superantigen group. Among them were many of the genes that were previously found to be upregulated during neuroinflammation in MS (19) or in EAE (13).

SUPERANTIGENS AND OLIGOCLONAL IMMUNOGLOBULIN SYNTHESIS IN THE CNS

Taken together different lines of evidence support the concept that T-cell superantigens expressed in the CNS may induce a cellular perivascular inflammatory reaction. While superantigen encephalitis may also be of pathogenetic relevance in bacterial or viral encephalitis or meningitis, its similarities with neuroinflammation in MS constitute a

Table 1. Gene expression of superantigen encephalitis (amplified by 10^7 ConA-blast i.v.) in CNS 7 days after SEA injection, at least 2-fold increase

Stage	Gene product
Antigen processing and presentation	MHC class II (multiple genes)
	MHC class I (multiple genes)
	Fc gamma receptor
	CD3, CD3d, CD48
	Proteasome subunit R-Ring 12
	Proteasome subunit RC1
	DORA
	Moesin
T-lymphocyte activation/apoptosis	S100A4
	CD5, CD13, CD37, CD38, CD39
	T-cell differentiation antigen
	OX-8 antigen
	Sak-a konase
	Ets-1
	RAS2
	Granzyme K
	Galectin
Cytokines and receptors	Mob-1
	rNFIL-6
	RANTES
	CCR1
	CCR5
	STAT1
	Galectin-3
	Gfi-zink-finger protein
	TGFβ-1
	gro
	Osteopontin
	Vav
	Interferon regulatory factor 1
	TNF receptor; TNF1 receptor
	RGS1
	P21 (cip)
	SOCS-3
	PLC-β3
	CD2-p59
	Gal/Galnac
	Ly-6b
	LyF-1
	Calpastatin
	Caspase 1
	drs
Cell contact or migration	TenascinC
	Rho-Protein
	Integrin alpha
	MCP-1
	uPAR, uPAR1
	LCA
	ICAM-1
	CD44
	MMP2, MMP9

Table 1. *Continued*

Stage	Gene product
Cell contact or migration—cont'd	CapG
	Syndecan
	Fibronectin
	BMK1/ERK5
	Granzyme
	Tyrosine kinase
	Protein tyrosine kinase
	SHP-1
Monocyte activation/complement system	Adipsin
	AIF-1
	aP2
	S100-related
	Lipocalin-2
	Lyn-kinase
	AnnexinI, Annexin II, Annexin III
	CD14
	ADRP
	BMP-2, BMP-7
	BMRP
	Osteocalcin
	Decorin
	β_2-microglobulin
	ARP2/3
Astrocyte reaction	GFAP
	GFAP, alternatively spliced
	HSP-27
	Alpha-2-macroglobulin
	Insulin-like growth factor-1
	TIMP-1
	Neurocan
	RDC-1 protein
	Atrial natriuretic factor
	C1-inhibitor
	Vimentin
Microglial reaction/phagocytosis	C1q, C3, C4
	P2-purinoceptor
	aP2
	CapG
	Lysozyme
	CathepsinD
	ADRP
Neuronal stress reaction	Neurotransmitter reporter rB21a
	Rat Prolactin gene
	Retinol dehydrogenase type II
	MKP3
	SBK signaling in brain development
Gene expression	Polypyrimidine tract-binding protein
	CREM
	CELF

Table continues

Table 1. *Continued*

Stage	Gene product
Gene expression—*continued*	Histone Hd1
	DNS topoisomerase IIa
	Chromosomal protein HMG-2
	Synaptonemal complex lateral element protein
Vascular reaction/extracellular matrix	Syndecan
	mRNA expressed in carotid artery tissue
	ACLP
	Lysyl oxidase
	Fibronectin
	Alpha-1 type 1 collagen
	Ceruloplasmin
	Hexokinase, hexokinase II
	Lysozyme
	Ornithine carbamoyltransferase
	Glycerol-3-phosphate acyltransferase mRNA
	GM2-activating protein
	Glyceraldehyde-3-phosphate dehydrogenase
	ASM15
	Rpe-65
	Immediate early serum response JE gene
	Brain factor 2
	Pro alpha 1 collagen type III
	PEST interacting protein
	Tropoelastin
Oxidative stress reaction	Cytochrome b558
	Cytochrome P450
	Gp91-phox
	Hemeoxygenase, hemeozygenase 1
	Metallothionein
	SOD-2

powerful explanation for the immune part of this disease. However, at least one important feature of MS cannot be explained by T-cell superantigen, namely the local and oligoclonal expression of immunoglobulins (Igs). Oligoclonal IgG which is a frequent and diagnostically relevant finding in MS could not be detected in cerebrospinal fluid (CSF) specimens taken from rats by suboccipital puncture after intracerebral exposure to SE (15). Ig genes were not found to be differentially expressed between controls or SEA-treated animals as outlined above. In fact, formation of Ig can hardly be expected in the CNS by use of T-cell superantigen. When the Ig synthesis in the nervous system in MS is considered, the following facts have to be taken into consideration: Ig is found in CSF but not in blood. Among the oligoclonal Igs there are specificities against multiple epitopes, and only a small minority of the Ig is specific for antigens present in the CNS (14). In fact there is a multitude of antigen specificities among the immunoglobulins in CSF from MS patients (25).

JOINT ACTION OF B-CELL SUPERANTIGENS AND T-CELL SUPERANTIGENS IN MS?

The known facts do not support a role for T-cell superantigen in Ig synthesis within the CNS. Furthermore, superantigen in the periphery is not essential in maintaining inflammation in the CNS, although systemic effects of superantigens may contribute to the activation of T or B cells outside the CNS. Antibody synthesis in B cells can be driven by conventional antigens or, e.g., by B-cell superantigens. Remarkably, potent B-cell superantigens are encoded by bacteria (e.g., staphylococcal protein A, SPA) or by viruses (e.g., the gp120 protein of HIV). Actually, oligoclonal Ig is frequently detected in the CSF of patients with HIV encephalopathy. Thus, it is not too far to speculate that oligoclonal Ig in MS may be due to B-cell superantigenic stimulation within the nervous system (16).

After intracerebral injection of the B-cell superantigen SPA into Lewis rats followed by intravenous loading of 10^7 ConA splenocyte blasts, we could not detect any inflammatory reaction in the brain nor were there oligoclonal CSF bands on agarose gels by isoelectric focussing (unpublished observations). These negative results were to be expected, since B-cell superantigens exert their effects after binding to Ig epitopes. But different from constitutively expressed MHC molecules on microglial cells to which T-cell superantigens bind, Ig epitopes are not commonly present in the CNS. Either the B-cell superantigens stay in the CNS over long times and activate the few B cells passing the blood-brain barrier by chance or they act on B cells that enter the CNS during periods of inflammation. As part of B-cell functions need costimulation from T cells, B-cell superantigens do not likely act per se. Rather they specifically stimulate part of those B cells that were attracted into cerebral tissue by a T-cell-driven inflammatory process (see above). When the combined action of T- and B-cell superantigens is taken into consideration, their effects may vary due to individual differences of the human immune system. There may be a preponderance of T- or B-cell responses or even a weak or almost absent inflammatory reaction as in primary progressive MS. Differences in the immune reaction may be reflected by the diverse appearance of inflammatory plaques of MS patients by histopathologic methods (20).

WHICH FEATURES OF MS CAN BE EXPLAINED BY THE NEW MODEL?

MS as a Viral Disease

The presumably viral origin of MS explains acquisition early in childhood (5). As in other bacterial or viral diseases of the nervous system such as borreliosis or measles panencephalitis or as in Theiler's virus disease of rodents, it is possible that only a few of the individuals originally infected will finally develop cerebral metadisease. This fact would explain that transmission of MS is seldom if at all observed. The presumably viral pathogenesis of MS is in accord with the fact that subtle degeneration (11) and sometimes even pronounced oligodendrocyte apoptosis (2) precede the inflammatory transformation of MS plaques. Remyelination is incomplete in MS (12). It may be impeded by viral presence in the CNS. Diffuse neurodegeneration is present at the earliest clinical stages of the disease (8, 9) and progresses during its entire course independently from the presence of immune phenomena or their treatment (6, 22, 24). On NMRI, correlates of neurodegeneration comprise diffuse atrophy or subtle alterations of cerebral tissue as identified, e.g., by magnetization transfer imaging (10). Substances that suppress or modify inflammation in MS do not necessarily suppress viral activities. Therefore, the failure of immunotherapy to inhibit silent progression in MS is in accord with a viral pathogenesis.

MS and T-Cell Superantigens

Inflammatory plaques in MS consist mainly of T cells. Unlike in many rodent autoimmune models, the cellular immune response in MS is predominantly of the T-suppressor/cytotoxic phenotype, sometimes with expansion of only few clones of T cells. Although it cannot be completely ruled out that the outlined findings in MS plaques are due to myelin-autoantigen-specific T cells, the similarities with the perivascular infiltrates seen in the brain after local expression of superantigen are striking. The antigen specificities of T-cell infiltrates in MS plaques are not known. When T-cell superantigen is involved, myelin-specific T cells are expected to play a minor role if at all.

It is well known that relapsing-remitting MS patients with frequent relapses progress faster than patients with less frequent relapses (6). The correlation between frequency of relapses and progression of the disease need not necessarily reflect a causal relation. When intracerebral expression of a viral superantigen is taken into consideration, its expression will depend on viral activity. This would mean that superantigen-driven relapses occur more frequently with faster progression of viral degeneration. Finally, HLA associations identified in patients with a relapsing-remitting course of MS may be due to MHC-specific binding properties of T-cell superantigens.

MS and B-Cell Superantigens

Oligoclonal Ig found in CSF or in plaques of MS patients displays a broad diversity of non-myelin specificities. Although not formally proven, this pattern is well explained by the action of a B-cell superantigen. It can hardly be due to myelin autoantigen or to T-cell super-antigen. Whether a pure B-cell superantigen acts in combination with a pure T-cell superantigen or whether there are substances combining both properties remains to be elucidated.

Up to now all evidence in favor of the presence of superantigen in MS is indirect. Actually, it will be hard to establish the presence of superantigen in MS directly, since these substances stimulate immune cells at concentrations 10^3 to 10^4 times lower than those of conventional antigens. Perhaps it might be easier to draw conclusions from sequence information of MS-specific viruses, once they are established.

It is quite clear that different pathogenetic principles may lead to autoimmune diseases of the CNS. Paraneoplastic encephalomyelitis or neuromyelitis optica (NMO) are examples for diseases that are initiated outside the CNS. Unlike in MS cerebrospinal fluid of patients with NMO usually does not contain oligoclonal IgG (34). Furthermore, in NMO specific serum antibodies against aquaporin-4 have been established recently (18).

SUPERANTIGENS AND NEUROMUSCULAR DISEASES

Different so-called autoimmune diseases involve nerves or muscles. Pathogens like bacteria or viruses are involved in part of them. Although it is likely that true autoimmune phenomena following molecular mimicry are of pathogenetic relevance in some of these diseases, it seems possible that superantigens are involved in parallel or alone in a subgroup of patients with autoimmune neuritis or myositis.

FURTHER RESEARCH STRATEGIES

The following points seem worth studying further: (i) The development of devices for the continuous expression of superantigen in nervous tissue is needed to set up a more realistic model for the immune part of MS. (ii) When continuous presence of superantigen is realized, discontinuous activation of the immune system in the periphery might parallel the relapsing-remitting type of course in MS in a predictable manner. (iii) It will be interesting to see whether the joint action of T- and B-cell superantigens may induce the expression of oligoclonal Ig in the CNS. (iv) Detection of superantigen in MS is a rewarding goal, although it does not seem easy to reach directly. (v) Because T-cell superantigen is capable of anergizing T cells, this might become a therapeutic strategy in MS.

Acknowledgment. We are grateful to R. Kiefer, Dept. of Neurology, Universitätsklinikum Münster (Germany), for valuable advice on immunocytochemistry.

REFERENCES

1. **Babbe, H., A. Roers, A. Waisman, H. Lassmann, N. Goebels, R. Hohlfeld, M. Friese, R. Schroeder, M. Deckert, S. Schmidt, R. Ravid, and K. Rajewski.** 2000. Clonal expansions of CD8(+) T cells dominate the T cell infiltrate in active multiple sclerosis lesions as shown by micromanipulation and single cell polymerase chain reaction. *J. Exp. Med.* **192:**393–404.
2. **Barnett, M. H., and J. W. Prineas.** 2004. Relapsing and remitting multiple sclerosis: pathology of the newly forming lesion. *Ann. Neurol.* **55:**458–468.
3. **Bieber, A. J., D. R. Ure, and M. Rodriguez.** 2005. Genetically dominant spinal cord repair in a murine model of chronic progressive multiple sclerosis. *J. Neuropathol. Exp. Neurol.* **64:**46–57.
4. **Brocke, S., A. Gaur, C. Piercy, A. Gautam, K. Gijbels, C. G. Fathman, and L. Steinman.** 1993. Induction of relapsing paralysis in experimental autoimmune encephalomyelitis by bacterial superantigen. *Nature* **365:**642–644.
5. **Cabre, P., A. Signate, S. Olindo, H. Merle, D. Caparros-Lefebvre, O. Bera, and D. Smadja.** 2005. Role of return migration in the emergence of multiple sclerosis in the French West Indies. *Brain* **128:**2899–2910.
6. **Confavreux, C., S. Vukusic, T. Moreau, and P. Adeleine.** 2000. Relapses and progression of disability in multiple sclerosis. *N. Engl. J. Med.* **343:**1430–1438.
7. **Das, M. R., A. Cohen, S. S. Zamvil, H. Offner, and V. K. Kuchroo.** 1996. Prior exposure to superantigen can inhibit or exacerbate autoimmune encephalomyelitis: T-cell repertoire engaged by the autoantigen determines clinical outcome. *J. Neuroimmunol.* **71:**3–10.
8. **De Stefano, N., S. Narayanan, S. J. Francis, S. Smith, M. Mortilla, M. C. Tartaglia, M. L. Bartolozzi, L. Guidi, A. Federico, and D. L. Arnold.** 2002. Diffuse axonal and tissue injury in patients with multiple sclerosis with low lesion load and no disability. *Arch. Neurol.* **59:**1565–1571.
9. **Filippi, M., M. Bozzali, M. Rovaris, O. Gonen, C. Kasevadas, A. Ghezi, V. Martinelli, R. I. Grossman, G. Scotti, G. Comi, and A. Falini.** 2003. Evidence for widespread axonal damage at the earliest clinic stage of multiple sclerosis. *Brain* **126:**433–437.
10. **Filippi, M., A. Campi, V. Dousset, C. Baratti, V. Martinelli, N. Canal, G. Scotti, and G. Comi.** 1995. A magnetization transfer imaging study of normal-appearing white matter in multiple sclerosis. *Neurology* **45:**478–482.
11. **Filippi, M., M. A. Rocca, G. Martino, M. A. Horsfield, and G. Comi.** 1998. Magnetization transfer changes in the normal appearing white matter precede the appearance of enhancing lesions in patients with multiple sclerosis. *Ann. Neurol.* **43:**809–814.
12. **Franklin, R. J.** 2002. Why does remyelination fail in multiple sclerosis. *Nat. Rev. Neurosci.* **3:**705–714.
13. **Jelinsky, S. A., J. S. Miyashiro, K. A. Saraf, C. Tunkey, P. Reddy, J. Newcombe, J. L. Oesreicher, E. Brown, W. L. Trepicchio, J. P. Leonard, and S. Marusic.** 2005. Exploiting genotypic differences to identify genes important for EAE development. *J. Neurol. Sci.* **239:**81–93.

14. **Kaiser, R., M. Obert, R. Kaufmann, and M. Czygan.** 1997. IgG-antibodies to CNS proteins in patients with multiple sclerosis. *Eur. J. Med. Res.* **2:**169–172.

15. **Kornhuber, M. E., C. Ganz, R. Lang, T. Brill, and W. Schmahl.** 2002. Focal encephalitis in the Lewis rat induced by intracerebral superantigen and amplified by activated intravenous splenocytes. *Neurosci. Lett.* **324:**93–96.

16. **Kornhuber, M. E., and S. Zierz.** 2003. Possibilities and limitations of immunotherapy in multiple sclerosis. Inflammatory and degenerative parts of the disease require a new pathogenetic effect. *Nervenarzt* **74:**537–538.

17. **Lee, S. J., K. W. Wucherpfennig, S. A. Brod, D. Benjamin, H. L. Weiner, and D. A. Hafler.** 1991. Common T-cell receptor V beta usage in oligoclonal T lymphocytes derived from cerebrospinal fluid and blood of patients with multiple sclerosis. *Ann. Neurol.* **29:**33–40.

18. **Lennon, V. A., D. M. Wingerchuk, T. J. Kryzer, S. J. Pittock, C. F. Jucchinetti, K. Fujihara, I. Nakashima, and B. G. Weinshenker.** 2004. A serum autoantibody marker of neuromyelitis optica: distinction from multiple sclerosis. *Lancet* **364:**2106–2112.

19. **Lock, C., G. Hermans, R. Pedotti, A. Brendolan, E. Schadt, H. Garren, A. Langer-Gould, S. Strober, B. Canella, J. Allard, P. Klonowski, A. Austin, N. Lad, N. Kaminski, S. J. Galli, J. R. Oksenberg, C. S. Raine, R. Heller, and L. Steinman.** 2002. Gene-microarray analysis of multiple sclerosis lesions yields new targets validated in autoimmune encephalomyelitis. *Nat. Med.* **8:**500–508.

20. **Lucchinetti, C., W. Brück, J. Parisi, B. Scheithauer, M. Rodriguez, and H. Lassmann.** 2000. Heterogeneity of multiple sclerosis lesions: implications for the pathogenesis of demyelination. *Ann. Neurol.* **47:**707–717.

21. **Meyer, O.** 1995. Superantigens and their implications in autoimmune diseases. *Presse Med.* **24:**1171–1177.

22. **Parry, A., R. Corkill, A. M. Blamire, J. Palace, S. Narayanan, D. Arnold, P. Styles, and P. M. Mathews.** 2003. Beta-Interferon treatment does not always slow the progression of axonal injury in multiple sclerosis. *J. Neurol.* **250:**171–178.

23. **Perron, H., J. A. Garson, F. Bedin, F. Beseme, G. Paranhos-Baccala, F. Komurian-Pradel, F. Mallet, P. W. Tuke, C. Voisset, J. L. Blond, B. Lalande, J. M. Seigneurin, and B. Mandrand.** 1997. Molecular identification of a novel retrovirus repeatedly isolated from patients with multiple sclerosis. The Collaborative Research Group on Multiple Sclerosis. *Proc. Natl. Acad. Sci. USA* **94:**7583–7588.

24. **PRISMS Study Group.** 1998. Randomized double-blind placebo-controlled study of interferon-1a in relapsing/remitting multiple sclerosis. *Lancet* **352:**1498–1504.

25. **Reiber, H., S. Ungefehr, and C. Jacobi.** 1998. The intrathecal, polyspecific and oligoclonal immune response in multiple sclerosis. *Mult. Scler.* **4:**111–117.

26. **Rott, O., H. Wekerle, and B. Fleischer.** 1992. Protection from experimental allergic encephalomyelitis by application of a bacterial superantigen. *Int. Immunol.* **4:**347–353.

27. **Rudge, P.** 1991. Does a retrovirally encoded superantigen cause multiple sclerosis? *J. Neurol. Neurosurg. Psychiatry* **54:**853–855.

28. **Schiffenbauer, J., H. M. Johnson, E. J. Butfiloski, L. Wegrzyn, and J. M. Soos.** 1993. Staphylococcal superantigens can reactivate experimental allergic encephalomyelitis. *Proc. Natl. Acad. Sci. USA* **90:**8543-8546.

29. **Skulina, C., S. Schmidt, K. Dornmair, H. Babbe, A. Roers, K. Rajewski, H. Wekerle, R. Hohlfeld, and N. Goebels.** 2004. Multiple sclerosis: brain-infiltrating CD8+ T cells persist as clonal expansions in the cerebrospinal fluid and blood. *Proc. Natl. Acad. Sci. USA* **101:**2428–2433.

30. **Soos, J. M., J. Schiffenbauer, and H. M. Johnson.** 1993. Treatment of PL/J mice with the superantigen, staphylococcal enterotoxin B, prevents development of experimental allergic encephalomyelitis. *J. Neuroimmunol.* **43:**39–43.

31. **Torres, B. A., S. Kominsky, G. Q. Perrin, A. C. Hobeika, and H. M. Johnston.** 2001. Superantigens: the good, the bad, and the ugly. *Exp. Biol. Med.* **226:**164–176.

32. **Vandevelde, M., and A. Zurbriggen.** 2005. Demyelination in canine distemper virus infection: a review. *Acta Neuropathol.* **109:**56–58.

33. **Wekerle, H., C. Linington, H. Lassmann, and R. Meyermann.** 1986. Cellular immune reactivity within the CNS. *Trends Neurosci.* **9:**271–277.

34. **Wingerchuk, D. M., W. F. Hogancamp, P. C. O'Brien, and B. G. Weinshenker.** 1999. The clinical course of neuromyelitis optica (Devic's syndrome). *Neurology* **53:**1107–1114.

35. **Yoshimoto, T., H. Nagase, H. Nakano, A. Matsuzuwa, and H. Nariuchi.** 1996. Deletion of CD4+ T cells by mouse mammary tumor virus (FM) superantigen with broad specificity of T cell receptor beta-chain variable region. *Virology* **223:**387–391.

Chapter 12

Novel Experimental Models for Dissecting Genetic Susceptibility of Superantigen-Mediated Diseases

Eva Medina

INTRODUCTION

The uncontrolled immunological response triggered by microbial superantigens has been implicated in the etiology of numerous human disorders. The observations that superantigens can differentially activate T cells from different individuals suggested that genetic heterogeneity contributes to the clinical phenotype following exposure to superantigens (7, 49). Given the central role played by the major histocompatibility complex (MHC) class II molecules on presentation of superantigens to T cells, the possibility that susceptibility or resistance to superantigen-induced diseases can be associated with particular MHC class II alleles constitutes the main focus of the ongoing research in this area. The influence of allelic polymorphism at the H-2 locus on the presentation of staphylococcal and streptococcal superantigens to T cells was noted years ago (31, 37, 50, 55, 59, 73). By studying these associations in patients that are clinically and genetically heterogeneous, it has been possible to identify genotypes that cosegregate with specific clinical features. The work of Kotb et al. (33) about the immunogenetics of immune responses to group A streptococcus has provided an elegant example of how allelic variations of the MHC class II antigens may contribute to susceptibility to (DRB1*14/DQB1*0503 or DRB1*07/DQB1*0201) or protection from (DRB1*1501/DQB1*0602) severe streptococcal diseases. Although the molecular basis for this difference remains unclear, several mechanisms have been proposed. Thus, it was suggested that an interaction between the T-cell receptor (TCR) and the MHC molecule takes place during superantigen recognition, and the strength of this interaction varies with the overall avidity of the TCR/superantigen/MHC complex (72). More recently, the findings that differences in the avidity of HLA molecules to bind superantigens and present them to T cells could dictate the strength and quality of the cytokine response (37) have provided perhaps the strongest evidence about the contribution of the HLA haplotype to susceptibility or resistance to superantigen-induced disorders.

Eva Medina • Department of Microbial Pathogenesis and Vaccine Research, Infection Immunology Research Group, HZI-Helmholtz Centre for Infection Research, 38124 Braunschweig, Germany.

The influence of genetic factors on host response to microbial superantigens has been hampered largely by the fact that, until recently, it has not been possible to compare the contribution of specific genes in isolation, under experimental conditions where the remainder of the genome is fixed. In recent years, however, the revolutionary techniques of modern molecular biology have provided powerful systems for investigating the extent of the host genetic contribution to variation in susceptibility to superantigen-mediated diseases. This has been achieved either by using cell lines transfected with different human HLA molecules in in vitro studies or in in vivo studies using congenic or transgenic mouse models expressing different human HLA haplotypes.

The use of laboratory mice to investigate correlates of infectious diseases, including the influence of host genetics and immune responses in the context of an intact host, has expanded exponentially in the past decade. A marked increase in the availability of transgenic mice and research tools developed specifically for the mouse has enhanced this research. A selected number of these experimental strategies will be described in detail in this chapter.

IN VITRO EXPERIMENTAL SYSTEMS

To study the relative ability of distinct isotypes of human HLA to bind microbial superantigens, many researchers have employed tissue culture models, most frequently cell lines transfected with different human *hla* genes. Thus, the relationships among the class II binding affinities of staphylococcal exotoxins were initially investigated by a direct binding assay of ^{125}I-labeled exotoxins to a mouse fibroblast cell line transfected with the genes encoding the α- and β-chains of the HLA-DR1. In this pioneer study (46), Mollick and colleagues provided the first evidence that these superantigens bind class II molecules with different affinities that reflect their abilities to stimulate T cells.

A more straightforward approach has been the use of a panel of HLA homozygous B lymphoblastoid cell lines to screen a range of HLA molecules for differences in superantigen binding (37, 50). BLS-1 cells derived from patients with bare lymphocyte syndrome and transfected with various HLA class II alleles have also been used for this type of study. BLS-1 is an HLA class II-null, Epstein-Barr virus-transformed B-lymphoblastoid cell line (32). Using a panel of BLS-1 cells transfected with various HLA class II alleles, including DRA1*0101/DRB1*0101 (DR1), DRA*0101/DRB1*0401 (DR4), DRA1*0101/DRB1* 01101 (DR5), DQA1*0501/DQB1*0302 (DQ2α3β), and DQA1*0301/DQB1*0302 (DQ3.2), Norrby-Teglund and colleagues (50) demonstrated a direct influence of the class II allelic variation on the magnitude of cytokine and proliferative responses induced by superantigens produced by *Streptococcus pyogenes*. An important finding of these studies is that the magnitude of the inflammatory responses triggered by streptococcal superantigens was a combination of the superantigen expression profile of the infecting isolate and the HLA class II haplotype of the host. This, in turn, influenced the severity of systemic manifestation during invasive infection with *S. pyogenes*.

Using a similar approach, Llewelyn et al. (37) have shown that polymorphisms in the DQ α-chain influenced the binding of streptococcal pyrogenic exotoxin A (SpeA) to HLA-DQ molecules. The differential binding affinity of SpeA to the different HLA-DQ molecules resulted in quantitative and qualitative differences in the cytokine responses.

Although these approaches enable a direct and quantitative assessment of superantigen stimulation driven by different HLA haplotypes, they constitute only a first-level analysis of the complex immunogenetics of superantigen-induced immune responses.

IN VIVO EXPERIMENTAL SYSTEMS

Murine models have proven to be excellent tools in supporting studies of the influence of host genetics in the course of infectious diseases. The use of murine models for studying the pathogenesis of superantigen-mediated diseases has been limited by the relatively weak response of mice to superantigens in comparison with humans (6, 44, 45, 65). Mouse resistance to microbial superantigen toxicity is believed to be due to a significantly lower affinity of the toxins for murine MHC class II molecules, which lack a critical lysine residue in the α-chain (20). As an exception, the presentation of superantigens produced by *Mycoplasma arthritidis* is much less active for human peripheral blood lymphocytes than for mouse splenocytes (9).

The sensitivity of mice to superantigens could be substantially increased after a potentiating dose of lipopolysaccharide (65). Other compounds, such as D-galactosamine, have been shown to enhance staphylococcal enterotoxin B (SEB) toxicity (45), possibly by impairing RNA synthesis and increasing sensitivity to tumor necrosis factor alpha (TNF-α) (36). Because the outcome of these treatments is a combination of both bacterial superantigens and potentiating components, these artificial models for toxic shock may have severe limitations and a clear lack of relevance to human responses.

The development of HLA class II transgenic murine models that are superantigen sensitive has been a critical step toward understanding the effect of HLA polymorphism on superantigen-mediated disease expression. Additionally, HLA-transgenic mice can also be instrumental for in vivo screening and identification of new immunomodulatory therapies, accepting the usual limitations associated with the extrapolation of results from murine to human disease.

The *M. arthritidis* Mitogen (MAM) Model

M. arthritidis, which can cause a chronic inflammatory polyarthritis in genetically susceptible strains of rodents (11), produces a soluble factor designated *M. arthritidis* mitogen (MAM) with superantigenic properties (9, 10, 12). This particular superantigen has the unique ability to induce a spontaneous, chronic form of arthritis in genetically susceptible strains of rodents that histologically resembles rheumatoid arthritis in humans (9, 11).

Although MAM has also been shown to be involved in the pathogenesis of rheumatoid arthritis in some patients (57), MAM is much less active for human peripheral blood lymphocytes than for mouse splenocytes (9). It was suggested that a difference in MAM binding affinity between human and mouse MHC class II molecules may account for their different MAM activities. Due to the high affinity of MAM for murine cells, the *M. arthritidis* model has been extremely useful for studying the influence of polymorphisms in the H-2 region in the host responses to superantigens in the murine system. Studies using inbred, congenic, and recombinant mice demonstrated that polymorphism at the locus encoding the H-2A molecule strongly influenced MAM reactivity (13).

As mentioned above, *M. arthritidis* can also bind to human HLA-DQ and can activate T cells but to a much lesser extent than staphylococcal or streptococcal superantigens. By using human HLA-transgenic mice, it was further demonstrated that polymorphisms of HLA-DQ molecules influenced the reactivity to MAM (13). Curiously, the pattern of reactivity to MAM for lymphocytes expressing various H-2A or HLA-DQ molecules was different from the pattern observed with staphylococcal SEB and SEA, suggesting that these three superantigens use unique binding sites on the MHC class II molecules. These data support the hypothesis proposed earlier by Fleischer and colleagues (19) that there has been an evolutionary adaptation between a parasite, its superantigens, and the manner in which it interacts with the immune system of its host.

MHC Class II-Congenic Murine Models

Recombinant congenic mice are a valuable resource for complex trait analysis. Two strains of mice are congenic if they are genetically identical except at a single genetic locus or region. The standard procedure for developing congenic mouse strains involves serial backcrossing to transfer a gene (allele) from a donor strain to a recipient host inbred strain. Following ten generations of backcrossing (N10) with accompanying selection for the gene of interest. A congenic strain is theoretically 99.9% identical to the host inbred strain at all loci except those linked to the transferred gene of interest. Intercrossing of heterozygous N10 mice and selection of mice homozygous for the gene of interest completes the congenic strain development. MHC class II-congenic mice have been instrumental in defining the MHC region and its role in infection (1, 5, 18, 42, 60), transplantation (53, 70), and autoimmunity (47).

MHC class II-congenic mice have been used to investigate the direct effect of haplotype differences within the MHC class II molecules on staphylococcal superantigen presentation to a panel of responsive Vβ-bearing T cells. The results from the studies of Taub and colleagues (67) clearly demonstrated that staphylococcal superantigen presentation by MHC class II-bearing accessory cells to murine T cells was greatly affected by polymorphisms within the MHC complex.

The influence of MHC class II allele polymorphisms in the responses of mice to infection with mouse mammary tumor viruses (MMTVs) has also been investigated using MHC class II-congenic mouse strains. Superantigens encoded by MMTVs play a crucial role in the viral life cycle (16). Presentation of these viral superantigens by B cells induces proliferative responses by superantigen-reactive T cells that amplify MMTV infection (16). It was observed that the levels of MMTV infection differed remarkably between the different MHC class II-congenic mouse strains, indicating that the differential ability of polymorphic MHC class II molecules to form a functional complex with MMTV superantigens determined the magnitude of the proliferative response of superantigen-reactive T cells (30). This differential activation strongly influenced the degree of T-cell help provided to infected B cells and therefore the efficiency of amplification of MMTV infection (30).

Mouse models of streptococcal infection have proven to be especially important in demonstrating the influence of genetic factors on the host response to *S. pyogenes*. Different inbred mouse strains show marked genetic differences in their resistance or susceptibility to infection with *S. pyogenes* (25, 43). Thus, while C3H/HeN (H-2^k haplotype) mice are very susceptible, BALB/c (H-2^d haplotype) mice are very resistant to streptococcal infection (25, 43). As *S. pyogenes* produces several superantigens that have been suggested to be major mediators of the systemic effects observed in severe invasive streptococcal infections (51, 62, 64), MHC class II-congenic mice have been used to determine the extent to which polymorphism of the MHC molecule influenced the overall resistance or susceptibility of mice to infection with *S. pyogenes*.

Using congenic BALB mice from a resistant background (BALB/c) but carrying the *H2^k* haplotype region of the susceptible C3H/HeN strain (BALB/k mice), it has been possible to show that, while the haplotype of the MHC class II might influence the extent of the inflammatory response taking place during severe streptococcal infection, non-*H2*-encoded genes present in the neighboring chromosomal region seem to make a more critical contribution to the overall susceptibility of mice to *S. pyogenes* (26).

Therefore, the outcome from studies where MHC class II-congenic mouse strains have been used to determine the influence of the MHC haplotype on the particular disease phenotype should be interpreted with caution since the observed effect may be due to other genes linked to this complex. Nevertheless, the commercial availability of MHC class II-congenic inbred mice with different genetic backgrounds (Table 1) provides a good incentive for using these mouse models as a first screening tool.

Human HLA-Transgenic Mice

The generation of transgenic mice expressing human HLA molecules has been an important step toward the creation of in vivo models for investigating the function of disease-associated HLA class II. HLA-transgenic mice provide a unique opportunity to establish the pathogenetic roles of alleles associated with superantigen-induced human diseases and should also facilitate the in vivo screening and identification of new immunotherapeutic strategies, prior to designing clinical trials.

Table 1. MHC class II-congenic mouse strains

Nomenclature	H-2 donor strain	H-2 locus[a]
B10.A	A/WySn	*H-2^a*
B10.A(2R)	A/WySn	*H-2^{h2}*
B10.A(3R)	A/WySn	*H-2^{i3}*
B10.A(4R)	A/WySn	*H-2^{h4}*
B10.A(5R)	A/WySn	*H-2^{i5}*
B10.BR	C57BR/cd	*H-2^k*
B10.D2	DBA/2	*H-2^d*
B10.G	Grey-lethal linkage, testing stock	*H-2^q*
B10.M	Noninbred stock M	*H-2^f*
B10.RIII	RIII/WyJ	*H-2^r*
B10.S	A.SW	*H-2^s*
BALB.B	C57BL/10Sn	*H-2^b*
BALB.k	C3H	*H-2^k*

[a]For mice, the MHC haplotypes are abbreviated with letters.

The process of generating humanized HLA-transgenic mouse models is not trivial and poses several problems. The first concern is how physiological the pattern of HLA expression produced by the HLA transgene is. The introduction of an HLA gene under a murine promoter ensures more physiological patterns of expression in the mouse (22). However, subtle differences exist between mice and humans in the expression of MHC class II molecules. The promoter regions of HLA genes determine the temporal pattern and tissue specificity of expression, as well as the modulation of expression during inflammation (39, 68). In addition, differences in regulation between alleles of HLA genes as well as promoter polymorphisms may result in allelic differences in expression (3, 38). To overcome these difficulties, HLA-transgenic lines have been established by introducing the HLA genes into mice under the control of their native human promoter (48).

The level and pattern of expression of the HLA molecule can also be influenced by the copy number and integration site of the transgene. The MHC class II overexpression syndrome, described in A^{k}_{β} transgenic mice, is often related to the integration of more than 50 copies of the transgene. It manifests as inflammatory diseases with low levels of cell surface MHC class II molecules, progressive B-cell deficiency, and abnormal extramedulary granulopoiesis with eosinophilia (24). This nonspecific effect resulting from the overexpression of any MHC class II allele phenotype can easily be mistaken for an HLA-related model of human inflammatory disease.

An additional problem posed by this system is that the presence of murine MHC molecules in an HLA-transgenic model may confuse attempts to study the function of the human MHC molecule and complicate the interpretation of such experiments. Therefore, the human HLA molecules needed to be expressed in the complete absence of their murine counterparts. Mice lacking MHC molecules provide the means by which the transgenic HLA molecule can be isolated as the sole restriction element in a murine model. Thus, MHC-II knockout mouse lines harboring a deletion of all classical MHC-II genes have been generated (41). By disrupting the Aβ genes, Cosgrove et al. (14) generated mice that could not express H-2-A molecule ($A\beta^{0}$). Because these mice were of the $H-2^{b}$ haplotype and lacked functional H-2-E molecule, no class II molecules were expressed on the cell surface. Transgenic mice were then generated expressing a functional HLA-DQ8 (DQA1*0301, DQB1*0302) molecule on the class II-deficient $A\beta^{0}$ background (8). The only class II molecule expressed in these transgenic mice was encoded by the HLA-DQ8 α and β genes. In the absence of endogenous class II molecules, the human class II molecules become the self-MHC in these mice and there is no risk of generating chimeric MHC-II molecules.

Sriskandan and colleagues (63) have shown that HLA-DQ8 but not HLA-DR transgenic mice were highly sensitive to streptococcal SpeA both in vitro and in vivo. Thus, HLA-DQ transgenic mice exhibited increased mortality after administration of SpeA or infection with *S. pyogenes* (63).

HLA-transgenic mice have been used to investigate the role played by the ubiquitous streptococcal superantigen SMEZ in pathogen-host interactions. SMEZ binds exclusively to the MHC class II β-chain (4). A strong influence of the HLA haplotype was evidenced by the higher responsiveness to rSMEZ-13 observed in spleen cells isolated from HLA-DQ8-transgenic mice expressing HLA-DQ-B1*0302 than in those isolated from transgenic mice expressing HLA-DR1 (69).

Transgenic Mice Expressing Both Human HLA and CD4 Molecules

The formation of the MHC class II-superantigen-TCR complex is a prerequisite for T-cell activation and proliferation. Although murine CD4 appears to perform adequately as coreceptor of the HLA molecule in some systems (2), in other cases the immune response of HLA transgenic mice has been rescued or augmented by the introduction of transgenic human CD4 (52, 74). Mice expressing human CD4 and human MHC class II molecules have been used to study humanlike responses to bacterial superantigens as well as for the evaluation of therapeutic vaccines (56, 71). An early multiple transgenic mouse model consisted in the introduction of the human CD4 transgene under the control of the murine CD3δ promoter, resulting in human CD4 molecule expression on all CD3+ cells, both CD4+ and CD8+ subsets (22). In the CD4/DR1 transgenic mouse model developed by Altmann et al. (2), CD4 expression was controlled by mouse MHC H-2^K promoters leading to the CD4 expression in all cells. Promoters with more lymphocyte specificity were used for CD4 expression in models with transgenic HLA-DR4, or HLA-DQ6 (23, 74). These transgenic mice expressed human CD4 on all T cells, and in the case of DQ6 mice, also on B cells. Yeung and colleagues (74) have shown that both human CD4 and MHC class II molecules can render mice supersensitive to superantigen-induced septic shock syndrome. The T lymphocytes from these double-transgenic humanized mice reacted to smaller amounts of staphylococcal SEB than control mice in vitro (74). In in vivo experiments, the double-transgenic mice succumbed to normally sublethal amounts of SEB (74). This high sensitivity to SEB was due to increased production of TNF-α by T cells, therefore mimicking the progression of septic shock in humans.

An additional feature of the HLA/CD4 transgenic mouse model that closely resembles the human system is that transgenic CD4 is expressed in antigen-presenting cells (monocytes and dendritic cells). While human antigen-presenting cells express CD4, mouse antigen-presenting cells are devoid of this marker (15). In mouse monocytes, *cd4* gene transcription is prevented because of missing binding sites for monocyte-specific regulatory factors upstream of the *cd4* gene (29). The CD4 transgene supplied CD4/DR3 mice with these missing elements, thus permitting expression of CD4 on mouse accessory cells. Therefore, the overall expression of CD4 resembles very closely that of human cells.

More recently, Laub et al. (35) developed a multiple transgenic mouse model expressing human CD4 and HLA-DR3 on a murine CD4-deficient background. Phenotypic analysis suggested an expression pattern of the transgenic CD4 very similar to that of humans which is unique among comparable mouse models. In this model, the human CD4+ cells in the periphery accurately replaced the mouse CD4+ T cells, and CD4/DR3 mice clearly showed individual CD4 and CD8 single positive T-cell subsets.

HLA/human CD4 (HLA-DQ8 or HLA-DR3) double-transgenic mice lacking endogenous MHC class II and murine CD4 expression have been shown to be extremely sensitive to bacterial superantigens, strongly emulating humanlike responses (17, 71). Welcher et al. (71) used these double-transgenic CD4/HLA-DQ8 or CD4/HLA-DR3 mice to evaluate the biological effects of SpeA produced by *S. pyogenes*. The typical response to SpeA observed in humans was triggered in the transgenic mice, including rapid cytokine release, proliferation of T cells, and selection of specific Vβ-expressing T cells. The intensity of the immune response triggered by SpeA was dependent on the HLA haplotype expressed by the transgenic mice. Thus, the response of CD4/HLA-DQ8 transgenic mice to SpeA was significantly higher than that of CD4/HLA-DR3 mice.

Mouse Models To Study the Role of Superantigens in the Development of Autoimmune Diseases

Genetic susceptibility to autoimmunity in humans and experimental animal models is due to the presence of multiple disease loci (54). Since particular combinations of genes confer susceptibility, only a relatively small fraction of the population appears to be genetically susceptible to a given autoimmune disease. In addition, increasing evidence has suggested that bacterial and viral superantigens are also involved in the development of autoimmune disorders (21, 40, 58). Although superantigens per se cannot trigger the autoimmune reaction, they may be important for activation and expansion of autoreactive lymphocytes. Thus, in most cases of autoimmune diseases, the mere existence of self-reactive cells is not sufficient to cause disease and, in general, an additional insult such as superantigen stimulation is required. Therefore, a particular autoimmune disease may only develop in a few genetically predisposed individuals who encounter a certain infectious agent. The epidemiology of several autoimmune diseases that are associated with specific infectious agents support this notion.

An example of this comes from the experiments showing that superantigens can induce relapses and exacerbations of a T-cell-mediated autoimmune process in murine models of experimental allergic encephalomyelitis (EAE), which is a murine model for multiple sclerosis (61, 66). EAE can be induced in PL/J mice after immunization with the N-terminal peptide of myelin basic protein (MBP) (75). Transgenic mice expressing a TCR derived from an encephalitogenic CD4 clone expressed enhanced susceptibility to the induction of central nervous system autoimmune disease following injection of MBP peptide (28). It was observed that a proportion of these transgenic mice spontaneously developed autoimmunity in early adulthood, but this was dependent on the microbial status of the mouse facility in which they were housed (27, 28). Mice maintained under specific pathogen-free conditions rarely developed the disease suggesting the contribution of microbial factors as a triggering mechanism.

Superantigens such as the staphylococcal enterotoxins can play an important role in exacerbation of autoimmune disorders such as EAE in mice. It has been shown that these superantigens are capable of reactivating EAE in PL/J mice that have been sensitized to MBP. The T-cell subset predominantly responsible for disease in PL/J mice bears the Vβ8+ T-cell antigen receptor (TCR). Soos and colleagues (61) have shown that two of the staphylococcal enterotoxins, SEA and SEB, are able to reactivate paralysis in PL/J mice that had been immunized with MBP and resolved an initial episode of paralysis.

Superantigens can also trigger the reactivation of bacterial cell wall or collagen-induced arthritis. The *M. arthritidis* superantigen (MAM) is derived from a naturally occurring murine arthritogenic mycoplasm and is a potent superantigen for Vβ5.1-, Vβ6-, and Vβ8-positive T cells. MAM can cause severe exacerbation of arthritis when administered during the chronic stage of the disease (9). The arthritis process induced by MAM can be even more severe than the initial arthritis induced by type II collagen. The superantigen can also trigger arthritis in mice that did not develop clinical disease following the initial immunization with type II collagen (11).

Other diseases for which a role of superantigens in the autoimmune process has been identified include psoriasis, lupuslike disease, and lymphoproliferative diseases (34).

These examples illustrate the relationship between superantigens and the development of autoimmune diseases in a genetically predisposed host. For many common autoimmune diseases little is known about the potential role of superantigens. Prospective studies using humanized mouse models may help to advance our knowledge about the exact role of superantigens and the specific mechanisms by which they contribute to disease mechanisms. A better understanding of the relationship between genetic factors, infection, and autoimmunity may lead to better prevention of disease development by early intervention.

REFERENCES

1. **Abdelnour, A., Y. X. Zhao, R. Holmdahl, and A. Tarkowski.** 1997. Major histocompatibility complex class II region confers susceptibility to *Staphylococcus aureus* arthritis. *Scand. J. Immunol.* **45:**301–307.
2. **Altmann, D. M., D. C. Douek, A. J. Frater, C. M. Hetherington, H. Inoko, and J. I. Elliott.** 1995. The T cell response of HLA-DR transgenic mice to human myelin basic protein and other antigens in the presence and absence of human CD4. *J. Exp. Med.* **181:**867–875.
3. **Andersen, L. C., J. S. Beaty, J. W. Nettles, C. E. Seyfried, G. T. Nepom, and B. S. Nepoom.** 1991. Allelic polymorphism in transcriptional regulatory regions of HLA-DQB genes. *J. Exp. Med.* **173:**181–192.
4. **Arcus, V. L., T. Proft, J. A. Sigrell, H. M. Baker, J. D. Fraser, and E. N. Baker.** 2000. Conservation and variation in superantigen structure and activity highlighted by the three-dimensional structures of two new superantigens from *Streptococcus pyogenes. J. Mol. Biol.* **299:**157–168.
5. **Blackwell, J. M., C. W. Roberts, and J. Alexander.** 1993. Influence of genes within the MHC on mortality and brain cyst development in mice infected with *Toxoplasma gondii*: kinetics of immune regulation in BALB H-2 congenic mice. *Parasite Immunol.* **15:**317–324.
6. **Blank, C., A. Luz, S. Bendigs, A. Erdmann, H. Wagner, and K. Heeg.** 1997. Superantigen and endotoxin synergize in the induction of lethal shock. *Eur. J. Immunol.* **27:**825–833.
7. **Chatellier, S., N. Ihendyane, R. G. Kansal, F. Khambaty, H. Basma, A. Norrby-Teglund, D. E. Low, A. McGeer, and M. Kotb.** 2000. Genetic relatedness and superantigen expression in group A streptococcus serotype M1 isolates from patients with severe and nonsevere invasive diseases. *Infect. Immun.* **68:**3523–3534.
8. **Cheng, S., J. Baisch, C. Krco, S. Savarirayan, J. Hanson, K. Hodgson, M. Smart, and C. David.** 1996. Expression and function of HLA-DQ8 (DQA1*0301/DQB1*0302) genes in transgenic mice. *Eur. J. Immunogenet.* **23:**15–20.
9. **Cole, B. C., and C. L. Atkin.** 1991. The *Mycoplasma arthritidis* T-cell mitogen, MAM: a model superantigen. *Immunol. Today* **12:**271–276.
10. **Cole, B. C., R. A. Daynes, and J. R. Ward.** 1982. Stimulation of mouse lymphocytes by a mitogen derived from Mycoplasma arthritidis. III. Ir gene control of lymphocyte transformation correlates with binding of the mitogen to specific Ia-bearing cells. *J. Immunol.* **129:**1352–1359.
11. **Cole, B. C., and M. M. Griffiths.** 1993. Triggering and exacerbation of autoimmune arthritis by the *Mycoplasma arthritidis* superantigen MAM. *Arthritis Rheum.* **36:**994–1002.
12. **Cole, B. C., D. R. Kartchner, and D. J. Wells.** 1990. Stimulation of mouse lymphocytes by a mitogen derived from Mycoplasma arthritidis (MAM). VIII. Selective activation of T cells expressing distinct V beta T cell receptors from various strains of mice by the "superantigen" MAM. *J. Immunol.* **144:**425–431.
13. **Cole, B. C., A. D. Sawitzke, E. A. Ahmed, C. L. Atkin, and C. S. David.** 1997. Allelic polymorphisms at the H-2A and HLA-DQ loci influence the response of murine lymphocytes to the *Mycoplasma arthritidis* superantigen MAM. *Infect. Immun.* **65:**4190–4198.
14. **Cosgrove, D., D. Gray, A. Dierich, J. Kaufman, C. Benoist, and D. Mathis.** 1991. Mice lacking MHC class II molecules. *Cell* **66:**1051–1066.
15. **Crocker, P. R., W. A. Jefferies, S. J. Clark, L. P. Chung, and S. Gordon.** 1987. Species heterogeneity in macrophage expression of the CD4 antigen. *J. Exp. Med.* **166:**613–618.
16. **Czarneski, J., J. C. Rassa, and S. R. Ross.** 2003. Mouse mammary tumor virus and the immune system. *Immunol. Res.* **27:**469–480.

17. DaSilva, L., B. C. Welcher, R. G. Ulrich, M. J. Aman, C. S. David, and S. Bavari. 2002. Humanlike immune response of human leukocyte antigen-DR3 transgenic mice to staphylococcal enterotoxins: a novel model for superantigen vaccines. *J. Infect. Dis.* **185:**1754–1760.

18. Fischer, H. G., R. Dorfler, B. Schade, and U. Hadding. 1999. Differential CD86/B7-2 expression and cytokine secretion induced by *Toxoplasma gondii* in macrophages from resistant or susceptible BALB H-2 congenic mice. *Int. Immunol.* **11:**341–349.

19. Fleischer, B., R. Gerardy-Schahn, B. Metzroth, S. Carrel, D. Gerlach, and W. Kohler. 1991. An evolutionary conserved mechanism of T cell activation by microbial toxins. Evidence for different affinities of T cell receptor-toxin interaction. *J. Immunol.* **146:**11–17.

20. Fremont, D. H., W. A. Hendrickson, P. Marrack, and J. Kappler. 1996. Structures of an MHC class II molecule with covalently bound single peptides. *Science* **272:**1001–1004.

21. Friedman, S. M., D. N. Posnett, J. R. Tumang, B. C. Cole, and M. K. Crow. 1991. A potential role for microbial superantigens in the pathogenesis of systemic autoimmune disease. *Arthritis Rheum.* **34:**468–480.

22. Fugger, L., S. A. Michie, I. Rulifson, C. B. Lock, and G. S. McDevitt. 1994. Expression of HLA-DR4 and human CD4 transgenes in mice determines the variable region beta-chain T-cell repertoire and mediates an HLA-DR-restricted immune response. *Proc. Natl. Acad. Sci. USA* **91:**6151–6155.

23. Fugger, L., J. B. Rothbard, and G. Sonderstrup-McDevitt. 1996. Specificity of an HLA-DRB1*0401-restricted T cell response to type II collagen. *Eur. J. Immunol.* **26:**928–933.

24. Gilfillan, S., S. Aiso, S. A. Michie, and H. O. McDevitt. 1990. Immune deficiency due to high copy numbers of an A^k beta transgene. *Proc. Natl. Acad. Sci. USA* **87:**7319–7323.

25. Goldmann, O., G. S. Chhatwal, and E. Medina. 2003. Immune mechanisms underlying host susceptibility to infection with group A streptococci. *J. Infect. Dis.* **187:**854–861.

26. Goldmann, O., A. Lengeling, J. Bose, H. Bloecker, R. Geffers, G. S. Chhatwal, and E. Medina. 2005. The role of the MHC on resistance to group a streptococci in mice. *J. Immunol.* **175:**3862–3872.

27. Goverman, J. 1999. Tolerance and autoimmunity in TCR transgenic mice specific for myelin basic protein. *Immunol. Rev.* **169:**147–159.

28. Goverman, J., A. Woods, L. Larson, L. P. Weiner, L. Hood, and D. M. Zaller. 1993. Transgenic mice that express a myelin basic protein specific T cell receptor develop spontaneous autoimmunity. *Cell* **72:**551–560.

29. Hanna, Z., C. Simard, A. Laperriere, and P. Jolicoeur. 1994. Specific expression of the human CD4 gene in mature CD4+ CD8- and immature CD4+ CD8+ T cells and in macrophages of transgenic mice. *Mol. Cell. Biol.* **14:**1084–1094.

30. Held, W., G. A. Waanders, H. R. MacDonald, and H. Acha-Orbea. 1994. MHC class II hierarchy of superantigen presentation predicts efficiency of infection with mouse mammary tumor virus. *Int. Immunol.* **6:**1403–1407.

31. Herman, A., G. Croteau, R. P. Sekaly, J. Kappler, and P. Marrack. 1990. HLA-DR alleles differ in their ability to present staphylococcal enterotoxins to T cells. *J. Exp. Med.* **172:**709–717.

32. Hume, C. R., L. A. Shookster, N. Collins, R. O'Reilly, and J. S. Lee. 1989. Bare lymphocyte syndrome: altered HLA class II expression in B cell lines derived from two patients. *Hum. Immunol.* **25:**1–11.

33. Kotb, M., A. Norrby-Teglund, A. McGeer, H. El-Sherbini, M. T. Dorak, A. Khurshid, K. Green, J. Peeples, J. Wade, G. Thomson, B. Schwartz, and D. E. Low. 2002. An immunogenetic and molecular basis for differences in outcomes of invasive group A streptococcal infections. *Nat. Med.* **8:**1398–1404.

34. Kotzin, B. L., D. Y. Leung, J. Kappler, and P. Marrack. 1993. Superantigens and their potential role in human disease. *Adv. Immunol.* **54:**99–166.

35. Laub, R., M. Dorsch, D. Meyer, J. Ermann, H. J. Hedrich, and F. Emmrich. 2000. A multiple transgenic mouse model with a partially humanized activation pathway for helper T cell responses. *J. Immunol. Methods* **246:**37–50.

36. Lehmann, V., M. A. Freudenberg, and C. Galanos. 1987. Lethal toxicity of lipopolysaccharide and tumor necrosis factor in normal and D-galactosamine-treated mice. *J. Exp. Med.* **165:**657–663.

37. Llewelyn, M., S. Sriskandan, M. Peakman, D. R. Ambrozak, D. C. Douek, W. W. Kwok, J. Cohen, and D. M. Altmann. 2004. HLA class II polymorphisms determine responses to bacterial superantigens. *J. Immunol.* **172:**1719–1726.

38. Louis, P., R. Vincent, P. Cavadore, J. Clot, and J. F. Eliaou. 1994. Differential transcriptional activities of HLA-DR genes in the various haplotypes. *J. Immunol.* **153:**5059–5067.

39. Mach, B., V. Steimle, E. Martinez-Soria, and W. Reith. 1996. Regulation of MHC class II genes: lessons from a disease. *Annu. Rev. Immunol.* **14:**301–331.

40. **Macphail, S.** 1999. Superantigens: mechanisms by which they may induce, exacerbate and control autoimmune diseases. *Int. Rev. Immunol.* **18:**141–180.

41. **Madsen, L., N. Labrecque, J. Engberg, A. Dierich, A. Svejgaard, C. Benoist, D. Mathis, and L. Fugger.** 1999. Mice lacking all conventional MHC class II genes. *Proc. Natl. Acad. Sci. USA* **96:**10338–10343.

42. **McClelland, E. E., D. L. Granger, and W. K. Potts.** 2003. Major histocompatibility complex-dependent susceptibility to *Cryptococcus neoformans* in mice. *Infect. Immun.* **71:**4815–4817.

43. **Medina, E., O. Goldmann, M. Rohde, A. Lengeling, and G. S. Chhatwal.** 2001. Genetic control of susceptibility to group A streptococcal infection in mice. *J. Infect. Dis.* **184:**846–852.

44. **Miethke, T., H. Gaus, C. Wahl, K. Heeg, and H. Wagner.** 1992. T-cell-dependent shock induced by a bacterial superantigen. *Chem. Immunol.* **55:**172–184.

45. **Miethke, T., C. Wahl, K. Heeg, B. Echtenacher, P. H. Krammer, and H. Wagner.** 1992. T cell-mediated lethal shock triggered in mice by the superantigen staphylococcal enterotoxin B: critical role of tumor necrosis factor. *J. Exp. Med.* **175:**91–98.

46. **Mollick, J. A., M. Chintagumpala, R. G. Cook, and R. R. Rich.** 1991. Staphylococcal exotoxin activation of T cells. Role of exotoxin-MHC class II binding affinity and class II isotype. *J. Immunol.* **146:**463–468.

47. **Morahan, G., and L. Morel.** 2002. Genetics of autoimmune diseases in humans and in animal models. *Curr. Opin. Immunol.* **14:**803–811.

48. **Nishimura, Y., T. Iwanaga, T. Inamitsu, Y. Yanagawa, M. Yasunami, A. Kimura, K. Hirokawa, and T. Sasazuki.** 1990. Expression of the human MHC HLA-DQw6 genes alters the immune response in C57BL/6 mice. *J. Immunol.* **145:**353–360.

49. **Norrby-Teglund, A., S. Chatellier, D. E. Low, A. McGeer, K. Green, and M. Kotb.** 2000. Host variation in cytokine responses to superantigens determines the severity of invasive group A streptococcal infection. *Eur. J. Immunol.* **30:**3247–3255.

50. **Norrby-Teglund, A., G. T. Nepom, and M. Kotb.** 2002. Differential presentation of group A streptococcal superantigens by HLA class II DQ and DR alleles. *Eur. J. Immunol.* **32:**2570–2577.

51. **Norrby-Teglund, A., P. Thulin, B. S. Gan, M. Kotb, A. McGeer, J. Andersson, and D. E. Low.** 2001. Evidence for superantigen involvement in severe group a streptococcal tissue infections. *J. Infect. Dis.* **184:**853–860.

52. **Patel, S. D., A. P. Cope, M. Congia, T. T. Chen, E. Kim, L. Fugger, D. Wherrett, and G. Sonderstrup-McDevitt.** 1997. Identification of immunodominant T cell epitopes of human glutamic acid decarboxylase 65 by using HLA-DR(alpha1*0101,beta1*0401) transgenic mice. *Proc. Natl. Acad. Sci. USA* **94:**8082–8087.

53. **Peugh, W. N., R. A. Superina, K. J. Wood, and P. J. Morris.** 1986. The role of H-2 and non-H-2 antigens and genes in the rejection of murine cardiac allografts. *Immunogenetics* **23:**30–37.

54. **Rioux, J. D., and A. K. Abbas.** 2005. Paths to understanding the genetic basis of autoimmune disease. *Nature* **435:**584–589.

55. **Robinson, J. H., G. Pyle, and M. A. Kehoe.** 1991. Influence of major histocompatibility complex haplotype on the mitogenic response of T cells to staphylococcal enterotoxin B. *Infect. Immun.* **59:**3667–3672.

56. **Roy, C. J., K. L. Warfield, B. C. Welcher, R. F. Gonzales, T. Larsen, J. Hanson, C. S. David, T. Krakauer, and S. Bavari.** 2005. Human leukocyte antigen-DQ8 transgenic mice: a model to examine the toxicity of aerosolized staphylococcal enterotoxin B. *Infect. Immun.* **73:**2452–2460.

57. **Sawitzke, A., D. Joyner, K. Knudtson, H. H. Mu, and B. Cole.** 2000. Anti-MAM antibodies in rheumatic disease: evidence for a MAM-like superantigen in rheumatoid arthritis? *J. Rheumatol.* **27:**358–364.

58. **Schiffenbauer, J., J. Soos, and H. Johnson.** 1998. The possible role of bacterial superantigens in the pathogenesis of autoimmune disorders. *Immunol. Today* **19:**117–120.

59. **Scholl, P. R., A. Diez, R. Karr, R. P. Sekaly, J. Trowsdale, and R. S. Geha.** 1990. Effect of isotypes and allelic polymorphism on the binding of staphylococcal exotoxins to MHC class II molecules. *J. Immunol.* **144:**226–230.

60. **Simmons, A.** 1989. H-2-linked genes influence the severity of herpes simplex virus infection of the peripheral nervous system. *J. Exp. Med.* **169:**1503–1507.

61. **Soos, J. M., A. C. Hobeika, E. J. Butfiloski, J. Schiffenbauer, and H. M. Johnson.** 1995. Accelerated induction of experimental allergic encephalomyelitis in PL/J mice by a non-V beta 8-specific superantigen. *Proc. Natl. Acad. Sci. USA* **92:**6082–6086.

62. **Sriskandan, S., D. Moyes, and J. Cohen.** 1996. Detection of circulating bacterial superantigen and lymphotoxin-alpha in patients with streptococcal toxic-shock syndrome. *Lancet* **348:**1315–1316.

63. **Sriskandan, S., M. Unnikrishnan, T. Krausz, H. Dewchand, S. Van Noorden, J. Cohen, and D. M. Altmann.** 2001. Enhanced susceptibility to superantigen-associated streptococcal sepsis in human leukocyte antigen-DQ transgenic mice. *J. Infect. Dis.* **184:**166–173.

64. **Stevens, D. L., M. H. Tanner, J. Winship, R. Swarts, K. M. Ries, P. M. Schlievert, and E. Kaplan.** 1989. Severe group A streptococcal infections associated with a toxic shock-like syndrome and scarlet fever toxin A. *N. Engl. J. Med.* **321:**1–7.

65. **Stiles, B. G., S. Bavari, T. Krakauer, and R. G. Ulrich.** 1993. Toxicity of staphylococcal enterotoxins potentiated by lipopolysaccharide: major histocompatibility complex class II molecule dependency and cytokine release. *Infect. Immun.* **61:**5333–5338.

66. **Stinissen, P., J. Raus, and J. Zhang.** 1997. Autoimmune pathogenesis of multiple sclerosis: role of autoreactive T lymphocytes and new immunotherapeutic strategies. *Crit. Rev. Immunol.* **17:**33–75.

67. **Taub, D. D., J. R. Newcomb, and T. J. Rogers.** 1992. Effect of isotypic and allotypic variations of MHC class II molecules on staphylococcal enterotoxin presentation to murine T cells. *Cell. Immunol.* **141:**263–278.

68. **Ting, J. P., and A. S. Baldwin.** 1993. Regulation of MHC gene expression. *Curr. Opin. Immunol.* **5:**8–16.

69. **Unnikrishnan, M., D. M. Altmann, T. Proft, F. Wahid, J. Cohen, J. D. Fraser, and S. Sriskandan.** 2002. The bacterial superantigen streptococcal mitogenic exotoxin Z is the major immunoactive agent of *Streptococcus pyogenes*. *J. Immunol.* **169:**2561–2569.

70. **Vermeer, B. J., B. Santerse, B. A. Van De Kerckhove, A. A. Schothorst, and F. H. Claas.** 1988. Differential immune response of congenic mice to ultraviolet-treated major histocompatibility complex class II-incompatible skin grafts. *Transplantation* **45:**607–610.

71. **Welcher, B. C., J. H. Carra, L. DaSilva, J. Hanson, C. S. David, M. J. Aman, and S. Bavari.** 2002. Lethal shock induced by streptococcal pyrogenic exotoxin A in mice transgenic for human leukocyte antigen-DQ8 and human CD4 receptors: implications for development of vaccines and therapeutics. *J. Infect. Dis.* **186:**501–510.

72. **Wen, R., M. A. Blackman, and D. L. Woodland.** 1995. Variable influence of MHC polymorphism on the recognition of bacterial superantigens by T cells. *J. Immunol.* **155:**1884–1892.

73. **Yagi, J. J., S. Rath, and C. A. Janeway, Jr.** 1991. Control of T cell responses to staphylococcal enterotoxins by stimulator cell MHC class II polymorphism. *J. Immunol.* **147:**1398–1405.

74. **Yeung, R. S., J. M. Penninger, T. M. Kundig, Y. Law, K. Yamamoto, N. Kamikawaji, L. Burkly, T. Sasazuki, R. Flavell, P. S. Ohashi, and T. W. Mak.** 1994. Human CD4-major histocompatibility complex class II (DQw6) transgenic mice in an endogenous CD4/CD8-deficient background: reconstitution of phenotype and human-restricted function. *J. Exp. Med.* **180:**1911–1920.

75. **Zamvil, S., P. Nelson, J. Trotter, D. Mitchell, R. Knobler, R. Fritz, and L. Steinman.** 1985. T-cell clones specific for myelin basic protein induce chronic relapsing paralysis and demyelination. *Nature* **317:**355–358.

Section V

THERAPEUTIC INTERVENTIONS IN SUPERANTIGEN-MEDIATED DISEASES

Superantigens: Molecular Basis for Their Role in Human Diseases
Edited by Malak Kotb and John D. Fraser
© 2007 ASM Press, Washington, D.C.

Chapter 13

Intravenous Immunoglobulin Therapy in Superantigen-Mediated Toxic Shock Syndrome

Anna Norrby-Teglund, Donald E. Low, and Malak Kotb

INTRODUCTION

Toxic shock syndrome (TSS) is a serious acute bacterial disease characterized by fever, diffuse erythematous rash, hypotension, multiorgan involvement, and desquamation of the skin one to two weeks after onset. It reflects the most severe clinical manifestation caused by *Streptococcus pyogenes* and *Staphylococcus aureus,* and is mediated by the superantigens expressed by these microbes. *S. pyogenes* and *S. aureus* both secrete several exotoxins with superantigenic activity which trigger an excessive proinflammatory response that is believed to result in the systemic features characterizing TSS. TSS was recognized early on as a superantigen disease and it was realized that intervention needed to focus not only on antimicrobials, but also on the toxemia itself. Various immunomodulatory agents and antisuperantigen therapeutic strategies have been proposed. One such strategy includes the administration of intravenous polyspecific immunoglobulin (IVIG). In this chapter we will review the mechanistic actions and use of IVIG as adjunctive therapy for TSS. In doing so, we first need to describe the clinical and pathogenic aspects of these infections.

TSS: CLINICAL AND EPIDEMIOLOGICAL ASPECTS

TSS Caused by *S. aureus*

TSS was formally described by Todd et al. (100) in 1978 as an infection caused by *S. aureus.* TSS is characterized as an acute-onset febrile, exanthematous illness associated with hypotension and multisystem failure, including shock, renal failure, myocardial suppression, and adult respiratory distress syndrome (ARDS). The illness usually presents with fever,

Anna Norrby-Teglund • Karolinska Institutet, Center for Infectious Medicine, Karolinska University Hospital, Huddinge, S-141 86 Stockholm, Sweden. *Donald E. Low* • Department of Microbiology, Mount Sinai Hospital and University of Toronto, Toronto, Ontario M5G 1X5, Canada. *Malak Kotb* • University of Tennessee Health Science Center, 930 Madison, Suite 468, Memphis, TN 38163.

Table 1. Clinical and epidemiologic aspects of streptococcal and staphylococcal toxic shock syndrome (TSS)[a]

Parameter	Streptococcal TSS	Staphylococcal TSS[b]	
		Menstrual	Nonmenstrual
Incidence	~0.5/100,000	~0.5/100,000	~0.5/100,000
Bacteremia	70–100%	Rare	Rare
Case fatality rate (%)	36–60	3	5
Implicated superantigens	SpeA-F, SSA, SmeZ	TSST-1	TSST-1, SEB, SEC
Soft-tissue infections	Common	No	Common

[a]Spe, streptococcal pyrogenic exotoxin; SSA, streptococcal superantigen; SmeZ, streptococcal mitogenic exotoxin Z; TSST-1, toxic shock syndrome toxin 1; SEB, staphylococcal enterotoxin B.
[b]Staphylococcal TSS exists in two forms, menstrual and nonmenstrual.

pharyngitis, diarrhea, vomiting, myalgia, and a scarlet fever rash, and may progress rapidly to hypovolemic hypotension. Staphylococcal TSS is subdivided into two major categories, menstrual and nonmenstrual (Table 1). The latter form of TSS can occur in association with nearly any *S. aureus* infection, but it is most commonly reported in postsurgical or burn patients, recalcitrant erythematous desquamating syndrome of AIDS patients, and postrespiratory viral infections (29, 38). The incidence of staphylococcal TSS is estimated to approximately 0.5/100,000 population, and overall fatality rates of 3% for menstrual cases and 5% for nonmenstrual cases (Table 1) (63).

TSS Caused by *S. pyogenes*

Streptococcal TSS was introduced in the late 1980s in response to a significant resurgence of severe invasive streptococcal infections. Beginning in the early 1980s, reports began to appear that described not only an increased mortality due to *S. pyogenes,* i.e., group A streptococcus, bacteremia (35 to 48%), but also a syndrome of toxic shock and multiorgan failure and in many cases rapidly progressive soft-tissue infection (Table 1) (9, 20, 27, 36, 95, 97). This clinical entity was described as streptococcal TSS due to similarities in pathogenesis and clinical features with staphylococcal TSS (20), and a consensus definition was established by The Working Group on Severe Streptococcal Infections (99). Patients were considered to have streptococcal TSS if they had hypotension in combination with two or more of the following: acute renal failure, coagulation abnormalities, liver abnormalities, ARDS, generalized rash, and necrotizing fasciitis. Severe pain out of proportion to clinical findings has been reported as one of the earliest complaints noted in a majority of patients with streptococcal TSS. Other initial signs include influenza-like symptoms such as fever, chills, myalgia, and diarrhea. Patients with streptococcal TSS often present with soft-tissue infections, including among others necrotizing fasciitis, cellulitis, myositis, and erysipelas. Streptococcal TSS has also been described after infection with group B, C, and G streptococci. An enhanced surveillance of invasive streptococcal infections in Denmark from 1999 to 2002 identified 1,260 cases caused by group A (40%), followed by group C (32%), group B (23%), and group G streptococci (6%) (30). Streptococcal TSS was significantly more frequent among group A streptococcal patients (10%), as compared with group C (4%), B (2%), or G (2%) streptococci.

Epidemiological analyses have revealed associations between clinical manifestation and certain serotypes of *S. pyogenes*. Serotypes M1 and M3 are commonly seen in association with the severe invasive streptococcal infections, including streptococcal TSS and necrotizing fasciitis (reviewed in reference 58). However, this association is far from exclusive; many other serotypes, including some nontypable strains, are known to cause these diseases (93).

TSS AND SUPERANTIGENS

The observation that staphylococcal TSS patients normally do not have detectable bacteremia, yet the patients demonstrate significant systemic features, suggested that TSS was the result of a toxemia. The report by Todd et al. in 1978 was one of the first to describe the association between TSS and an exotoxin (100). It was realized that the agents responsible for both streptococcal and staphylococcal TSS were a group of exotoxins, collectively referred to as pyrogenic exotoxins, which shared several important biological characteristics. However, it was not until 1990 that these exotoxins were found to belong to the same family of bacterial toxins, i.e., the superantigen family described in the landmark paper of Marrack and Kappler (61). This paper describes how superantigens cause a remarkable T-cell expansion by simultaneous engagement of the major histocompatibility complex (human leukocyte antigen, HLA) class II on antigen-presenting cells and specific variable regions of the Vβ-chain of the T-cell receptors on T cells. This is described in detail in other chapters of this book.

Staphylococcal Superantigens

S. aureus express a vast number of exotoxins, which belong to the superantigen family (Table 2). The classical staphylococcal superantigens include the staphylococcal enterotoxins (SE) A–C, as well as the toxic shock syndrome toxin-1 (TSST-1). However, whole-genome sequencing of *S. aureus* clinical isolates revealed a new cluster of staphylococcal superantigens, i.e., the *egc*-encoded superantigens including SEG, SEI, SEM, and SEO (52). The staphylococcal exotoxin TSST-1, formerly called staphylococcal enterotoxin (SE) F or staphylococcal pyrogenic exotoxin C, is responsible for the vast majority of menstrual TSS cases (12, 13, 86). The exclusive association between TSST-1 and menstrual TSS is believed to be contributed by the unique ability of TSST-1 to cross the mucosal surface, which is not a property of the other staphylococcal superantigens. Nonmenstrual TSS may be caused by any of the staphylococcal superantigens, but is most often associated with TSST-1, SEB, or SEC (85).

Streptococcal Superantigens

S. pyogenes produces several superantigens including the streptococcal pyrogenic exotoxins (Spe) A, B, C, F, G, H, I, J, L, and M (50, 83, 90), streptococcal superantigen (SSA) (64), and the streptococcal mitogenic exotoxin Z (Table 2) (47, 82). Most *S. pyogenes* strains express several different superantigens, and strains harbor in general genes encoding three to five of the superantigens, but the repertoire of genes varies between strains. It has not been possible to implicate a particular superantigen as the cause of streptococcal TSS, but the data rather indicate that several different superantigens are able to trigger severe systemic inflammation

Table 2. Virulence factors of *S. aureus* and *S. pyogenes* grouped according to function

Function	Virulence factors[a] of:	
	S. aureus	*S. pyogenes*
Adherence/colonization/invasion	Fibronectin-binding protein A and B	Capsule
	Fibrinogen-binding protein (Efb)	M protein
	Clumping factor A and B	Protein F/Sfb1
	Collagen-binding protein	Fibronectin-binding protein
	Elastin-binding protein	Glyceraldehyde-3-phosphate dehydrogenase
	Extracellular adherence protein (EAP)	Fibronectin-binding protein
		Vitronectin-binding protein
		Collagen-binding protein
Antiphagocytic mechanisms	Capsule	Capsule
	Protein A	M protein
	Clumping factor A	M-like proteins
	Efb	*Streptococcus* inhibitor of complement (SIC)
	Staphylococcal complement inhibitor (SNIN)	*Streptococcus* cysteine protease (SpeB)
	Staphylokinase	Cell envelope proteinase (SpyCEP)
	Chemotaxis inhibitory protein (CHIPS)	
	EAP	
Resistance to antimicrobial peptides	DltABCD	SIC
	MprF proteins	GRAB/SpeB
	Aureolysin	
Dissemination of infection	Spreading factors (lipase, hyaluronidase)	Spreading factors (DNases, hyaluronidase)
	Staphylokinase	Plasminogen-binding proteins
	Coagulase	Streptokinase

	Staphylococcus aureus	*Streptococcus pyogenes*
Killing of host leukocytes	α-Hemolysin γ-Hemolysin Panton-Valentine leukocidin Leukocidin E/D Leukocidin M/F-PV-like	Streptolysin O Streptolysin S
Inhibition of proteolysis	Staphostatin A Staphostatin B	GRAB α$_2$-Macroglobulin-binding proteins
Induction of vascular leakage	Staphopain A and B	M protein SpeB

Proinflammatory activities	*Superantigens*
	  Staphylococcal enterotoxins A–E, G–Q
	  TSST-1
	Toll-like receptor ligands
	  Peptidoglycan
	  Lipoteichoic acid
	  CpG DNA
	TNFR1 ligand
	  Protein A
		Superantigens
		  SpeA–C, F–M
		  SmeZ
		  SSA
		Toll-like receptor ligands
		  Peptidoglycan
		  Lipoteichoic acid
		  CpG DNA

*a*Spe, streptococcal pyrogenic exotoxins; SmeZ, streptococcal mitogenic; TNFR1, TNF receptor 1.

and, most likely, that these superantigens synergize with each other as well as with other streptococcal virulence factors in inducing severe disease.

Superantigen-Mediated Inflammation and Shock

One of the initial events in sepsis is the bacterial antigenemia that causes a release of proinflammatory cytokines, which trigger cytokine cascades, causes the activation of the complement and coagulation systems, induces endothelium and vessel injury, and elicits the release of proteases, arachidonic acid metabolites, and nitric oxide (16, 45). The cytokines that are most commonly associated with sepsis include interleukin 1 (IL1), tumor necrosis factor alpha (TNFα), IL6, IL8, IL12, gamma interferon (IFNγ), macrophage migration inhibitory factor (MIF), and high-mobility group 1 (HMGB-1) (4, 14, 17, 104). However, several additional cytokines are released during sepsis, and together with the abovementioned ones they interact in a complex network involving several crossover points and feedback loops.

The simultaneous binding of a superantigen to T cells and antigen-presenting cells results in potent activation of these cells and subsequent massive cytokine production. The superantigen-induction profile includes a wide array of cytokines, i.e., IL1α, IL1, IL1ra, IL6, IL8, IL12, MIF, TNFα, IL2, TNFβ, and IFNγ (49, 63, 81). The most pronounced and distinctive superantigen-induced cytokine production is seen for the Th1 cytokines TNFβ and IFNγ, which can be detected in up to 20% of peripheral blood mononuclear cells following 72 to 96 hours of superantigen stimulation in vitro (1, 71, 73). In contrast, the Th2 cytokines are produced at low frequencies (1, 71, 73).

A high degree of interindividual variation in mitogenic and cytokine responses induced by superantigens has been reported in several studies (1, 71, 73). Some individuals responded consistently high to superantigens with elevated IL1, TNFβ, and IFNγ but low Th2 cytokines, whereas the reverse was true for a "low-responder" (71). This interindividual variation between high and low responders was found to be attributed to host immunogenetic factors, i.e., the HLA class II haplotype of the individual, and to significantly affect disease severity (51). The study by Kotb et al. (51) identified both risk and protective HLA class II haplotypes in patients with severe or nonsevere invasive *S. pyogenes* infections, and provided evidence that this was associated with the ability of the HLA class II molecules to promote a high or a low superantigen-mediated T-cell response.

OTHER PATHOGENIC MECHANISMS IN STREPTOCOCCAL AND STAPHYLOCOCCAL INFECTIONS

Although superantigens are central mediators for the systemic effects seen in TSS, many additional virulence factors contribute to disease potential and fitness of the bacteria (Table 2). *S. pyogenes* and *S. aureus* are major human pathogens largely due to their ability to modulate and exploit the host defense mechanisms. This is contributed by a wide array of virulence factors that act in a complex network to promote colonization, growth, and immune escape within the human host. The pathogenesis of streptococcal and staphylococcal invasive infections demonstrates many similarities, as well as unique pathogen-specific mechanisms. Both pathogens express several virulence factors, cell associated or secreted, which in various ways interact with human cells to promote growth, dissemination, and survival of the organism. Most of the membrane-bound molecules are important for evasion and modulation of the innate immunity, as well as bacterial adherence to host cells and tissue, whereas several of the secreted proteins such as peptidases, streptolysins, superantigens, and proteases are important for spread and growth of the bacteria and result in induction of inflammatory responses (21, 28, 32, 59, 74).

LACK OF PROTECTIVE HUMORAL IMMUNITY IN TSS

Lack of humoral immunity appears to be a key risk factor for the development of staphylococcal and streptococcal TSS. Lack of detectable antibodies to TSS-associated superantigens in the acute-phase serum was predictable of susceptibility to staphylococcal TSS (96, 102), and was such a prominent finding that a revision of the case definition of staphylococcal TSS to include this factor was suggested (77). More than 90% of healthy men and women aged 25 years had protective antibody titers against TSST-1, as compared with only 9.5% in patients with menstrual TSS during the acute phase of infection (102).

It was established in 1962 that opsonic antibodies against the M protein confer resistance against infection; however, the protection is serotype specific and the individual remains susceptible to infection by other serotypes (54). To date 124 different serotypes of *S. pyogenes* have been described (46). Analyses of the recent outbreaks in the late 1980s, which were caused predominantly by M1T1 strains, revealed that invasive cases lacked protective antibodies against the M1 protein (11, 42).

Antibody levels against different superantigens were also assessed in patient materials collected during the recent outbreaks with somewhat discrepant results (10, 31, 42, 62, 75). The different studies revealed lack of protective immunity against specific superantigens, but which superantigen(s) differed between the countries. This likely reflects the involvement of different strains with varying superantigen profiles, but uniformly the studies demonstrate that lack of protective immunity is associated with susceptibility to invasive disease.

CONVENTIONAL THERAPY OF TSS

Streptococcal TSS should be treated with clindamycin and penicillin (94). The rationale for prescribing clindamycin is based on in vitro studies demonstrating both toxin suppression and modulation of cytokine (i.e., TNF) production, on animal studies demonstrating superior efficacy versus that of penicillin, and on two observational studies demonstrating greater efficacy for clindamycin than for β-lactam antibiotics (66, 108). This effect has also been demonstrated in vitro with linezolid, which may be an alternative agent to use for those patients who are at high risk for toxic shock caused by strains of methicillin-resistant *S. aureus* (94).

Conventional therapy of invasive *S. pyogenes* infections has consisted of antimicrobials and, when necessary in severe invasive disease, support of vital functions for those patients with streptococcal TSS and surgery for those patients with necrotizing fasciitis. *S. pyogenes* is uniformly susceptible to benzylpenicillin and other β-lactam antibiotics, and penicillin remains the cornerstone in antibiotic treatment of these infections. However, patients with severe *S. pyogenes,* such as myositis, necrotizing fasciitis, and/or TSS should be treated with clindamycin and penicillin (94). Although *S. pyogenes* has remained exquisitely sensitive to penicillin, resistance to the macrolides and clindamycin has emerged worldwide. Therefore, an approach for severe invasive *S. pyogenes* infections has been to utilize a combination of penicillin and clindamycin, since the penicillin provides coverage against 100% of *S. pyogenes* strains.

Patients with streptococcal TSS require supportive therapy to manage their hypotension and multiorgan failure, but despite improvement in intensive care units and improved awareness of this disease, the mortality from streptococcal TSS has not changed significantly (26, 44, 94). Often patients succumb to their infection before antimicrobials can have any beneficial effect, emphasizing the importance of research in immune modulation therapy.

IVIG AS ADJUNCTIVE THERAPY

The finding that lack of protective humoral immunity is a significant risk factor for development of TSS suggested that immunoglobulins might be a potential adjunctive therapy (10, 42, 62, 75). For an immunoglobulin therapy to be efficacious for TSS, a broad antibody specificity would be required to cover all the different serotypes of streptococci as well as the whole spectrum of streptococcal and staphylococcal superantigens and other important virulence factors. IVIG exhibits high polyspecificity as it consists of antibodies pooled from several thousands of donors. IVIG is commonly used as therapy in various autoimmune and immunodeficiency diseases, as well as in Kawasaki disease (reviewed in references 7, 65, and 88). The proven efficacy of IVIG in Kawasaki disease is of special interest since this disease has been suggested to be a superantigen-mediated disorder that shares several clinical features with TSS (55).

Mechanistic Actions of IVIG

Several different modes of actions that contribute to the beneficial effect in autoimmune and systemic inflammatory diseases have been ascribed to IVIG. These include blockade of Fc receptors on the reticuloendothelial cell system and phagocytic cells, modulation of Fc-receptor expression, interference with activated complement, modulation of cytokine responses, modulation of immune cell functions, interaction with the idiotype-antiidiotypic network, antigen neutralization, and selection of immune repertoires (reviewed in references 7 and 65).

Mechanistic actions directly related to the pathogenesis of staphylococcal and streptococcal TSS include antigen neutralization, bacterial opsonization, as well as cytokine modulation (Fig. 1). IVIG contains opsonizing antibodies that promote phagocytosis and bacterial clearance of several pathogenic microorganisms, including *S. pyogenes* and *S. aureus* (11, 33, 41, 105, 106). Antibodies against streptococcal M proteins and against the staphylococcal adhesins clumping factor A and EAP have been demonstrated in IVIG preparations (11, 37, 103). Analyses of patient plasma obtained pre- and post-IVIG therapy from patients with invasive streptococcal infections showed that these opsonizing anti-M1 antibodies were conferred to the patients upon IVIG therapy (11). Thus, increased bacterial clearance through opsonizing antibodies against the pathogens represents a likely mechanistic action of IVIG contributing to clinical efficacy (Fig. 1). However, an experimental murine model

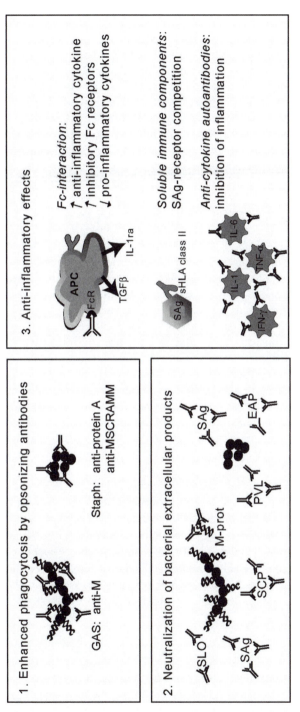

Figure 1. Proposed mechanisms of action of intravenous immunoglobulin in TSS caused by *S. pyogenes* or *S. aureus*. Intravenous immunoglobulin interacts at different stages in the bacterial pathogenesis to improve bacterial clearance and to neutralize toxins, superantigens, and proteases, as well as to improve immunosuppression through various immunomulatory effects. MSCRAMM, microbial surface components recognizing adhesive matrix molecules; SAg, superantigens; SCP, streptococcal cysteine protease, i.e., SpeB; SLO, streptolysin O; EAP, extracellular adherence protein; PVL, Panton-valentine leukocidin; APC, antigen-presenting cell; FcR, Fc receptor.

of necrotizing fasciitis that compared the efficacy of clindamycin, penicillin, and IVIG, alone or in combination, failed to support this hypothesis (78). Efficacy of the various treatment regimens was based on quantitative bacterial clearance, and IVIG did not enhance killing of the M3 *S. pyogenes* strain used. However, the lack of benefit may well be because human immunoglobulins are not efficient opsonins for mouse phagocytes.

Another theoretical benefit of the M-specific antibodies could be inhibition of the M-protein-mediated activation of neutrophils (40), but this remains to be tested. IVIG also contains neutralizing antibodies against a wide spectrum of staphylococcal and streptococcal superantigens. These antibodies are potent inhibitors of the proliferative and cytokine-inducing capacity of these superantigens in vitro at physiological concentrations of IVIG (23, 24, 69, 70, 89, 98). All superantigens that have been tested have been inhibited by IVIG, but the IVIG inhibitory concentrations varied somewhat depending on the superantigen. In a comparative study of IVIG neutralization of streptococcal and staphylococcal superantigens, IVIGs were more potent in inhibiting the streptococcal than the staphylococcal superantigens (23). This study used crude mixtures of superantigens present in bacterial stationary culture supernatants, and hence did not allow for assessment of IVIG-mediated neutralization of individual superantigens. A recent study by Holtfreter et al. (43) demonstrated that human sera neutralized *egc*-encoded superantigens from *S. aureus* much less efficiently than the classical staphylococcal enterotoxins or TSST-1. Hence, less efficient inhibition of *egc*-superantigens may have contributed to the reduced efficacy of IVIG against staphylococcal superantigens. These studies have shown that IVIG preparations may differ in their neutralizing activity but considering that at physiological concentrations the vast majority of superantigens are 100% inhibited by a wide range of different IVIG preparations, this is unlikely to affect the clinical efficacy of the therapy if high doses (1 to 2 g/kg body weight) are used. The data rather demonstrate that IVIG exhibits an extraordinarily broad specificity against staphylococcal and streptococcal virulence factors that is efficiently conferred to the patients upon intravenous infusion. Furthermore, antibodies against other important virulence factors, such as the streptococcal DNaseB and streptolysin O as well as the staphylococcal Panton-Valentine leukocidin, have also been found in IVIG preparations (34, 57, 91).

Most studies mentioned above have used IVIG composed of IgG. However, analyses of different IVIG preparations containing varying concentrations of IgG, IgA, and/or IgM revealed that they varied in opsonizing and toxin-neutralizing capacity, and variation in inhibitory activity was even observed between lots of the same preparation (41, 68). IgA and IgM were found to be potent inhibitors of streptococcal superantigens, and in the case of SpeA the most efficient neutralization was achieved by a preparation containing a mixture of IgG, IgA, and IgM (68). These findings suggest that optimization of IVIG therapy may be achieved by changing the type or lot of IVIG preparation; however, this remains to be proven in a clinical setting.

IVIG Modulation of Cytokine Responses

IVIG exerts anti-inflammatory effects through modulation of cytokine expression, not only via direct antigen neutralizing, but also Fc interactions, soluble immune components, and induction of regulatory cytokines (reviewed in references 7 and 65). Coculture of human monocytes with adherent IgG or IVIG results in strong induction of IL1 receptor antagonist (IL1ra), which serves as antagonist to IL1 signaling (3, 5, 80). Also IL8 production is upregulated by coculture with human monocytes and IVIG (2, 84). IL8 is usually considered a mediator of proinflammation due to its chemotactic properties, but it has been suggested that IL8 release systemically could have an anti-inflammatory effect due to a reduction in accumulation of neutrophils in the inflammatory sites (6).

IVIG has been shown in vitro to be a powerful inhibitor of superantigen-induced T-cell activation and subsequent lymphokine production, with the strongest suppression seen for the Th1 cytokines IFNγ and TNFβ, as their production was almost completely abolished (3, 23, 68, 70, 89). This inhibitory effect was seen, although to a lesser extent, even when addition of IVIG was delayed 24 hours poststimulation with superantigen (3, 89). A differential effect of IVIG was noted on superantigen-induced monokine production with upregulated IL8 and decreased IL6 production (3). Studies on the effect of IVIG on superantigen-induced IL1 production have reported conflicting results, as one study demonstrated no effect on IL1 production (89), whereas the other reported a significant reduction of IL1 (68). Thus, the effect of IVIG on superantigen-induced monokines remains to be elucidated. Most importantly, the production of the Th1 type of cytokines that are characteristic of a superantigen response is completely inhibited by IVIG, which likely represents a major mechanistic action of IVIG contributing to clinical efficacy.

Cytokine modulation by IVIG has also been shown in vivo in several diseases, including, among others, severe invasive *S. pyogenes* infections where patients showed decreased levels of TNFα and IL6 (48, 67); Guillain-Barré syndrome patients showed a selective downregulation of proinflammatory cytokines (87), and Kawasaki patients demonstrated elevated IL1ra and IL8, as well as decreased proinflammatory cytokines following IVIG therapy (56).

Clinical Studies

Only limited clinical data are available for IVIG as adjunctive therapy in staphylococcal TSS with three case reports (Table 3) (25, 39, 76). The most recent case report describes a 14-year-old boy with septicemia and disseminated foci of infection, including necrotizing fasciitis, septic arthritis, and deep vein thrombosis of the leg. The infection was caused by a Panton-Valentine leukocidin (PVL)-producing strain of community-acquired methicillin-resistant *S. aureus* (MRSA) (39), an emergent cause of severe, rapidly progressing systemic manifestations including soft-tissue infections and necrotizing pneumonia with mortality rates as high as 75% (35, 101). The current case received empirical antibiotics (intravenous cefuroxime, flucloxacillin, and metronidazole) and clindamycin was added at 48 h. Antibiotics were then changed to linezolide in combination with rifampicin to which the isolate was susceptible. Despite this, the boy failed to improve clinically and at day 7, IVIG was given. This was followed by clinical improvement and a marked reduction in inflammatory markers. The boy was discharged from intensive care 5 days later.

The documentation of the clinical efficacy of IVIG in streptococcal TSS includes several case reports (8, 18, 19, 53, 60, 67, 79, 91, 107), as well as two observational cohort studies (72, 91), one case-control study (48), and one multicenter placebo-controlled trial (22) (Table 3). The case-control study was designed to evaluate the efficacy of IVIG therapy in patients with streptococcal TSS and included 21 cases that were treated with IVIG

Table 3. Intravenous polyspecific immunoglobulin (IVIG) as adjunctive therapy in streptococcal and staphylococcal TSS[a]

Patients	No. of patients[b]	Infectious agents[c]	Case fatality rate (%)
Case reports			
TSS + pneumonia (76)	1	*S. aureus*	0
TSS + necrotizing pneumonia (39)	1	PVL + CA-MRSA	0
TSS (25)	2	*S. aureus*	0
TSS + NM (53)	1	*S. pyogenes*, M1	0
TSS + NF (79)	1	*S. pyogenes*	0
TSS + NF (18)	1	*S. pyogenes*	0
TSS + NF (107)	1	*S. pyogenes*	0
TSS (60)	1	*S. pyogenes*, M1	0
TSS (8)	1	*S. pyogenes*, M49	0
TSS (67)	1	*S. pyogenes*, M1	0
TSS (19)	1	*S. pyogenes*, M74	0
Observational cohort study			
TSS (91)	5	*S. pyogenes*, M1	20
TSS + severe soft-tissue infections (72)	6	*S. pyogenes*, M1 (50%), 5, 28, 31	0
Case-control study			
TSS (48)		*S. pyogenes*	
IVIG	21	48% M1, 19% M3	33
No IVIG	32	6% M1, 28% M3	66
Multicenter, placebo-controlled trial			
TSS[d] (22)		*S. pyogenes*	
IVIG	10	T1 (14%), T12 (43%)	10
Placebo	11	T1 (70%)	36

[a]PVL, Panton-Valentine leukocidin; CA-MRSA, community-acquired methicillin-resistant *S. aureus;* NM, necrotizing myositis; NF, necrotizing fasciitis.
[b]All received IVIG unless otherwise specified.
[c]The M or T serotype of *S. pyogenes* strains is indicated for known cases.
[d]Trial prematurely terminated due to slow patient recruitment (22).

from 1994 to 1995 and 32 nontreated controls identified through active surveillance of invasive *S. pyogenes* infections from 1992 through 1995 (48). Multivariate analysis revealed that IVIG therapy and a lower acute physiology and chronic health evaluation II (APACHE) score were significantly associated with survival. One confounding factor in the material was that IVIG-treated cases were more likely to have received clindamycin therapy than the controls. Therefore, a secondary multivariate analysis considering only cases and controls that had received clindamycin was performed, and APACHE II score and IVIG therapy remained the two variables associated with survival. Further support for the use of IVIG was provided by in vitro studies of blood samples collected pre- and post-IVIG therapy, which showed an increased superantigen-neutralizing activity in plasma collected posttherapy (48). The majority of patients' post-IVIG plasma caused 80 to 100% inhibition of the bacterial supernatants. Considering that the material included patients infected with *S. pyogenes* strains of varying serotype (Table 3), this demonstrates that

IVIG has a very broad spectrum of superantigen-neutralizing antibodies. IVIG therapy also resulted in a significantly reduced TNFα and IL6 production in peripheral blood mononuclear cells in four patients tested (48). Thus, together these data suggest that the clinical improvement achieved by IVIG therapy may be partly attributed to inhibition of the superantigens produced by the clinical isolates, and a reduction in the proinflammatory response. Although the results of this study demonstrated a significant benefit of IVIG, the study had two confounding factors, i.e., historical controls and difference in antibiotic therapy, which could potentially affect the mortality rate. To further document the safety and efficacy of this adjunctive therapy, a multicenter placebo-controlled trial of IVIG in streptococcal TSS was initiated in Europe (22). The trial was prematurely terminated due to a low incidence of disease in the participating countries and consequently a slow patient recruitment. Results were obtained from 21 enrolled patients (10 IVIG recipients and 11 placebo recipients). The primary end point was mortality at 28 days, and a 3.6-fold higher mortality rate was found in the placebo group (Table 3). This trend to improved survival was strengthened by the significant improvement in organ function revealed by the reduction in the sepsis-related organ failure assessment score after treatment, which was evident in the IVIG group but not in the placebo group. Furthermore, a significant increase in plasma-neutralizing activity against superantigens expressed by autologous isolates was noted in the IVIG group after treatment.

Streptococcal TSS is often seen in combination with necrotizing fasciitis and the mortality is even higher among these patients. The treatment of necrotizing fasciitis has emphasized the importance of early aggressive surgical intervention to reduce the systemic inflammatory response and the spread of local infection (15, 92). Unfortunately, this procedure usually occurs at a time when the patient is most unstable and therefore interferes with monitoring and treatment. In an observational case study (72), the use of an aggressive medical regimen including high-dose IVIG together with a conservative surgical approach was studied. The report describes seven patients with severe soft-tissue infection caused by S. pyogenes, in whom surgery was not performed or only limited exploration was carried out. Six of the patients had TSS, and they all received effective antimicrobials and high-dose IVIG. All patients survived. This observational study, although limited in numbers, suggests that an initial conservative surgical approach combined with the use of immune modulators, such as IVIG, may reduce the morbidity associated with extensive surgical exploration in hemodynamically unstable patients without increasing mortality.

CONCLUDING REMARKS

TSS is a superantigen-mediated disease, and the systemic features and severity of infection are associated with the magnitude of cytokine release. Hence, adjunctive therapy needs to target superantigens and the proinflammatory response. Not one toxin is solely responsible for development of TSS, but rather a repertoire of the many superantigens produced by S. pyogenes and S. aureus, respectively. The data suggest that IVIG is efficacious against a wide variety of strains of varying serotypes and with different superantigen production, and that the efficacy contributes to direct antigen neutralization, suppression of proinflammatory responses, and bacterial opsonization. Although it would be desirable to have a controlled trial to provide definite proof of the clinical efficacy of IVIG in these diseases, considering the high mortality and morbidity of streptococcal TSS and necrotizing fasciitis, it seems reasonable that IVIG be used in conjunction with conventional therapy in the severe cases. The efficacy of IVIG in staphylococcal TSS has not yet been documented, but the functional data as well as the few case reports available suggest that it should be considered in the severe cases.

REFERENCES

1. **Andersson, J., S. Nagy, L. Björk, J. Abrams, S. Holm, and U. Andersson.** 1992. Bacterial toxin-induced cytokine production studied at the single-cell level. *Immunol. Rev.* **127:**69–96.
2. **Andersson, J., U. Skansén-Saphir, E. Sparrelid, and U. Andersson.** 1994. Intravenous immune globulin affects cytokine production in T lymphocytes and monocytes/macrophages. *Clin. Exp. Immunol.* **104**(Suppl.):10–20.
3. **Andersson, U., L. Björck, U. Skansén-Saphir, and J. Andersson.** 1994. Pooled human IgG modulates cytokine production in lymphocytes and monocytes. *Immunol. Rev.* **139:**21–43.
4. **Andersson, U., and K. J. Tracey.** 2003. HMGB-1 in sepsis. *Scand. J. Infect. Dis.* **35:**577.
5. **Arend, W. P., M. F. J. Smith, R. W. Janson, and F. G. Joslin.** 1991. IL-1 receptor antagonist and IL-1 beta production in human monocytes are regulated differently. *J. Immunol.* **147:**1530–1536.
6. **Asano, T., and S. Ogawa.** 2000. Expression of IL-8 in Kawasaki disease. *Clin. Exp. Immunol.* **122:**514–519.
7. **Ballow, M.** 1997. Mechanisms of action of intravenous immune serum globulin in autoimmune and inflammatory diseases. *Allergy Clin. Immunol.* **100:**151–157.
8. **Barry, W., L. Hudgins, S. T. Donta, and E. L. Pesanti.** 1992. Intravenous immunoglobulin therapy for toxic shock syndrome. *JAMA* **267:**3315–3316.
9. **Bartter, T., A. Dascal, K. Carroll, and F. J. Curley.** 1988. 'Toxic strep syndrome'. A manifestation of group A streptococcal infection. *Arch. Intern. Med.* **148:**1421–1424.
10. **Basma, H., A. Norrby-Teglund, Y. Guedez, A. McGeer, D. E. Low, O. El-Ahmedy, B. Schwartz, and M. Kotb.** 1999. Risk factors in the pathogenesis of invasive group A streptococcal infections: Role of protective humoral immunity. *Infect. Immun.* **67:**1871–1877.
11. **Basma, H., A. Norrby-Teglund, A. McGeer, D. E. Low, O. El-Ahmedy, J. B. Dale, B. Schwartz, and M. Kotb.** 1998. Opsonic antibodies to the surface M protein, present in pooled normal immunoglobulins (IVIG), may contribute to its clinical efficacy in severe invasive group A streptococcal infections. *Infect. Immun.* **66:**2279–2283.
12. **Bergdoll, M. S., B. A. Crass, R. F. Reiser, R. N. Robbins, and J. P. Davis.** 1981. A new staphylococcal enterotoxin, enterotoxin F, associated with toxic-shock-syndrome *Staphylococcus aureus* isolates. *Lancet* **1:**1017–1021.
13. **Bergdoll, M. S., and P. M. Schlievert.** 1984. Toxic-shock syndrome toxin. *Lancet* **2:**691.
14. **Bernhagen, J., T. Calandra, and R. Bucala.** 1998. Regulation of the immune response by macrophage migration inhibitory factor: biological and structural features. *J. Mol. Med.* **76:**151–161.
15. **Bisno, A. L., and D. L. Stevens.** 1996. Streptococcal infections of skin and soft tissues. *N. Engl. J. Med.* **334:**240–245.
16. **Bone, R. C.** 1991. The pathogenesis of sepsis. *Ann. Intern. Med.* **115:**457–469.
17. **Cavaillon, J. M., M. Adib-Conquy, C. Fitting, C. Adrie, and D. Payen.** 2003. Cytokine cascades in sepsis. *Scand. J. Infect. Dis.* **35:**535–544.
18. **Cawley, M. J., M. Briggs, L. R. J. Haith, K. J. Reilly, R. E. Guilday, G. R. Braxton, and M. L. Patton.** 1999. Intravenous immunoglobulin as adjunctive treatment for streptococcal toxic shock syndrome associated with necrotizing fasciitis: case report and review. *Pharmacotherapy* **19:**1094–1098.
19. **Chiu, C. H., J. T. Ou, K. S. Chang, and T. Y. Lin.** 1997. Successful treatment of severe streptococcal toxic shock syndrome with a combination of intravenous immunoglobulin, dexamethasone and antibiotics. *Infection* **25:**47–48.
20. **Cone, L. A., D. R. Woodard, P. M. Schlievert, and G. S. Tomory.** 1987. Clinical and bacteriological observations of a toxic shock-like syndrome due to *Streptococcus pyogenes*. *N. Engl. J. Med.* **317:**146–149.
21. **Cunningham, M. W.** 2000. Pathogenesis of group A streptococcal infections. *Clin. Microbiol. Rev.* **13:**470–511.
22. **Darenberg, J., N. Ihendyane, J. Sjölin, E. Aufwerber, S. Haidl, P. Follin, J. Andersson, A. Norrby-Teglund, and the StreptIg Study Group.** 2003. Intravenous immunoglobulin G therapy in streptococcal toxic shock syndrome: a European randomized double-blind placebo-controlled trial. *Clin. Infect. Dis.* **37:**333–340.

23. **Darenberg, J., B. Söderquist, B. Henriques Normark, and A. Norrby-Teglund.** 2004. Differences in potency of intravenous polyspecific immunoglobulin G against streptococcal and staphylococcal superantigens: implications for therapy of toxic shock syndrome. *Clin. Infect. Dis.* **38:**836–842.

24. **Darville, T., L. B. Milligan, and K. K. Laffoon.** 1997. Intravenous immunoglobulin inhibits staphylococcal toxin-induced human mononuclear phagocyte tumor necrosis factor alpha production. *Infect. Immun.* **65:**366–372.

25. **Dass, R., P. Nishad, and S. Singhi.** 2004. Toxic shock syndrome. *Indian J. Pediatr.* **71:**433–435.

26. **Davies, D. H., A. McGeer, B. Schwartz, K. Green, D. Cann, A. E. Simor, D. E. Low, and the Ontario Group A Streptococcal Study Group.** 1996. Invasive group A streptococcal infections in Ontario, Canada. *N. Engl. J. Med.* **135:**547–554.

27. **Demers, B., A. E. Simor, H. Vellend, P. M. Schlievert, S. Byrne, F. Jamieson, S. Walmsley, and D. E. Low.** 1993. Severe invasive group A streptococcal infections in Ontario, Canada: 1987–1991. *Clin. Infect. Dis.* **16:**792–800.

28. **Dinges, M. M., P. M. Orwin, and P. M. Schlievert.** 2000. Exotoxins of *Staphylococcus aureus. Clin. Microbiol. Rev.* **13:**16–34.

29. **Edwards-Jones, V., M. M. Dawson, and C. Childs.** 2000. A survey into toxic shock syndrome (TSS) in UK burns units. *Burns* **26:**323–333.

30. **Ekelund, K., P. Skinhoj, J. Madsen, and H. B. Konradsen.** 2005. Invasive group A, B, C and G streptococcal infections in Denmark 1999-2002: epidemiological and clinical aspects. *Clin. Microbiol. Infect.* **11:**569–576.

31. **Eriksson, B. K., J. Andersson, S. E. Holm, and M. Norgren.** 1999. Invasive group A streptococcal infections: T1M1 isolates expressing pyrogenic exotoxins A and B in combination with selective lack of toxin-neutralizing antibodies are associated with increased risk of streptococcal toxic shock syndrome. *J. Infect. Dis.* **180:**410–418.

32. **Ferry, T., T. Perpoint, F. Vandanesch, and J. Etienne.** 2005. Virulence determinants in *Staphylococcus aureus* and their involvement in clinical syndromes. *Curr. Infect. Dis. Rep.* **7:**420–428.

33. **Fisher, G. W., T. J. Cieslak, S. R. Wilson, L. E. Weisman, and V. G. Heeming.** 1994. Opsonic antibodies to *Staphylococcus epidermis*: in vitro and in vivo studies using human intravenous immune globulin. *J. Infect. Dis.* **169:**324–329.

34. **Gauduchon, V., G. Cozon, F. Vandenesch, A. L. Genestier, N. Eyssade, S. Peyrol, J. Etienne, and G. Lina.** 2004. Neutralization of *Staphylococcus aureus* Panton Valentine leukocidin by intravenous immunoglobulin in vitro. *J. Infect. Dis.* **189:**346–353.

35. **Gillet, Y., B. Issartel, P. Vanhems, J. C. Fournet, G. Lina, M. Bes, F. Vandenesch, Y. Piemont, N. Brousse, D. Floret, and J. Etienne.** 2002. Association between *Staphylococcus aureus* strains carrying gene for Panton-Valentine leukocidin and highly lethal necrotising pneumonia in young immunocompetent patients. *Lancet* **359:**753–759.

36. **Goepel, J. R., D. G. Richards, D. M. Harris, and L. Henry.** 1980. Fulminant *Streptococcus pyogenes* infection. *Brit. Med. J.* **281:**1412.

37. **Haggar, A., O. Shannon, A. Norrby-Teglund, and J.-I. Flock.** 2005. Dual effects of extracellular adherence protein from *Staphylococcus aureus* on peripheral blood mononuclear cells. *J. Infect. Dis.* **192:**210–217.

38. **Hajjeh, R. A., A. Reingold, A. Weil, K. Shutt, A. Schuchat, and B. A. Perkins.** 1999. Toxic shock syndrome in the United States: surveillance update, 1979–1996. *Emerg. Infect. Dis.* **5:**807–810.

39. **Hampson, F. G., S. W. Hancock, and R. A. Primhak.** 2006. Disseminated sepsis due to a Panton-Valentine leukocidin producing strain of community acquired meticillin resistant *Staphylococcus aureus* and use of intravenous immunoglobulin therapy. *Arch. Dis. Child.* **91:**201.

40. **Herwald, H., H. Cramer, M. Mörgelin, W. Russell, U. Sollenberg, A. Norrby-Teglund, H. Flodgaard, L. Lindblom, and L. Björck.** 2004. M protein, a classical bacterial virulence determinant, forms complexes with fibrinogen that induce vascular leakage. *Cell* **116:**367–379.

41. **Hiemstra, P. S., J. Brands-Tajouiti, and R. van Furth.** 1994. Comparison of antibody activity against various microorganisms in intravenous immunoglobulin preparations determined by ELISA and opsonic assay. *J. Lab. Clin. Med.* **123:**241–246.

42. **Holm, S. E., A. Norrby, A.-M. Bergholm, and M. Norgren.** 1992. Aspects of the pathogenesis in serious group A streptococcal infections in Sweden 1988-1989. *J. Infect. Dis.* **166:**31–37.

43. **Holtfreter, S., K. Bauer, D. Thomas, C. Feig, V. Lorenz, K. Roschack, E. Friebe, K. Selleng, S. Lövenich, T. Greve, A. Greinacher, B. Panzig, S. Engelmann, G. Lina, and B. M. Bröker.** 2004. *egc*-encoded super-

antigens from *Staphylococcus aureus* are neutralized by human sera much less efficiently than are classical staphylococcal enterotoxins or toxic shock syndrome toxin. *Infect. Immun.* **72:**4061–4071.

44. **Hook, E. W., C. A. Horton, and D. R. Schaberg.** 1983. Failure of intensive care unit support to influence mortality from pneumococcal bacteremia. *JAMA* **249:**1055–1057.

45. **Hotchkiss, R. S., and I. E. Karl.** 2003. The pathophysiology and treatment of sepsis. *N. Engl. J. Med.* **348:**138–150.

46. **Johnson, D. R., E. L. Kaplan, A. VanGheem, R. R. Facklam, and B. Beall.** 2006. Characterization of group A streptococci (*Streptococcus pyogenes*): correlation of M-protein and *emm*-gene type with T-protein agglutination pattern and serum opacity factor. *J. Med. Microbiol.* **55:**157–164.

47. **Kamezawa, Y., T. Nakahara, S. Nakano, Y. Abe, J. Nozaki-Renard, and T. Isono.** 1997. Streptococcal mitogenic exotoxin Z, a novel acidic superantigenic toxin produced by a T1 strain of *Streptococcus pyogenes*. *Infect. Immun.* **65:**3828–3833.

48. **Kaul, R., A. McGeer, A. Norrby-Teglund, M. Kotb, B. Schwartz, K. O'Rourke, J. Talbot, D. E. Low, and the Canadian Streptococcal Study Group.** 1999. Intravenous immunoglobulin therapy for streptococcal toxic shock syndrome—a comparative observational study. *Clin. Infect. Dis.* **28:**800–807.

49. **Kotb, M.** 1995. Bacterial pyrogenic exotoxins as superantigens. *Clin. Microbiol. Rev.* **8:**411–426.

50. **Kotb, M.** 1998. Superantigens of gram-positive bacteria: structure-function analyses and their implications for biological activity. *Curr. Opin. Microbiol.* **1:**56–65.

51. **Kotb, M., A. Norrby-Teglund, A. McGeer, M. K. Dorak, A. Khurshid, H. El-Shirbini, K. Green, J. Peeples, J. Wade, G. Thomson, B. Schwartz, and D. E. Low.** 2002. Immunogenetic and molecular basis for the differences in outcomes of invasive group A streptococcal infections. *Nat. Med.* **8:**1398–1404.

52. **Kuroda, M., T. Ohta, I. Uchiyama, T. Baba, H. Yuzawa, I. Kobayashi, L. Cui, A. Oguchi, K. Aoki, Y. Nagai, J. Lian, T. Ito, M. Kanamori, H. Matsumaru, A. Maruyama, H. Murakami, A. Hosoyama, Y. Mizutani-Ui, N. K. Takahashi, T. Sawano, R. Inoue, C. Kaito, K. Sekimizu, H. Hirakawa, S. Kuhara, S. Goto, J. Yabuzaki, M. Kanehisa, A. Yamashita, K. Oshima, K. Furuya, C. Yoshino, T. Shiba, M. Hattori, N. Ogasawara, H. Hayashi, and K. Hiramatsu.** 2001. Whole-genome sequencing of methicillin-resistant *Staphylococcus aureus*. *Lancet* **357:**1225–1240.

53. **Lamothe, F., P. D'Amico, P. Ghosn, C. Tremblay, J. Braidy, and J. Patenaude.** 1995. Clinical usefulness of intravenous human immunoglobulins in invasive group A streptococcal disease: case report and review. *J. Clin. Inf. Dis.* **21:**1469–1470.

54. **Lancefield, R. C.** 1962. Current knowledge of type-specific M antigen of group A streptococci. *J. Immunol.* **89:**307–313.

55. **Leung, D. Y.** 1996. Kawaski syndrome: immunomodulatory benefit and potential toxin neutralization by intravenous immune globulin. *Clin. Exp. Immunol.* **104**(Suppl. 1):49–54.

56. **Leung, D. Y., R. S. Cotran, E. Kurt-Jones, J. C. Burns, J. W. Newburger, and J. S. Pober.** 1989. Endothelial cell activation and high interleukin-1 secretion in the pathogenesis of acute Kawasaki disease. *Lancet* **2:**1298–1302.

57. **Lissner, R., W. G. Struff, I. B. Autenrieth, B. G. Woodcock, and H. Karch.** 1999. Efficacy and potential clinical applications of Pentaglobin, an IgM-enriched immunoglobulin concentrate suitable for intravenous infusion. *Eur. J. Surg.* **584**(Suppl.):17–25.

58. **Low, D. E., B. Schwartz, and A. McGeer.** 1998. The reemergance of severe group A streptococcal disease: An evolutionary perspective, p. 93–123. *In* W. M. Scheld, D. Armstrong, and J. M. Hughes (ed.), *Emerging infections,* vol. 7. ASM Press, Washington, D.C.

59. **Lowy, F. D.** 1998. *Staphylococcus aureus* infections. *N. Engl. J. Med.* **339:**520–532.

60. **Mahieu, L. M., S. E. Holm, H. J. Goossens, and K. J. Van Acker.** 1995. Congenital streptococcal toxic shock syndrome with absence of antibodies against streptococcal pyrogenic exotoxins. *J. Pediatr.* **127:**987–989.

61. **Marrack, P., and J. Kappler.** 1990. The staphylococcal enterotoxins and their relatives. *Science* **248:**705–711.

62. **Mascini, E. M., M. Jansze, J. F. Schellekens, J. M. Musser, J. A. Faber, L. A. Verhoef-Verhage, L. Schouls, W. J. van Leeuwen, J. Verhoef, and H. van Dijk.** 2000. Invasive group A streptococcal disease in the Netherlands: evidence for a protective role of anti-exotoxin A antibodies. *J. Infect. Dis.* **181:**631–638.

63. **McCormick, J. K., J. M. Yarwood, and P. M. Schlievert.** 2001. Toxic shock syndrome and bacterial superantigens: an update. *Annu. Rev. Microbiol.* **55:**77–104.

64. **Mollick, J. A., G. G. Miller, J. Musser, R. G. Cook, D. Grossman, and R. R. Rich.** 1993. A novel super-antigen isolated from pathogenic strains of *S. pyogenes* with aminoterminal homology to staphylococcal enterotoxins B and C. *J. Clin. Invest.* **92:**710–719.

65. **Mouthon, L., S. V. Kaveri, S. H. Spalter, S. Lacroix-Desmazes, C. Lefranc, R. Desai, and M. D. Kazatchkine.** 1996. Mechanisms of action of intravenous immune globulin in immune-mediated diseases. *Clin. Exp. Immunol.* **104**(Suppl. 1)**:**3–9.

66. **Mulla, Z. D., P. E. Leaverton, and S. T. Wiersma.** 2003. Invasive group A streptococcal infections in Florida. *South. Med. J.* **96:**968–973.

67. **Nadal, D., R. P. Lauener, C. P. Braegger, A. Kaufhold, B. Simma, R. Lutticken, and R. A. Seger.** 1993. T cell activation and cytokine release in streptococcal toxic shock-like syndrome. *J. Pediatr.* **122:**727–729.

68. **Norrby-Teglund, A., N. Ihendyane, R. Kansal, H. Basma, M. Kotb, J. Andersson, and L. Hammarström.** 2000. Relative neutralizing activity in polyspecific IgM, IgA, and IgG preparations against group A streptococcal superantigens. *Clin. Infect. Dis.* **31:**1175–1182.

69. **Norrby-Teglund, A., R. Kaul, D. E. Low, A. McGeer, J. Andersson, U. Andersson, and M. Kotb.** 1996. Evidence for the presence of streptococcal superantigen neutralizing antibodies in normal polyspecific IgG (IVIG). *Infect. Immun.* **64:**5395–5398.

70. **Norrby-Teglund, A., R. Kaul, D. E. Low, A. McGeer, D. Newton, J. Andersson, U. Andersson, and M. Kotb.** 1996. Plasma from patients with severe invasive group A streptococcal infections treated with normal polyspecific IgG inhibits streptococcal superantigen-induced T cell proliferation and cytokine production. *J. Immunol.* **156:**3057–3064.

71. **Norrby-Teglund, A., R. Lustig, and M. Kotb.** 1997. Differential induction of Th1 versus Th2 cytokines by group A streptococcal toxic shock syndrome isolates. *Infect. Immun.* **65:**5209–5215.

72. **Norrby-Teglund, A., M. P. Muller, A. McGeer, B. S. Gan, V. Guru, J. Bohnen, P. Thulin, and D. E. Low.** 2005. Successful management of severe group A streptococcal soft tissue infections using intravenous polyspecific immunoglobulin and a conservative surgical approach. *Scand. J. Infect. Dis.* **37:**166–172.

73. **Norrby-Teglund, A., M. Norgren, S. E. Holm, U. Andersson, and J. Andersson.** 1994. Similar cytokine induction profiles of a novel streptococcal exotoxin, MF, and pyrogenic exotoxins A and B. *Infect. Immun.* **62:**3731–3738.

74. **Norrby-Teglund, A., R. Norrby, and D. E. Low.** 2003. The treatment of severe group A streptococcal infections. *Curr. Infect. Dis. Rep.* **5:**28–37.

75. **Norrby-Teglund, A., K. Pauksens, S. E. Holm, and M. Norgren.** 1994. Relation between low capacity of human sera to inhibit streptococcal mitogens and serious manifestation of disease. *J. Infect. Dis.* **170:**585-591.

76. **Ogawa, M., S. Ueda, N. Anzai, K. Ito, and M. Ohto.** 1995. Toxic shock syndrome after staphylococcal pneumonia treated with intravenous immunoglobulin. *Vox Sang.* **68:**59–60.

77. **Parsonnet, J.** 1997. Case definition of staphylococcal TSS: a proposed revision incorporating laboratory findings, p. 15. *In* J. Arbuthnott and B. Furman (ed.), *International Congress Symposium Series European Conference on Toxic Shock Syndrome.* Royal Society of Medicine Press, London, United Kingdom.

78. **Patel, R., M. S. Rouse, M. V. Florez, K. E. Piper, F. R. Cockerill, W. R. Wilson, and J. M. Steckelberg.** 2000. Lack of benefit of intravenous immune globulin in a murine model of group A streptococcal necrotizing fasciitis. *J. Infect. Dis.* **181:**230–234.

79. **Perez, C. M., B. M. Kubak, H. G. Cryer, S. Salemugodam, P. Vespa, and D. Farmer.** 1997. Adjunctive treatment of streptococcal toxic shock syndrome with intravenous immunoglobulin: case report and review. *Am. J. Med.* **102:**111–113.

80. **Poutsiaka, D. D., B. D. Clark, E. Vannier, and C. A. Dinarello.** 1991. Production of interleukin-1 receptor antagonist and interleukin-1 beta by peripheral blood mononuclear cells is differentially regulated. *Blood* **78:**1275–1281.

81. **Proft, T., and J. D. Fraser.** 2003. Bacterial superantigens. *Clin. Exp. Immunol.* **133:**299–306.

82. **Proft, T., S. L. Moffatt, C. J. Berkahn, and J. D. Fraser.** 1999. Identification and characterization of novel superantigens from *Streptococcus pyogenes*. *J. Exp. Med.* **189:**89–102.

83. **Proft, T., S. L. Moffatt, K. D. Weller, A. Paterson, D. Martin, and J. D. Fraser.** 2000. The streptococcal superantigen SMEZ exhibits wide allelic variation, mosaic structure, and significant antigenic variation. *J. Exp. Med.* **191:**1765–1776.

84. **Ruiz de Souza, V., M. P. Carreno, S. V. Kaveri, A. Ledur, H. Sadeghi, J. M. Cavaillon, M. D. Kazatchkine, and N. Haeffner-Cavaillon.** 1995. Selective induction of interleukin-1 receptor antagonist and

interleukin-8 in human monocytes by normal polyspecific IgG (intravenous immunoglobulin). *Eur. J. Immunol.* **25:**1267–1273.

85. **Schlievert, P. M.** 1986. Staphylococcal enterotoxin B and toxic-shock syndrome toxin-1 are significantly associated with non-menstrual TSS. *Lancet* **i:**1149–1150.

86. **Schlievert, P. M., K. N. Shands, B. B. Dan, G. P. Schmid, and R. D. Nishimura.** 1981. Identification and characterization of an exotoxin from *Staphylococcus aureus* associated with toxic-shock syndrome. *J. Infect. Dis.* **143:**509–516.

87. **Sharief, M. K., D. A. Ingram, M. Swash, and E. J. Thompson.** 1999. IV immunoglobulin reduces circulating proinflammatory cytokines in Guillain-Barré syndrome. *Neurology* **52:**1833–1838.

88. **Shulman, S. R., and M. Bendet.** 1997. Kawasaki disease. *Compr. Ther.* **23:**13–18.

89. **Skansen-Saphir, U., J. Andersson, L. Björk, and U. Andersson.** 1994. Lymphokine production induced by streptococcal pyrogenic exotoxin-A is selectively down-regulated by pooled human IgG. *Eur. J. Immunol.* **24:**916–922.

90. **Smoot, L. M., J. K. McCormick, J. C. Smoot, N. P. Hoe, I. Strickland, R. L. Cole, K. D. Barbian, C. A. Earhart, D. H. Ohlendorf, L. G. Veasy, H. R. Hill, D. Y. Leung, P. M. Schlievert, and J. M. Musser.** 2002. Characterization of two novel pyrogenic toxin superantigens made by an acute rheumatic fever clone of *Streptococcus pyogenes* associated with multiple disease outbreaks. *Infect. Immun.* **72:**7095–7104.

91. **Stegmayr, B., S. Bjorck, S. Holm, J. Nisell, A. Rydvall, and B. Settergren.** 1992. Septic shock induced by group A streptococcal infection: clinical and therapeutic aspects. *Scand. J. Infect. Dis.* **24:**589–597.

92. **Stevens, D. L.** 1999. The flesh-eating bacterium: what's next? *J. Infect. Dis.* **179**(Suppl. 2)**:**S366–S374.

93. **Stevens, D. L.** 1992. Invasive group A streptococcus infections. *Clin. Infect. Dis.* **14:**2–13.

94. **Stevens, D. L., A. L. Bisno, H. F. Chambers, E. D. Everett, P. Dellinger, E. J. Goldstein, S. L. Gorbach, J. V. Hirschmann, E. L. Kaplan, J. G. Montoya, and J. C. Wade.** 2005. Practice guidelines for the diagnosis and management of skin and soft-tissue infections. *Clin. Infect. Dis.* **41:**1373–1406.

95. **Stevens, D. L., M. H. Tanner, J. Winship, R. Swarts, K. M. Ries, P. M. Schlievert, and E. Kaplan.** 1989. Severe group A streptococcal infections associated with a toxic shock-like syndrome and scarlet fever toxin A. *N. Engl. J. Med.* **321:**1–7.

96. **Stolz, S. J., J. P. Davis, J. M. Vergeron, B. A. Crass, P. J. Chesney, P. J. Wand, and M. S. Bergdoll.** 1985. Development of serum antibody to toxic shock toxin among individuals with toxic shock syndrome in Wisconsin. *J. Infect. Dis.* **151:**883–889.

97. **Strömberg, A., V. Romanus, and L. G. Burman.** 1991. Outbreak of group A streptococcal bacteremia in Sweden: an epidemiological and clinical study. *J. Infect. Dis.* **164:**595–598.

98. **Takei, S., Y. K. Arora, and S. M. Walker.** 1993. Intravenous immunoglobulin contains specific antibodies inhibitory to activation of T cells by staphylococcal toxin superantigens. *J. Clin. Invest.* **91:**602–607.

99. **The Working Group on Severe Streptococcal Infections.** 1993. Defining the group A streptococcal toxic shock syndrome. Rationale and consensus definition. *JAMA* **269:**390–391.

100. **Todd, J. K., F. A. Kapral, M. Fishaut, and T. R. Welch.** 1978. Toxic shock syndrome associated with phage group I staphylococci. *Lancet* **2:**1116–1118.

101. **Vandenesch, F., T. Naimi, M. C. Enright, G. Lina, G. R. Nimmo, H. Heffernan, N. Liassine, M. Bes, T. Greenland, M. E. Reverdy, and J. Etienne.** 2003. Community-acquired methicillin-resistant *Staphylococcus aureus* carrying Panton-Valentine leukocidin genes: worldwide emergence. *Emerg. Infect. Dis.* **9:**978–984.

102. **Vergeront, J., S. Stoltz, B. A. Crass, D. Nelson, J. P. Davis, and M. Bergdoll.** 1983. Prevalence of serum antibodies to staphylococcal enterotoxin F among Wisconsin residents: implication for toxic-shock syndrome. *J. Infect. Dis.* **4:**692–698.

103. **Vernachio, J. H., A. S. Bayer, B. Ames, D. Bryant, B. D. Prater, P. J. Syribeys, E. L. Gorovits, and J. M. Patti.** 2006. Human immunoglobulin G recognizing fibrinogen-binding surface proteins is protective against both *Staphylococcus aureus* and *Staphylococcus epidermis* infections in vivo. *Antimicrob. Agents Chemother.* **50:**511–518.

104. **Wang, H., O. Bloom, M. Zhang, J. M. Vishnubhakat, M. Ombrellino, J. Che, A. Frazier, H. Yang, S. Ivanova, L. Borovikova, K. R. Manogue, E. Faist, E. Abraham, J. Andersson, U. Andersson, P. E. Molina, N. N. Abumrad, A. Sama, and K. J. Tracey.** 1999. HMG-1 as a late mediator of endotoxin lethality in mice. *Science* **285:**248–251.

105. **Weisman, L. E., D. F. Cruess, and G. W. Fisher.** 1994. Opsonic activity of commercially available standard intravenous immunoglobulin preparations. *Pediatr. Infect. Dis.* **13:**1122–1125.

106. **Yang, K. D., J. M. Bathras, A. O. Shigeoka, J. James, S. H. Pincus, and H. R. Hill.** 1989. Mechanisms of bacterial opsonization by immune globulin intravenous: correlation of complement consumption with opsonic activity and protective efficacy. *J. Infect. Dis.* **159:**701-707.
107. **Yong, J. M.** 1994. Necrotising fasciitis. *Lancet* **343:**1427.
108. **Zimbelman, J., A. Palmer, and J. Todd.** 1999. Improved outcome of clindamycin compared with beta-lactam antibiotic treatment for invasive *Streptococcus pyogenes* infection. *Pediatr. Infect. Dis. J.* **18:**1096–1100.

Superantigens: Molecular Basis for Their Role in Human Diseases
Edited by Malak Kotb and John D. Fraser
© 2007 ASM Press, Washington, D.C.

Chapter 14

Broad-Spectrum Peptide Antagonists of Superantigen Toxins

Revital Levy, Iris Nasie, Dalia Hillman, Gila Arad, and Raymond Kaempfer

Bacterial superantigens are among the most lethal of toxins. These stable proteins bind directly to most major histocompatibility (MHC) class II molecules (29) and stimulate virtually all T cells bearing particular domains in the variable portion of the β-chain of the αβ T-cell receptor (TCR), without need for processing by antigen-presenting cells (9, 13–15, 19). The TCR interacts with superantigens via the outer face of its variable β-chain (Vβ) domain, a region not involved in ordinary antigen recognition (10). Bypassing the restricted presentation of conventional antigens, superantigens can activate up to 50% of T cells to divide and produce cytokines. Thus, superantigens activate the cellular immune response three orders of magnitude more strongly than do ordinary antigens. Toxic shock results from a sudden and massive induction of T-helper 1 (Th1) cell-derived cytokines that include interleukin-2 (IL-2), gamma interferon (IFN-γ), and tumor necrosis factor (TNF) (7, 20, 25). Death resulting from capillary leak syndrome occurs within 1 to 2 days, but even at concentrations several logs below lethal ones, these toxins can elicit severe and prolonged incapacitation in humans, manifested by nausea, vomiting, and diarrhea, symptoms of severe food poisoning (11). Lethal shock and widespread incapacitation by natural mixtures of these toxins constitute an as yet unsolved medical problem as well as a bioterror threat. The medical problem is compounded by the increasing incidence of methicillin-resistant *Staphylococcus aureus* (MRSA) infection. Currently, no antidote or vaccine is available against superantigen toxins.

The family of well over two dozen bacterial superantigens includes the staphylococcal enterotoxins (SEs) secreted by *S. aureus,* among which SEB and SEA are prominent, as well as toxic shock syndrome toxin 1 (TSST-1), and the streptococcal pyrogenic exotoxins produced by *Streptococcus pyogenes,* among them SPEA (25) and smeZ (27), causative agents of streptococcal toxic shock ("flesh-eating bacteria") (25). This toxin family is

Revital Levy, Iris Nasie, Dalia Hillman, Gila Arad, and Raymond Kaempfer • Department of Molecular Virology, The Hebrew University-Hadassah Medical School, 91120 Jerusalem, Israel.

growing, with new members being reported steadily (24, 27, 30). To compound the problem of protection, the amino acid sequences of the bacterial superantigens are highly divergent. Thus, SEB and SEA share 27% sequence homology (5) whereas TSST-1 is only 6% homologous with SEB (6). This molecular diversity demands the development of broad-spectrum countermeasures.

Previous efforts to develop antidotes against toxic shock concentrated on blocking downstream phenomena in the toxicity cascade, mainly by inhibiting the action of TNF with monoclonal antibodies or soluble receptors. However, the extremely high levels of Th1 cytokines produced in response to superantigens render this approach difficult and clinical trials to date have been largely ineffective.

The powerful ability of superantigens to activate T cells involves their effective binding to the TCR and MHC class II molecule (12, 16, 21, 23, 26, 33). A short, unstructured peptide would not be expected to exhibit that property, yet we conjectured that should it compete with the toxin for an essential ligand binding site, it might prevent cooperative interactions (3). We have shown that the lethal effect of widely different superantigens can be blocked with antagonist peptides that inhibit their action at the top of the toxicity cascade, before activation of T cells takes place. The peptides are capable of protecting mice from the lethal effects of superantigen toxins as widely different as SEB and TSST-1, and they can rescue animals already deeply into toxic shock (1, 3). The protected animals, moreover, rapidly develop a broad-spectrum, protective immunity against further lethal toxin challenges with the same superantigen and even with superantigen toxins that they have not encountered before.

The antagonist peptides bear homology to a novel domain in superantigens that, while conserved, is not involved in the binding of either of their known cellular receptors, MHC class II molecule and TCR. The peptides thus provide a tool for the identification of a novel cellular target that may interact with this superantigen domain.

SUPERANTIGEN ANTAGONIST PEPTIDES EFFECTIVE IN VIVO

To activate T cells, superantigens must bind to the TCR and MHC class II molecule and this binding is stabilized by interactions at multiple sites (12, 16, 21, 23, 26, 33). A short peptide would not be expected to mimic this property of the intact superantigen (for example, SEB is composed of 239 amino acids) but if it were to compete with the superantigen for an essential site, it might prevent the activation of the Th1 response. In an attempt to obtain antagonists of SEB, we synthesized short peptides consisting of amino acid sequences from various SEB domains. A dodecapeptide derived from the SEB$_{150-161}$ domain, p*SEB(150-161)* (TNKKKVTAQELD), antagonized SEB weakly as judged from its ability to block induction of IL-2, IFN-γ, and TNF-β mRNA in human peripheral blood mononuclear cells (PBMCs). However, a man-made variant of this peptide, p*12(150-161)* (YNKKKATVQELD; p*12*), proved to be a powerful antagonist (Fig. 1).

Introduction of the N-terminal Y residue instead of T in p*12(150-161)* significantly enhanced its antagonist activity. p*12(150-161)* blocked the induction of IL-2 and IFN-γ mRNA almost completely, whereas p*SEB(150-161),* even at a 10-fold higher concentration, inhibited no more than twofold (Fig. 1). Likewise, expression of TNF-β mRNA was strongly inhibited by p*12(150-161)* but only weakly by p*SEB(150-161)*. Antagonist activity of p*12(150-161)* could be further improved by abutting D-Ala residues to its N and C

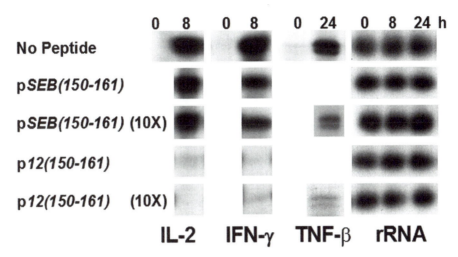

Figure 1. Peptide p*12(150-161)* is an antagonist of SEB. Inhibition of SEB-mediated induction of IL-2, IFN-γ, and TNF-β mRNA by p*12(150-161)* and p*SEB(150-161)* is shown. Aliquots of 3×10^7 PBMCs were incubated with SEB, in the absence (No peptide) or presence of the indicated peptide (10X: 10 μg/ml). At times shown, total RNA was extracted and subjected to RNase protection analysis, using a ^{32}P-labeled IL-2, IFN-γ, TNF-β, or ribosomal RNA (rRNA) antisense RNA probe. Autoradiograms show levels of mRNA; rRNA served as loading control. Reprinted from *Nature Medicine* (3) with permission of the publisher.

termini, to render it more resistant to proteolysis. This peptide, p*12A,* was a potent antagonist of SEB in vitro. Similar data were obtained with SEA, SPEA, and TSST-1 (3). Although the SEB$_{150-161}$ domain is conserved among superantigens (see below), it is not known to be involved in the binding of either TCR or MHC class II molecule (12, 16, 21, 23, 26, 33).

When present in up to 200-fold higher molar amounts than SEB, the antagonist peptide by itself was devoid of SEB agonist activity, shown by a lack of the ability to induce expression of IL-2 and IFN-γ mRNA (3). The antagonist effect was not generally directed against antigen-mediated Th1 cytokine gene activation since p*12(150-161)* inhibited the induction of IL-2 and IFN-γ mRNA by the superantigen SEB but not by a conventional antigen, bovine tuberculin PPD (3). Thus, although p*12(150-161)* interferes with the action of the superantigen, it is not a general TCR or MHC class II antagonist and does not have an immunosuppressive effect unrelated to superantigen action.

We next synthesized p*12B* (VQYNKKKATVQELD), a derivative of p*12A* that carries two extra N-terminal amino acids corresponding to SEB residues 148 to 149. This extension was based on the observation that removal of two N-terminal amino acids from the dodecamer motif led to a significant decline in antagonist activity whereas a pronounced increase in antagonist activity resulted from the T to Y substitution in p*12A* (Fig. 1), indicating that the N-terminal side of the peptide is critical. p*12B* was also abutted with D-Ala residues to render it more protease resistant. As an SEB antagonist, p*12B* was as active as p*12A* (1).

PROTECTION AND RESCUE OF MICE FROM LETHAL SHOCK

The D-galactosamine-sensitized mouse, an accepted model for studying lethality of super-antigens (3), was used to investigate protective activity of p12A and p12B. Mice exposed to antagonist peptide alone remained viable and showed no detectable side effects throughout two weeks after challenge. Of the mice challenged with SEB, only 30% were still alive at 24 h after toxin exposure and 20% at later times. However, all of the SEB-challenged mice were protected by p12B administered at 30 min before toxin ($P = 0.0003$) (Fig. 2A). Surviving animals showed no signs of distress and remained indistinguishable from healthy controls in behavior; they survived for as long as monitored, two weeks. Partial protection was obtained when administration of the antagonist peptide was delayed to 3 h ($P = 0.05$), 5 h ($P = 0.08$), or even 7 h after lethal challenge. A progressively decreasing protective effect of p12B was seen between 20 and 40 h, yielding 70%, 60%, and 50% survival, respectively (Fig. 2A). Thus, p12B was not only fully protective when given before SEB challenge but was able to rescue mice after they were exposed to toxin. Protection or rescue was observed when the antagonist peptide was in only a 20-fold molar excess over SEB, showing that the peptide is a potent superantigen antagonist in vivo.

Figure 2B shows a therapeutic effect as well, for TSST-1, at 3 and 18 h posttoxin. Even though TSST-1 exhibits a mere 6% overall sequence homology with SEB, p12A, which protects mice from SEB (3), was also protective against this toxin. TSST-1 killed the mice more slowly than SEB but all of the mice in the control group died ultimately, with half-maximal mortality reached by 40 h (Fig. 2B). p12A did not protect when administered just before TSST-1 but it afforded significant protection (up to 70%) when also injected after toxin challenge. The protective effect became progressively more pronounced with repeated administration at 3 and 18 h. Survival of mice from TSST-1-mediated toxic shock thus depends on sustained presence of the peptide, suggesting that although its half-life is

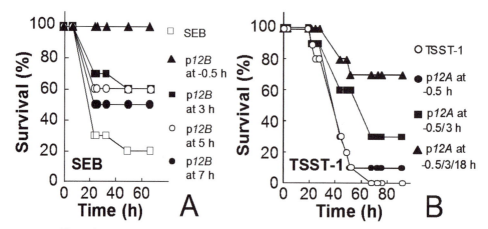

Figure 2. Antagonist peptide protects and rescues mice from SEB-induced lethal shock and protects mice from TSST-1-induced lethal shock. Groups of 10 BALB/c mice were challenged with 10 μg of SEB (A) or 5 μg of TSST-1 (B), alone or in the presence of antagonist peptide added at times shown. Reprinted from the *Journal of Leukocyte Biology* (1) (A) and *Nature Medicine* (3) (B) with permission of the publishers.

limited (estimated in the order of 2 to 4 h), it is long enough to protect the mice against death. Peptides p12A and p12B are broad-spectrum superantigen antagonists in vivo (1, 3).

Previously, it was assumed that a superantigen engages its receptors within a very brief interval, 30 min, beyond which its toxic action becomes irreversible. The ability of our antagonist peptides to rescue mice even several hours after their exposure to a superantigen toxin, demonstrated in Fig. 2, implies that it is possible to dislodge the superantigen from its cellular target even after it has bound. These data show that signaling by a superantigen through its receptors is not limited to a narrow time window, as it can be blocked hours later, and thus support the concept that the antagonist peptides may have clinical utility.

The mouse model is perhaps the most rigorous and challenging model to demonstrate a therapeutic effect as a lethal dose of superantigen is delivered at once by injection. In a biodefense scenario, exposure of humans is likely to be more gradual, both in terms of dose and rate of delivery, extending the therapeutic window. The same will hold true for intoxication of humans by superantigens released during staphylococcal or streptococcal bacterial infections.

BROAD-SPECTRUM, PROTECTIVE IMMUNITY WITHOUT IMMUNIZATION

Surviving mice rapidly developed a broad-spectrum, protective immunity against further lethal challenges with the same superantigen and even with superantigen toxins that they did not encounter before. In the experiment of Fig. 3A, mice that had survived a lethal challenge with SEB owing to protection by p12A were rechallenged 2 weeks later with a double dose of SEB, this time in the absence of antagonist peptide. All but one of the mice survived. The survivors had rapidly acquired cross-protection against different superantigens (Fig. 2A). These mice, once protected from SEB by a single dose of antagonist peptide, were able to survive through four subsequent lethal rechallenges: with SEB, with SPEA in two escalating doses, and finally with TSST-1. We could repeat this observation using lethal challenges with different superantigens and varying the order in which they are given (1).

Adoptive transfer of serum from the surviving mice was sufficient to protect naive mice against lethal challenge with SEB (Fig. 3B). By contrast, serum from mice that had been injected only with antagonist peptide p12A was not protective and serum from mice primed with SEB under nonlethal conditions, in the absence of D-galactosamine, protected only partially (Fig. 3B). Rapidly evolving resistance to toxin challenge thus is based on the generation of protective antibodies in animals surviving a first toxin exposure owing to the presence of the antagonist peptide. This protective immunity is long-lasting (3). Yet, we could not detect antibodies against the antagonist peptide. Indeed, the lack of immunogenicity and the relatively rapid clearance of a short peptide, 12 to 14 amino acids in length, constitute therapeutic advantages.

Immunoglobulin M (IgM) and IgG against SEB, SPEA, and TSST-1 were detected in the serum of the surviving mice in Fig. 3A even before rechallenge with the relevant toxin. IgM and IgG had developed against SEB after two SEB challenges, with IgG being higher in most mice, and were stable or increased thereafter. Before exposure to SPEA, antibodies against SPEA were already present albeit at low levels, yet these sufficed to protect mice completely from this toxin (Fig. 3A). Anti-SPEA antibody levels increased with each toxin challenge and were mainly IgM. Strikingly, before TSST-1 challenge, the survivor

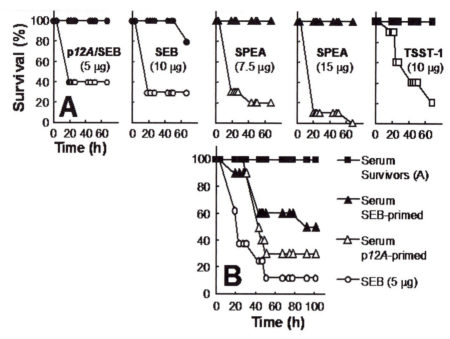

Figure 3. Antagonist-mediated acquisition of resistance to different superantigens. Five BALB/c mice received 5 μg SEB together with p*12A* (A, left panel). Without further injection of p*12A*, survivors were rechallenged successively at 2-week intervals with SEB and SPEA (twice) and after a 9-week interval with TSST-1. At each challenge, 10 naive mice served as toxin controls. (B) Adoptive transfer of protection. Serum collected 2 weeks after TSST-1 challenge was injected into ten naive mice 1 h before challenge with 5 μg SEB. Groups of ten naive mice received serum from mice injected 2 weeks earlier with p*12A* or with 10 μg SEB without D-galactosamine sensitization. Eight naive mice served as SEB challenge controls. Survival remained constant beyond the times shown. Modified from *Nature Medicine* (3) with permission of the publisher.

mice, which had never been exposed to TSST-1, harbored significant levels of anti-TSST-1 IgM and some even had IgG. In the period preceding TSST-1 challenge, levels of anti-TSST-1 IgM increased strongly (2).

Thus, when lethal toxic shock was prevented by antagonist peptide during exposure to a superantigen, mice swiftly acquired immunity against further toxin challenges, even with different toxins that they did not encounter before, and developed protective antitoxin antibodies (2, 3). By blocking the ability of the toxin to induce a cellular immune response leading to toxic shock, the antagonist peptide allows the superantigen to induce a vigorous humoral immune response directed against itself. Under these conditions, the superantigen acts as its own adjuvant to elicit protective antibodies that recognize a common feature among superantigens.

ANTAGONIST PEPTIDE DEFINES A NOVEL SUPERANTIGEN DOMAIN

Peptides deriving from the $SEB_{150-161}$ domain exhibit superantigen antagonist activity. This SEB domain is remote from the regions that participate in binding of TCR and/or MHC class II molecule. That is seen clearly from the crystallographic structures of the complexes formed by SEB with the human TCR Vβ8 chain and with the human MHC class II molecule, HLA DR1 (Color Plate 13A and B). Moreover, this SEB domain lies outside the region sufficient for mitogenic activity, the N-terminal 138 amino acids (8, 18). Therefore, the ability of p*12B* and p*12A* to act as SEB antagonists was surprising.

The $SEB_{150-161}$ "antagonist" domain showing homology to the antagonist peptides forms a central turn starting within a β-strand and connects it, via another short β-strand, to an α-helix (Color Plate 13B). This domain is conserved among pyrogenic toxins, with 10/12 amino acid sequence identities for SEA, SEC1, SEC2, SEC3, and SPEA, 9/12 for SEE and smeZ, and even 4/12 for TSST-1, the most remote member within the staphylococcal and streptococcal superantigen family (Color Plate 14, right). Though highly homologous with SEB in the 150 to 161 domain, SEA shows only 27% overall sequence homology with SEB; SPEA has 48% homology with SEB and TSST-1 merely 6% (5). Notwithstanding these differences in overall sequence, the three-dimensional structures of these superantigens are remarkably similar, especially in their right halves (Color Plate 14A). A β-strand-hinge-α-helix domain corresponding to residues 150 to 161 in SEB is found in each, including TSST-1.

The $SEB_{150-161}$ domain and its equivalents in SEA, SPEA, and TSST-1 show not only overall spatial conservation (Color Plate 14A) but also structural similarity (Color Plate 14B). In SEB, SEA, and SPEA, this domain forms a pocket in which T, K, and E residues are oriented to allow for hydrogen bonding. In TSST-1, the core of this pocket is hydrophobic in character, containing proximal F, L, and T residues, with the K residue extending away.

The sequence of p*12(150-161)* differs in several positions from the corresponding sequence in SEB. The KKK and QELD motifs are spaced equally but p*12(150-161)* contains the aromatic ring residue Y where SEB contains T, resembling more closely F at this position in TSST-1 (Color Plate 14, right). This may explain why the T to Y substitution rendered p*12(150-161)* a more potent antagonist (Fig. 1). The peptide combines features of the four superantigens in their corresponding domains, a plausible explanation for its broad-spectrum inhibitory activity. In TSST-1, this domain (FDKKQLAISTLD) shares only 33% sequence homology with the corresponding SEB domain (TNKKKVTAQELD), yet the domain folding is conserved. Although it shares far higher homology with SEB, the antagonist peptide was nevertheless capable of protecting against lethal shock induced by TSST-1 (Fig. 2B).

THE ANTAGONIST DOMAIN IN SEB IS ACCESSIBLE

It was already seen from crystallographic structures shown in Color Plate 13 that the antagonist domain in SEB is well removed from superantigen regions that participate in binding of TCR and/or MHC class II molecule. This renders the antagonist domain in principle accessible to another ligand. Within this domain, several amino acid residues are exposed to the environment whereas others are buried (Color Plate 15).

During their convergent evolution, the superantigen toxins from *S. aureus* and *S. pyogenes* have acquired molecular structures designed to recognize the receptors of the human immune system critical for their function, among them TCR and MHC class II molecule. Yet, superantigens differ substantially in the way they bind to these two ligands (22, 31, 32). Thus, whereas the binding site for the TCR Vβ-chain in SEB is within a cleft juxtaposed to the MHC II binding site, in TSST-1 the TCR Vβ-chain is bound by a domain on the other side of the toxin molecule. The MHC class II binding site in SEB (Color Plate 13) is a generic MHC class II α-chain binding site found in many superantigens near the N terminus. By contrast, SEA has a second, more powerful MHC class II β-chain binding site located in the β-grasp near its C terminus (corresponding to the far right in the structure shown for SEB in Color Plates 13B and 15), involving a Zn^{2+} atom; indeed, SEA binds far more tightly than SEB to the MHC class II molecule (28). The dual binding sites allow SEA to cross-link MHC class II molecules and this property may explain why SEA is even more toxic than SEB in humans; SEA has an 8-fold higher proliferative activity for human T cells than SEB (27). Despite the greater potency of SEA, antagonist peptide p*12* effectively blocked SEA-mediated induction of IL-2 and IFN-γ mRNA in human PBMC (3) and protected mice from lethal SEA challenge (1). This result agrees well with the fact that in the SEA structure, the antagonist domain (Color Plate 14A, top right) is not only remote from the generic MHC class II binding site as in the case of SEB, but also from the second binding site in the β-grasp. Based on these structural data, the antagonist activity of the peptide for SEA is not accounted for by a competitive inhibition of HLA binding.

A more recently discovered set of superantigens from *S. pyogenes* is the smeZ family, which also uses the β-grasp and Zn^{2+} atom for high-affinity binding of the MHC class II molecule but lacks the generic MHC class II binding site (4, 27). The superantigens smeZ, SPE-C, and SPE-H from *S. pyogenes* all have lost the generic binding site and solely use the β-grasp to bind to MHC class II molecules. Among the smeZ subset of superantigens, smeZ-2 is a variant that is about 40-fold more potent than SEB in stimulating human T-cell proliferation and the most potent superantigen discovered thus far. Although many smeZ variants are found among patients, they all retain the same MHC class II binding site structure (27). Based on structural considerations, our results with SEA suggest that smeZ will prove equally sensitive to antagonism by p*12* peptide.

HYPOTHESIS: THE ANTAGONIST DOMAIN BINDS TO A NOVEL LIGAND

When superantigen-mediated lethal toxic shock was prevented by a superantigen mimetic peptide, mice swiftly acquired immunity against further toxin challenges and developed broadly protective antibodies (Fig. 3). We reason that when the peptide blocks the Th1 cytokine response leading to lethal shock, it may leave the Th2 cytokine response intact, allowing for B-cell differentiation and the development of protective immunity. To explain such Th1 selectivity of the superantigen antagonist peptides, we postulate that activation of Th1 but not of Th2 cytokine gene expression by superantigen requires an additional receptor and that binding of superantigen to this receptor occurs through the antagonist domain, rendering it sensitive to the mimetic peptide (Fig. 4).

The antagonist peptides show homology to a superantigen domain consisting of a β-strand/hinge/β-strand/α-helix motif that is conserved spatially and in sequence among all bacterial superantigens studied. This provides a plausible explanation for the broad-spectrum antagonist activity against superantigens, despite their strong molecular diver-

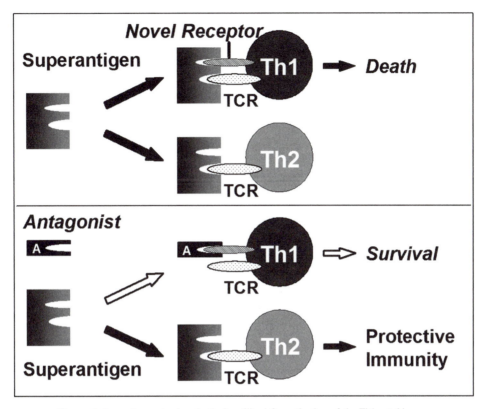

Figure 4. A novel receptor is selectively utilized for activation of the Th1 cytokine response to superantigen. In this proposed model, to activate Th1 cytokine gene expression, a superantigen must engage not only MHC-II and TCR but also a novel receptor that is dispensable for activation of Th2 cytokine genes. Binding of antagonist peptide to this receptor results in a selective block of Th1 activation, to yield survival as well as protective immunity mediated by the action of Th2 cytokines. For clarity, antigen-presenting cell and MHC-II were omitted.

sity. Most likely, superantigens use the conserved domain homologous to the antagonist to bind to a novel receptor on T cells or antigen-presenting cells critical for their action. By competing with superantigens in binding to this receptor, the antagonist peptide is able to block Th1 cell activation and the resulting toxicity. The superantigen antagonist peptides described here protect or rescue mice from lethal shock in a molar excess of as low as 20-fold over the toxin, implying that they bind tightly to a cellular target that is critical for superantigen action. In view of this high affinity, superantigen toxins are not likely to be amenable to facile improvement or to engineering of resistance against an antidote that disturbs a highly specific molecular interaction between the toxin and a target receptor whose nature in humans will remain constant. Thus, although these biological toxins pose a serious threat, countermeasures designed against them, as exemplified here, will also be more difficult to overcome.

The antagonist peptides described in this chapter provide a new molecular tool for understanding the mechanism of excessive human immune response activation by superantigens that occurs during toxic shock and for the identification of a novel target ligand that may interact with this superantigen domain. Structural analysis shows that this domain is well removed from the binding sites for MHC class II molecule and TCR and remains fully accessible even after these two ligands have been bound to SEB (Color Plate 13); it has not been implicated in the binding of either ligand (12, 16, 21, 23, 26, 33).

CONCLUSION

The diversity in MHC class II and TCR binding modes of superantigens (22, 31, 32) stands in contrast to the spatial and sequence conservation of the β-strand/hinge/β-strand/α-helix domain and supports the concept that this conserved domain is needed for a critical interaction with a third receptor during T-cell activation. The antagonist peptide most likely acts to bind that receptor by induced fit, although it is possible that through intramolecular bonding as illustrated in Color Plate 14B, it may assume a conformation similar to that found in the intact superantigen molecule. Removal of two amino acids from the dodecamer motif led to a significant decline in antagonist activity; this truncation may affect conformational stability or appropriate folding onto this putative receptor and reduce its affinity for the target.

Acknowledgments. We thank Hans Langedijk for help with structure rendering.

This research was supported in part by U.S. Defense Advanced Research Projects Agency (DARPA) grant N65236-98-1-5402.

REFERENCES

1. **Arad, G., D. Hillman, R. Levy, and R. Kaempfer.** 2001. Superantigen antagonist blocks Th1 cytokine gene induction and lethal shock. *J. Leukoc. Biol.* **69:**921–927.
2. **Arad, G., D. Hillman, R. Levy, and R. Kaempfer.** 2004. Broad-spectrum immunity against superantigens is elicited in mice protected from lethal shock by a superantigen antagonist peptide. *Immunol. Lett.* **91:**141–145.
3. **Arad, G., R. Levy, D. Hillman, and R. Kaempfer.** 2000. Superantigen antagonist protects against lethal shock and defines a new domain for T-cell activation. *Nat. Med.* **6:**414–421.
4. **Arcus, V. L., T. Proft, J. A. Sigrell, H. M. Baker, J. D. Fraser, and E. N. Baker.** 2000. Conservation and variation in superantigen structure and activity highlighted by the three-dimensional structures of two new superantigens from *Streptococcus pyogenes. J. Mol. Biol.* **299:**157–168.
5. **Betley, M. J., and J. J. Mekalanos.** 1988. Nucleotide sequence of the type A staphylococcal enterotoxin gene. *J. Bacteriol.* **170:**34–41.
6. **Blomster-Hautamaa, D. A., B. N. Kreiswirth, J. S. Kornblum, R. P. Novick, and P. M. Schlievert.** 1986. The nucleotide and partial amino acid sequence of toxic shock syndrome toxin-1. *J. Biol. Chem.* **261:**15783–15786.
7. **Bohach, G. A., D. J. Fast, R. D. Nelson, and P. M. Schlievert.** 1990. Staphylococcal and streptococcal pyrogenic toxins involved in toxic shock syndrome and related illnesses. *Crit. Rev. Microbiol.* **17:**251–272.
8. **Buelow, R., R. E. O'Hehir, R. Schreifels, T. J. Kummerehl, G. Riley, and J. R. Lamb.** 1992. Localization of the immunologic activity in the superantigen Staphylococcal enterotoxin B using truncated recombinant fusion proteins. *J. Immunol.* **148:**1–6.
9. **Choi, Y., A. Herman, D. DiGiusto, T. Wade, P. Marrack, and J. Kappler.** 1990. Residues of the variable region of the T-cell-receptor beta-chain that interact with *S. aureus* toxin superantigens. *Nature* **346:**471–473.
10. **Choi, Y. W., B. Kotzin, L. Herron, J. Callahan, P. Marrack, and J. Kappler.** 1989. Interaction of *Staphylococcus aureus* toxin "superantigens" with human T cells. *Proc. Natl. Acad. Sci. USA* **86:**8941–8945.
11. **Dinges, M. M., P. M. Orwin, and P. M. Schlievert.** 2000. Exotoxins of *Staphylococcus aureus. Clin. Microbiol. Rev.* **13:**16–34.
12. **Fields, B. A., E. L. Malchiodi, H. Li, X. Ysern, C. V. Stauffacher, P. M. Schlievert, K. Karjalainen, and R. A. Mariuzza.** 1996. Crystal structure of a T-cell receptor β-chain complexed with a superantigen. *Nature* **384:**188-192.

13. **Fraser, J. D.** 1989. High-affinity binding of staphylococcal enterotoxins A and B to HLA-DR. *Nature* **339:**221–223.

14. **Herman, A., J. W. Kappler, P. Marrack, and A. M. Pullen.** 1991. Superantigens: mechanisms of T-cell stimulation and role in immune responses. *Annu. Rev. Immunol.* **9:**745–772.

15. **Janeway, C. A., J. Yagi, M. E. Katz, B. Jones, S. Vregop, and S. Buxser.** 1989. T Cell responses to Mls and to bacterial proteins that mimic its behavior. *Immunol. Rev.* **107:**61–68.

16. **Jardetzky, T. S., J. H. Brown, J. C. Gorga, L. J. Stern, R. G. Urban, Y. I. Chi, C. Stauffacher, J. L. Strominger, and D. C. Wiley.** 1994. Three-dimensional structure of a human class II histocompatibility molecule complexed with superantigen. *Nature* **368:**711–718.

17. **Kaempfer, R.** 2004. Peptide antagonists of superantigen toxins. *Mol. Divers.* **8:**113–120.

18. **Kappler, J. W., A. Herman, J. Clements, and P. Marrack.** 1992. Mutations defining functional regions of the superantigen staphylococcal enterotoxin B. *J. Exp. Med.* **175:**387–389.

19. **Kappler, J., B. Kotzin, L. Herron, E. W. Gelfand, R. D. Bigler, A. Boylston, S. Carrel, C. D. Posneit, Y. Choi, and P. Marrack.** 1989. Vβ-specific stimulation of human T cells by staphylococcal toxins. *Science* **244:**811–814.

20. **Kotzin, B. L., D. Y. Leung, J. Kappler, and P. Marrack.** 1993. Superantigens and their potential role in human disease. *Adv. Immunol.* **54:**99–166.

21. **Leder, L., A. Llera, P. M. Lavoie, M. I. Lebedeva, H. Li, R. P. Sekaly, G. A. Bohach, P. J. Gahr, P. M. Schlievert, K. Karjalainen, and R. A. Mariuzza.** 1998. A mutational analysis of the binding of staphylococcal enterotoxins B and C3 to the T cell receptor β chain and major histocompatibility complex class II. *J. Exp. Med.* **187:**823–833.

22. **Li, H., A. Llera, and R. A. Mariuzza.** 1998. Structure-function studies of T-cell receptor-superantigen interactions. *Immunol. Rev.* **163:**177–186.

23. **Li, H., A. Llera, D. Tsuchiya, L. Leder, X. Ysern, P. M. Schlievert, K. Karjalainen, and R. A. Mariuzza.** 1998. Three-dimensional structure of the complex between a T cell receptor β chain and the superantigen staphylococcal enterotoxin B. *Immunity* **9:**807–816.

24. **McCormick, J. K., A. A. Pragman, J. C. Stolpa, D. Y. Leung, and P. M. Schlievert.** 2001. Functional characterization of streptococcal pyrogenic exotoxin J, a novel superantigen. *Infect. Immun.* **69:**1381–1388.

25. **McCormick, J. K., J. M. Yarwood, and P. M. Schlievert.** 2001. Toxic shock syndrome and bacterial superantigens: an update. *Annu. Rev. Microbiol.* **55:**77–104.

26. **Papageorgiou, A. C., H. S. Tranter, and K. R. Acharya.** 1998. Crystal structure of microbial superantigen staphylococcal enterotoxin B at 1.5 Å resolution: implications for superantigen recognition by MHC class II molecules and T-cell receptors. *J. Mol. Biol.* **277:**61–79.

27. **Proft, T., S. L. Moffatt, C. J. Berkahn, and J. D. Fraser.** 1999. Identification and characterization of novel superantigens from *Streptococcus pyogenes*. *J. Exp. Med.* **189:**89–102.

28. **Schad, E. M., I. Zaitseva, V. N. Zaitsev, M. Dohlsten, T. Kalland, P. M. Schlievert, D. H. Ohlendorf, and L. A. Svensson.** 1995. Crystal structure of the superantigen staphylococcal enterotoxin type A. *EMBO J.* **14:**3292–3301.

29. **Scholl, P., A. Diez, W. Mourad, J. Parsonnet, R. S. Geha, and T. Chatila.** 1989. Toxic shock syndrome toxin 1 binds to major histocompatibility complex class II molecules. *Proc. Natl. Acad. Sci. USA* **86:**4210–4214.

30. **Smoot, L. M., J. K. McCormick, J. C. Smoot, N. P. Hoe, I. Strickland, R. L. Cole, K. D. Barbian, C. A. Earhart, D. H. Ohlendorf, L. G. Veasy, H. R. Hill, D. Y. Leung, P. M. Schlievert, and J. M. Musser.** 2002. Characterization of two novel pyrogenic toxin superantigens made by an acute rheumatic fever clone of *Streptococcus pyogenes* associated with multiple disease outbreaks. *Infect. Immun.* **70:**7095–7104.

31. **Sundberg, E. J., H. Li, A. S. Llera, J. K. McCormick, J. Tormo, P. M. Schlievert, K. Karjalainen, and R. A. Mariuzza.** 2002. Structures of two streptococcal superantigens bound to TCR beta chains reveal diversity in the architecture of T cell signaling complexes. *Structure* **10:**687–699.

32. **Sundberg, E. J., Y. Li, and R. A. Mariuzza.** 2002. So many ways of getting in the way: diversity in the molecular architecture of superantigen-dependent T-cell signaling complexes. *Curr. Opin. Immunol.* **14:**36–44.

33. **Swaminathan, S., W. Furey, J. Pletcher, and M. Sax.** 1992. Crystal structure of staphylococcal enterotoxin B, a superantigen. *Nature* **359:**801–805.

Superantigens: Molecular Basis for Their Role in Human Diseases
Edited by Malak Kotb and John D. Fraser
© 2007 ASM Press, Washington, D.C.

Chapter 15

Small Nonpeptide Inhibitors of Staphylococcal Superantigen-Induced Cytokine Production and Toxic Shock

Teresa Krakauer

INTRODUCTION

Staphylococcus aureus is a ubiquitous gram-positive coccus that produces several exotoxins with potent immunostimulating activities which contribute to its ability to cause disease in humans and laboratory animals (reviewed in references 17, 24, 38, 39, 59, 64, 82). Staphylococcal enterotoxins A through R (SEA to SER) and toxic shock syndrome toxin 1 (TSST-1) are called superantigens because of their ability to polyclonally activate T cells at picomolar concentrations, thus stimulating a large proportion of T cells (5 to 30%), whereas a conventional antigen stimulates less than 0.01% of the T-cell population (19, 59). The interaction of superantigen with host cells differs from that of conventional antigens in that it binds outside the peptide-binding groove of major histocompatibility complex (MHC) class II, exerting its effect as an intact molecule without being "processed" (19, 59). The dual affinity of staphylococcal superantigens for MHC class II molecules and specific T-cell receptor (TCR) Vβ-chains enables these microbial toxins to perturb the immune system and induce high levels of proinflammatory cytokines, chemokines, tissue factor, lytic enzymes, and reactive oxygen species, activating both inflammation and coagulation (22, 36, 38–40, 42, 43, 44, 53, 62, 80, 92, 99, 102). Two key inflammatory cytokines, tumor necrosis factor alpha (TNF-α) and interleukin 1 (IL-1), are direct mediators of fever, hypotension, and shock (54). In addition, gamma interferon (IFN-γ) produced by activated T cells acts synergistically with TNF-α and IL-1 to enhance immune reaction and tissue injury.

Staphylococcal enterotoxins (SEs) and TSST-1 are 22- to 30-kDa single-chain proteins with well-characterized secondary and tertiary structures (79). SEB has historically been the most widely studied superantigen and is listed by the Centers for Disease Control and

Teresa Krakauer • Department of Immunology, Integrated Toxicology Division, United States Army Medical Research Institute of Infectious Diseases, Fort Detrick, Frederick, MD 21702-5011.

Prevention (CDC) as a category B priority agent, as it can be used as an airborne, food-borne and waterborne toxic agent. Depending on the dose and route of exposure, SEB and other SEs cause food poisoning, acute and fatal respiratory distress, and toxic shock (33, 39, 80).

SUPERANTIGEN BINDING TO HOST CELLS

Staphylococcal superantigens are grouped into three classes based on their primary sequence homology (64, 73, 82). SEA, SED, SEE, and SEH share the highest sequence homology, between 53% and 81%. The second group consists of SEB, the SECs, and SEG, which are 50% to 66% homologous. TSST-1 is distantly related (28% homology) as it has a distinct, shorter primary sequence of 194 amino acids with no cysteines and a missing "disulfide loop" commonly found in SEs. However, X-ray crystallography of SEB and TSST-1 reveals similarities in the secondary-tertiary structure with two tightly packed domains containing β-sheets and α-helices (reviewed in reference 79). The relatively conserved TCR-binding site is located in the shallow groove between these two domains (37, 79).

Superantigens bind to common, conserved elements of MHC class II molecules with high affinity ($K_d = 10^{-8}$ to 10^{-7} M) (72). However, each individual toxin displays preferential binding to distinct alleles of specific MHC isotypes, suggesting different modes of contact for superantigen with MHC class II (18, 29, 30, 72). In general, HLA-DR binds SE and TSST-1 better than HLA-DP or -DQ, and murine IE molecules bind better than IA (88, 100). Crystallographic studies indicate two distinct sites on MHC class II molecules for superantigen binding. A common, low-affinity binding site is located on the α-chain of MHC class II and a high-affinity, zinc-dependent binding site is found on the β-chain (79, 82, 104). Superantigens in the SEA subfamily bind to both sites, whereas SEB and TSST-1 bind only to the generic low-affinity site (34, 100, 104).

The interaction of each toxin on the TCR Vβ-chain is unique, as shown by the different Vβ specificities of each superantigen (19, 39, 59). The binding contacts are mostly between the side-chain atoms of the superantigen and the complementarity-determining regions 1 and 2 and the hypervariable region 4 within the Vβ-chain. The mitogenic potency of these toxins results from a cooperative process such that the superantigen/MHC complex binds the TCR with a higher affinity than toxin alone.

As with conventional antigens, expression of costimulatory molecules on antigen-presenting cells (APCs) and T cells provides additional signals for optimal cell activation by the ternary complex of superantigen/MHC/TCR and can influence T-cell differentiation into two subsets of T cells: T-helper type 1 (Th1) or type 2 (Th2). Expression of intercellular adhesion molecule (ICAM) on an APC promotes stable cell conjugate formation and provides costimulatory signals. The interactions of LFA-1/ICAM-1 and CD80/CD28 have both been implicated in SEA-mediated T-cell activation (40, 57, 85). Activation of the CD28-regulated signal transduction pathway during superantigen stimulation of T cells is reportedly necessary for IL-2 induction (25). In addition, zinc-binding superantigens like SEA persist on the surface of APC due to their ability to cross-link MHC class II thereby prolonging their exposure and effects on T cells (81). Costimulatory molecules such as CD40 on APC and CD154 on T cells are also important in modulating immune responses to conventional antigens and superantigens (66). Other cell surface molecules such as CD2, CD11a/ICAM-1, and ELAM are also required for optimal activation of endothelial cells and T cells by SEB (40).

SIGNAL TRANSDUCTION AND IMMUNE ACTIVATION

The main target cells of superantigens are the CD4+ T cells and mononuclear phagocytes bearing MHC class II molecules (4, 13, 59, 101). Interaction of superantigen with MHC class II and TCR on APC and T cells, respectively, activates intracellular signaling (14). High concentrations of SEB elicit phosphatidylinositol production and intracellular Ca^{2+} flux in T-cell clones without inducing proliferation (55). Similar to mitogenic activation of T cells, superantigens also activate protein kinase C (PKC) and protein tyrosine kinase (PTK) pathways (15, 89). Activation of PKC and PTK is also required for enhanced cell adhesion observed after lymphocyte activation with MHC class II ligands. Ultimately, activation of transcriptional factors NFκB and AP-1 by superantigens results in the expression of proinflammatory cytokines, chemokines, and adhesion molecules on macrophages and T cells (14, 89). Additionally, the mediators produced by these superantigen-activated cells exert potent effects on the immune and cardiovascular system, culminating in multiorgan dysfunction and lethal shock (Fig. 1).

The proinflammatory cytokines IL-1 and TNF-α can directly activate the transcriptional factor NFκB in many other cell types that include epithelial and endothelial cells, thus perpetuating the inflammatory response (54). IFN-γ from superantigen-activated T cells also synergizes with IL-1 and TNF-α to induce IL-6 and chemotactic cytokines in these cells. The synergistic action of these three cytokines on endothelial cells increases the expression of MHC class II, adhesion molecules, and tissue factor, culminating in disseminated intravascular coagulation. IL-1 and TNF-α also act synergistically on epithelial cells, ultimately causing cell damage and epithelial leakage that affects ion and protein transport. Inflammatory cytokines IL-1, TNF-α, and IL-6 from both macrophages and activated T cells act on the liver to release acute-phase proteins and down-regulate liver clearance function. Various chemokines from superantigen-activated cells attract neutrophils and sequester them to sites of tissue injury and inflammation. Cytokine- and chemokine-activated neutrophils produce reactive oxygen species (ROS) resulting in organ dysfunction. SEB can cause acute lung injury as systemic administration of SEB results in lung pathology characterized by increased expression of adhesion molecules ICAM-1 and VCAM, increased numbers of neutrophils and mononuclear cells, endothelial cell injury, and increased vascular permeability (75). Thus, systemic release of inflammatory mediators affects multiple organs and cell types culminating in decreased peripheral vascular resistance, multiorgan failure, hypotension, and shock.

IN VITRO CELLULAR RESPONSE

Human peripheral blood mononuclear cells (PBMCs) are used extensively to study the cellular requirements for activation by staphylococcal superantigen. Therapeutic agents have been tested in vitro to block these pathways used by superantigens (42, 44–47, 49, 50, 51, 53, 91). PBMCs secrete the cytokines IL-1, IL-2, IL-6, TNF-α, TNF-β, and IFN-γ and the chemokines IL-8, macrophage inflammatory protein 1α (MIP-1α), MIP-1β, and monocyte chemoattractant protein-1 (MCP-1) in response to SEB and TSST-1 (22, 36, 42, 44, 91, 92). Both monocytes and T cells are required for optimal induction of mediators, suggesting that cognate interaction of superantigen bound on APC with T cells contributes to the production of these cytokines and chemokines (13, 44, 92, 101). Most of the mediators are induced early, with mRNA expression appearing as early as 3 h after exposure to

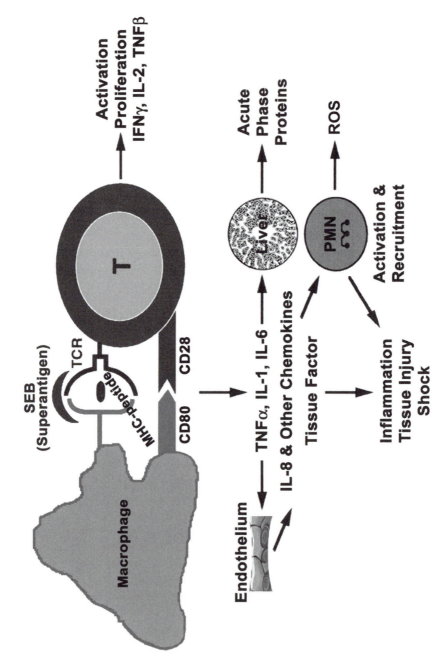

Figure 1. Cells and mediators participating in superantigen-induced toxic shock.

superantigen (51). Superantigen-driven T-cell proliferation appears later, reaching maximum levels at 48 to 72 h. Direct superantigen presentation to T cells in the absence of MHC class II molecules can induce an anergic response (31).

Other cell types responding directly to staphylococcal superantigen include B cells, synovial fibroblasts, intestinal epithelial cells, and mast cells (28, 74, 87). Stimulation of synovial fibroblasts with superantigens leads to the induction of chemokine gene expression, raising the possibility that superantigens can trigger chemotactic cytokines and initiate inflammatory arthritis (74). SEB can also transcytose across an intestinal epithelial cell line (28) although in human B cells internalized SEB can traffic to lysosomal compartments (81). However, the interactions of most superantigens with epithelial and endothelial cells are mostly indirect, via the release of IL-1, TNF-α, and IFN-γ from superantigen-activated APC and T cells (46, 65). IL-1, TNF-α, and IFN-γ are key mediators released by immune cells in response to many inflammatory stimuli such as lipopolysaccharide (LPS), other bacterial cell wall components, and pathogens. Both IL-1 and TNF-α are endogenous pyrogens that activate many cell types to enhance immune reactions and inflammation (54). IFN-γ produced by activated T cells augments immunological responses by increasing MHC class II and ICAM-1 molecules on APCs, as well as epithelial and endothelial cells (54). Additionally, IFN-γ upregulates TNF-α and IL-1 receptors, and acts synergistically with TNF-α and IL-1 to augment immunological reactions and promote tissue injury. The chemokines, IL-8, MCP-1, MIP-1α, and MIP-1β, are induced directly by SEB or TSST-1 and selectively act as chemoattractants and activate leukocytes (44, 54, 99).

ANIMAL MODELS

Current in vivo investigations with the SEs have relied heavily on murine models of lethal shock. Humans are much more sensitive to SEB intoxication and low doses are enough to cause lethal shock without the use of synergistic agents. In humans and monkeys, SEs induce an emetic response and toxic shock at submicrogram concentrations (32). Mast cell stimulation and the release of cysteinyl leukotrienes contribute to the emetic response (87). Microgram levels of aerosolized SEB in monkeys resulted in emesis and diarrhea that developed within 24 h of exposure, followed by the abrupt onset of lethargy, difficult breathing, hypotension, fever, and finally death from toxic shock (61). Because of the synergistic action of SEs with other agents, such as bacterial endotoxin and viruses, the effective lethal dose of each of these agents can be much lower. Inhalation of lower, nanogram levels of SEB causes severe incapacitation. TNF-α was completely absent when non-human primates were given a sublethal dose of aerosolized SEB that causes incapacitation (52).

A major problem of in vivo testing of therapeutics against SEB, in particular SEB-induced toxic shock, is finding a relevant model that mimics human disease. The rabbit model of subcutaneous or continuous infusion of superantigen-induced shock mimics human disease closely (64), but lack of immunological reagents hampers its use for routine testing of therapeutic efficacy. In general, mice are preferred as models for drug testing because of their inbred homogeneity, and large numbers of animals can be used with results available in a relatively short time. However, mice are poor responders to SEB as the affinity of these toxins to mouse MHC class II is much lower than that for human MHC class II (88, 95) and thus they are naturally resistant to superantigen-induced toxic shock. The mouse models commonly used today rely on the use of sensitizing agents such as D-galactosamine, actinomycin D, LPS, or viruses to induce toxic shock (10, 16, 86, 95, 96, 106, 108). Recently transgenic mice with human MHC class II were found to be an ideal animal model for examining the biological effects of superantigens, as they respond to much lower doses of toxins due to the higher-affinity binding of SEs to human MHC class II molecules (21). Subsequent studies (84; unpublished observations) indicate that two doses of relatively high amounts of SEB (30 to 100 μg/mouse) are necessary to induce toxic shock in these transgenics, and in some cases, sensitizing agents such as D-galactosamine are still required.

LPS naturally synergizes with superantigens to induce the proinflammatory cytokine cascade (10, 95). In the mouse models that use potentiating agents, a correlation exists between increased serum levels of IL-1, IL-2, TNF-α, and IFN-γ with SEB-induced shock (10, 27, 56, 95). It is likely that the shock syndrome induced by superantigens results from the culmination of biological effects of these proinflammatory cytokines. It is difficult to determine whether any one particular cytokine and at what serum concentration is required to cause SEB-induced toxic shock, as the sensitizing agents induce the same proinflammatory cytokines as superantigens. Moreover, sensitizing agents like LPS potentiate the induction of cytokines by superantigens, and some of the cytokines produced (TNF-α, IL-1, and IFN-γ) synergize with each other to promote the deleterious effects. None of the existing mouse models faithfully reproduces all of the complex events of human toxic shock syndrome. Mouse models used for therapeutic efficacy studies may offer a higher stringency than is applicable in a setting where LPS and infections are present naturally with superantigens (76, 83, 94). Bacterial superantigens cause toxic shock and contribute to septic complications during infection (83, 94). In addition, toxic shock syndrome represents a spectrum and progression of clinical features including multiorgan failure in humans exposed to bacterial toxins and/or concurrent bacterial infection, pathogenic features seemingly absent in most mouse models.

In both humans and mice, an early T-cell cytokine profile includes TNF-α and IFN-γ, which are cytokines generally associated with a Th1-type response (9, 69, 70). These activated T cells subsequently produce IL-2, IL-10, and TNF-β (12, 23, 97). However, the typical Th2 type cytokine IL-10 was detected in vivo after repeated superantigen stimulation (23, 97). IL-10 knockout mice showed increased levels of IL-2, IFN-γ, TNF-α after SEB stimulation, and they are more susceptible to SEB-induced lethal shock, suggesting that IL-10 dampens the response of superantigen-induced Th1-type cytokines in vivo. Repeated superantigen exposure also generates immunosuppressive regulatory T cells with attendant IL-10 secretion and inhibited IL-2 production (71, 97), accompanied by clonal deletion and apoptosis of some of these activated T cells (31, 63).

ROLE OF KEY CYTOKINES

In vitro results indicate that IL-1, TNF-α, and IFN-γ are key mediators produced by superantigen-stimulated human PBMC. Because IFN-γ acts in synergy with IL-1 and TNF-α, small amounts of IFN-γ can profoundly affect the potentiation of proinflammatory effects of these two cytokines (54). In vivo neutralization of IFN-γ either protects or harms the host, depending on the mouse model and dose of sensitizing D-galactosamine used (23, 60). It is likely that IFN-γ is only effective as a synergistic agent and exerts immunopotentiating effects together with TNF-α and IL-1.

The in vivo effects of IL-1 alone have not been examined carefully in animal models but, in most cases, there is a correlation between increased survival and decreased serum IL-1 levels when various therapeutics are used to mitigate toxic shock (27, 50, 53). IL-1 exists in multiple isoforms, with IL-1β being the predominant form in humans and IL-1α most often encountered in mice. Antibodies to each form of IL-1 are species specific, which hampers research on its role in pathogenesis. IL-1 is an endogenous pyrogen that interacts with IL-1 receptor 1 (IL-1R1) subsequently activating downstream signaling molecules, the adaptor myeloid differentiation factor (MyD88), IL-1R1 associated protein kinase (IRAK), and TNF receptor-associated factor 6 (TRAF-6) (54). The similarity between the IL-1R and the toll-like receptor (TLR) intracellular signaling pathways used by pathogens to stimulate innate immunity underscores the importance of controlling the cytokine cascade for disease prevention.

TNF-α is considered the key mediator in the pathogenesis of toxic shock, as neutralization of TNF-α by anti-TNF-α or soluble TNF receptor 1 in vivo completely abrogates superantigen-mediated lethality (69, 70). TNF-α induction occurs early with peak serum levels reached at 90 min and seemingly originates from activated T cells, whereas macrophages appear to produce TNF-α at a later time in vivo (9). Most of the biological effects of TNF-α and IL-1 are similar and each can induce the production of other cytokines, chemokines, and cell adhesion molecules with potent immunological and vascular effects (54). TNF-α and IL-1 also synergistically interact with each other and with IFN-γ, resulting in amplification of their biological effects.

HUMAN DISEASES CAUSED BY STAPHYLOCOCCAL SUPERANTIGENS

Food Poisoning

Staphylococcal food poisoning is most often associated with ingestion of SEs (33). Nausea, vomiting, and diarrhea are seen within 6 h of toxin ingestion. TSST-1 causes systemic toxic shock but not emesis (17). The separation of the emetic and superantigenic domains of SEs remains controversial but some studies indicate that the disulfide loop of SEs, which is absent in TSST-1, may be the region responsible for the emetic activity of SEs (2, 73). Carboxymethylation of histidine residues in SEB eliminates its emetic activity but not superantigenicity (2). Little is known about how SEs induce enteric effects and specific receptors in the intestinal tract responsible for emesis have not been identified. Oral administration of SEB induces activation and expansion of murine Vβ8[+] T cells in Peyer's patches, accompanied by increased IFN-γ and IL-2 mRNA expression (93). IL-2 from activated T cells might be responsible for the enteric effects of SEs as IL-2 given to cancer patients produces side effects similar to staphylococcal food poisoning. Other mediators include cysteinyl leukotrienes from mast cells and substance P from sensory neurons (3, 87).

Toxic Shock Syndrome

Staphylococcal toxic shock syndrome (TSS) is characterized by fever, hypotension, desquamation of skin, fever, and dysfunction of three or more organ systems (17). Superantigens from both *S. aureus* and *Streptococcus pyogenes* are the causative agents of staphylococcal and streptococcal toxic shock (82). These bacterial toxins have profound effects on the immune system through the action of proinflammatory cytokines which affect local and distant sites of infection. Toxin effects on endothelial cell function and homeostasis are mostly through these host-produced mediators. Increased adhesion molecules, chemotactic cytokines, and procoagulant activities from endothelial cells can alter the activities of extravascular cells and leukocytes.

Autoimmunity

Microbial superantigens are also causative agents of autoimmune diseases as they can stimulate the immune system by activating APC and normally quiescent, autoreactive T and B cells (1, 11, 90, 107). Several animal models show that staphylococcal superantigens are arthrogenic (1, 90). TSST-1 is known to exacerbate bacterial cell wall-induced arthritis in rats and is possibly linked to accumulation of $V\beta 11^+$ T cells and IFN-γ production in arthritic joints (90, 109). TSST-1 also plays a pivotal role in murine septic arthritis, as the frequency and severity of arthritis is increased after intravenously administered TSST-1-secreting *S. aureus* (1). In humans, a good correlation exists between the presence of SEB-specific IgM and arthritis, suggesting a role for this toxin in disease (77). How exogenously administered toxin can trigger the development of these autoimmune processes is not known at present. It is likely that the cytokines and chemokines produced in response to superantigens can facilitate specific recruitment and migration of reactive T cells to synovial tissue and joints. In the presence of minor tissue injury or inflammation and its attendant release of potential autoantigens, the increased presence of immune cells might initiate the autoimmune process.

The evidence is accumulating that TSST-1 is the causative agent for Kawasaki syndrome, a disease with immunoregulatory abnormalities (67, 68). The hypothesis proposed is that a superantigen-producing organism (TSST-producing *S. aureus,* or other superantigen-producing microbes) colonizes the mucous membranes of the gastrointestinal tract of a genetically susceptible individual and the absorbed superantigen stimulates local or circulating mononuclear cells to produce proinflammatory cytokines that induce fever, vasculitis, and the clinical picture of Kawasaki syndrome (68). Psoriasis and atopic dermatitis (AD) are also autoimmune diseases linked to staphylococcal and streptococcal colonization of skin and subsequent production of exotoxins like SEA, SEB, SEC, TSST-1, and streptococcal pyrogenic exotoxins (SPEs) (39, 107). Patients with AD have increased numbers of peripheral blood $CD4^+CD25^+$ T regulatory cells (T_{reg}) with normal immunosuppressive activity. Unlike T_{reg} from healthy patients, T_{reg} from AD patients can be reactivated by superantigen and lose their immunosuppressive activity (78).

THERAPEUTICS

At present, there is no available therapeutic for treating staphylococcal exotoxin-induced shock except for the use of intravenous immunoglobulins (20). Antibody-based therapy targeting direct neutralization of SEB or other superantigens is most suitable at the early stages of exposure before cell activation and release of proinflammatory cytokines. Some of these neutralizing antibodies against superantigens cross-react with different superantigens (7). Recombinant mutants of SEB with attenuated binding to MHC class II and devoid of superantigenicity were also used successfully to vaccinate mice and monkeys against SEB-induced disease (6). Given the complex pathophysiology of toxic shock, an understanding of the interaction of cellular receptors and signaling pathways used by these staphylococcal superantigens and the biological mediators they induce provides invaluable insight into selecting appropriate therapeutic targets. Potential targets to prevent the toxic effects of SEs include blocking the interaction of SEs with MHC or TCR (14, 26), or other costimulatory molecules (40, 57, 85); inhibiting signal transduction pathways used by SEs (15, 50, 91); inhibiting cytokine and chemokine production (44, 45, 50, 51, 53); and blocking the downstream signaling pathways used by proinflammatory cytokines and chemokines.

Inhibitors of Cell Receptor-Toxin Interaction

Because the binding regions of SEB to MHC class II and TCR are known, small overlapping peptides of SEB were examined as antagonists to block the initial step of receptor-toxin interactions (5, 105). Conserved peptides corresponding to residues 150 to 161 of SEB can act as an antagonist and prevent SEA-, SEB-, or TSST-1-induced lethal shock in mice when given intravenously 30 min after an intraperitoneal toxin dose (5). This segment of SEB is not associated with the classically defined MHC class II or TCR binding domains, but it may block costimulatory signals necessary for T-cell activation. A subsequent study reported recently indicates that these peptides are ineffective inhibitors of SEB-induced effects both in vitro and in vivo (84). Recently, bispecific chimeric inhibitors composed of the DRα1 domain of MHC class II and Vβ domain of the TCR connected by a flexible GSTAPPA$_2$ linker were reported to bind SEB competitively and prevent its binding to MHC class II of APC and TCR on T cells (26). Initial cellular activation was blocked by the use of these chimeras and IL-2 release was inhibited in SEB-stimulated PBMC. Blockade of the CD28 costimulatory receptor by its synthetic ligand, CTLA4-Ig, prevented TSST-1-induced proliferation of T cells in vitro as well as lethal toxic shock in vivo (85).

Inhibitors of Signal Transduction

Other therapeutic compounds to be considered are those that can block SEB signal transduction pathways, as these events are postexposure and may be more amenable to suppression and manipulation. In vitro and in vivo studies have shown that many of the genes (i.e., cell adhesion molecules, cytokines, chemokines, acute-phase proteins, and inducible nitric oxide synthase) that are implicated in superantigen-induced lethal shock contain NFκB binding sites in the promotor/enhancer region (98). The activation of NFκB therefore leads to the inducible expression of many of the mediators involved in inflammatory diseases (48). NFκB binding activity is increased in patients with acute inflammation and sepsis, and can be correlated with clinical severity and mortality (reviewed in reference 98). Transient interruption of the NFκB pathway may therefore be beneficial for superantigen-induced shock. The nuclear import of NFκB allows transcriptional activation of over 100 genes that encode mediators of inflammatory and immune responses. Accordingly, a cell-permeable cyclic peptide targeting NFκB nuclear transport attenuated SEB-induced T-cell responses and inflammatory cytokine production (58). The extent of liver apoptosis and hemorrhagic necrosis was also reduced in mice given D-galactosamine plus SEB along with this NFκB inhibitor, which can be correlated with significantly decreased mortality rates (58).

Another potent NFκB inhibitor is dexamethasone, a well-known immunosuppressive drug used clinically to treat various inflammatory diseases. In vitro, dexamethasone potently inhibited staphylococcal exotoxin-induced T-cell proliferation, cytokine release, and activation markers in human PBMC (41, 42). In vivo, dexamethasone also significantly reduced serum levels of TNF-α, IFN-γ, IL-1α, IL-2, and IL-6 in the LPS-potentiated model of SEB-induced shock (50). Furthermore, dexamethasone attenuated the hypothermic response to SEB and improved survival of mice by 90% even when administered hours after SEB.

Other signal transduction inhibitors include those directed against protein kinase C (PKC) and protein tyrosine kinase. H7, a PKC inhibitor, and genistein, a tyrosine kinase inhibitor, each blocked TNF-α but not IL-1 production from TSST-1-stimulated PBMC (91). D609, an inhibitor of phospholipase C, which is an upstream activator of PKC, blocked SE-induced effects both in vitro and in vivo (45, 103). Curiously, the serum level of TNF-α in mice treated with D609 and superantigen remained high (103). A list of small nonpeptide inhibitors effective in blocking the effects of superantigens is shown in Table 1.

Table 1. Small nonpeptide therapeutics for SEB-induced shock

Pharmacologic agent	Target	Biological effects against SEB

Dexamethasone
  FDA-approved for treating
  inflammatory diseases
	NFκB	Inhibited SEB-induced proinflammatory
		  cytokines and chemokines in PBMC (42)
		Blocked cell adhesion molecules (ICAM,
		  ELAM, VCAM) on endothelial cells (41)
		Reduced serum levels of cytokines,
		  attenuated hypothermia due to SEB,
		  improved survival of mice (50)

Pentoxifylline
  FDA-approved for treating
  peripheral arterial disease
	Phosphodiesterase	Attenuated SEB-induced proinflammatory
		  cytokines and chemokines in PBMC
		  (44, 53)
		Blocked cytokine release in vivo and
		  prevented SEB-induced lethal shock in
		  mice (53)

Baicalin
  Herbal medicine used for
  treating infectious diseases
  in China
	NFκB	Inhibited SEB-induced cytokines and
		  chemokines at the transcriptional level
		  (51)
		Blocked SEB-induced T-cell proliferation
		  (51)

Pirfenidone	Inhibition of TGF-β
	  (exact mechanism
	  unknown)
		Inhibited SEB-stimulated cytokines in vitro
		  and in vivo (27)
		Improved survival of mice (27)

Niacinamide	Nitric oxide synthase	Inhibited serum IL-2 and IFN-γ (56) Prevented death of mice from SEB- mediated shock (56)

D609	Phospholipase C	Blocked SEB-stimulated cytokines,
		  chemokines, and proliferation in human
		  PBMc (45)
		Improved survival of mice (103)

Inhibitors of Cytokines

Due to the pathophysiological complexities of toxic shock resulting from excessive proinflammatory cytokine release from host cells responding to microbial products like superantigens, therapeutic strategies are aimed at inhibiting the release of multiple inflammatory mediators. Most therapeutic testing in animal models of SEB-induced shock have targeted proinflammatory cytokines, as there is a strong correlation between toxicity and increased serum levels of these inflammatory mediators (42, 44, 45, 47–51, 53). Neutralizing antibodies against TNF-α prevented SEB-induced lethality (69). The anti-inflammatory cytokine IL-10 was used to block the production of IL-1, TNF-α, and IFN-γ, resulting in reduced lethality to superantigen-induced toxic shock (8).

Another strategy to attenuate IL-1 release from superantigen-activated cells is to target caspase 1, a proteolytic enzyme that cleaves pro-IL-1 into active IL-1 (54). The caspase-1-specific inhibitor, Ac-YVAD-cmk, blocked IL-1 and MCP production in superantigen-stimulated PBMC cultures but had no effect on other cytokines or T-cell proliferation (47). Caspase 3 and caspase 8 inhibitors were also ineffective in down-regulating superantigen-activated cells. In contrast, a pan-caspase inhibitor, Z-D-CH$_2$-DCB, attenuated the production of IL-1β, TNF-α, IL-6, IFN-γ, MCP, MIP-1α, and MIP-1β and inhibited T-cell proliferation in SEB- and TSST-1-stimulated PBMC (47). Preliminary results indicate that pan-caspase inhibitor delayed the time of death in a lethal mouse model of SEB-mediated shock (unpublished observations).

Other drugs tested to block cytokine release from superantigen-activated cells include doxycycline, an antibiotic, and pentoxyfylline, a methylxanthine derivative. Doxycycline inhibited SEB-induced proinflammatory cytokines and chemokines and T-cell proliferation in human PBMC (49). Pentoxyfylline, a phosphodiesterase inhibitor, is used clinically to treat peripheral vascular disease. Its interference with intracellular regulator pathways affects leukocyte adhesion and cytokine production. Pentoxyfylline inhibited SEB- or TSST-1-induced toxic shock, as well as cytokine and chemokine release (44, 53). Dexamethasone, pentoxyfylline, and doxycycline are FDA-approved drugs used for other indications, and have been in clinical use for many years with a proven safety record.

Another compound, baicalin, is a flavone isolated from the Chinese medicinal herb *Scutellaria baicalensis,* and is a potent inhibitor of SEB-mediated effects in vitro (51). Niacinamide, a nitric oxide inhibitor, mitigated the effects of SEB by inhibiting the production of IL-2 and IFN-γ, and improved survival of mice given LPS plus SEB (56).

Blocking the signal transduction pathways used by inflammatory cytokines represents another means of inhibiting cellular responses to superantigens. One target is the suppressor of cytokine signal 3 (SOCS3) which regulates the signal transducer and activator of transcription family of proteins (35). In this regard, a cell-penetrating form of SOCS3 protected animals from lethal effects of SEB and LPS by reducing production of inflammatory cytokines and attenuating liver apoptosis and hemorrhagic necrosis (35).

SUMMARY

By binding to both MHC class II and TCR, superantigens stimulate T-cell proliferation and excessive release of multiple inflammatory cytokines and chemokines. Similar to other shock syndromes, extensive tissue injury is produced by this exaggerated activation of the host immune system to pathogens and their products. In particular, proinflammatory cytokines TNF-α, IL-1, and IFN-γ act synergistically on multiple cells and organs resulting in cardiovascular derangement, multiorgan failure, and shock. The ability to stop the inflammatory events initiated by superantigens early appears to be critical in preventing toxic shock. However, anti-inflammatory/immunosuppressive treatment has to be balanced by the fact that inflammation is the host's self-protective response to external challenges.

Acknowledgments. The views expressed in this publication are those of the author and do not reflect the official policy or position of the Department of the Army, the Department of Defense, or the U.S. Government.

REFERENCES

1. **Abdelnour, A. T., T. Bremell, and A. Tarkowski.** 1994. TSST-1 contributes to the arthritogenecity of *Staphylococcus aureus. J. Infect. Dis.* **170:**94–99.

2. **Alber, G., D. K. Hammer, and B. Fleischer.** 1990. Relationship between enterotoxic- and T lymphocyte-stimulating activity of staphylococcal enterotoxin B. *J. Immunol.* **144:**4501–4506.

3. **Alber, G., P. H. Scheuber, B. Reck, B. Sailer-Kramer, A. Hartmann, and D. K. Hammer.** 1989. Role of substance P in immediate-type skin reactions induced by staphylococcal enterotoxin B in unsensitized monkeys. *J. Allergy Clin. Immunol.* **84:**880–885.

4. **Anderson, M. R., and M. Tary-Lehmann.** 2001. Staphylococcal enterotoxin-B-induced lethal shock in mice is T-cell-dependent, but disease susceptibility is defined by the non-T-cell compartment. *Clin. Immunol.* **98:**85–94.

5. **Arad, G., R. Levy, D. Hillman, and R. Kaempfer.** 2000. Superantigen antagonist protects against lethal shock and defines a new domain for T-cell activation. *Nat. Med.* **6:**414–421.

6. **Bavari, S., B. Dyas, and R. G. Ulrich.** 1996. Superantigen vaccines: a comparative study of genetically attenuated receptor-binding mutants of staphylococcal enterotoxin A. *J. Infect. Dis.* **174:**338–345.

7. **Bavari, S., R. G. Ulrich, and R. D. LeClaire.** 1999. Cross-reactive antibodies prevent the lethal effects of *Staphylococcus aureus* superantigens. *J. Infect. Dis.* **180:**1365–1369.

8. **Bean, A. G., R. A. Freiberg, S. Andrade, S. Menon, and A. Zlotnik.** 1993. Interleukin 10 protects mice against staphylococcal enterotoxin B-induced lethal shock. *Infect. Immun.* **61:**4937–4939.

9. **Bette, M., M. K. Schafer, N. van Rooijen, E. Weihe, and B. Fleischer.** 1993. Distribution and kinetics of superantigen-induced cytokine gene expression in mouse spleen. *J. Exp. Med.* **178:**1531–1539.

10. **Blank, C., A. Luz, S. Bendigs, A. Erdmann, H. Wagner, and K. Heeg.** 1997. Superantigen and endotoxin synergize in the induction of lethal shock. *Eur. J. Immunol.* **27:**825–833.

11. **Brocke, S., S. Hausmann, L. Steinmam, and K. W. Wucherpfennig.** 1998. Microbial peptides and superantigens in the pathogenesis of autoimmune diseases of the central nervous system. *Semin. Immunol.* **10:**57–67.

12. **Cameron, S. B., M. C. Nawijn, W. W. Kum, H. F. Savelkoul, and A. W. Chow.** 2001. Regulation of helper T cell responses to staphylococcal superantigens. *Eur. Cytokine Netw.* **12:**210–222.

13. **Carlsson R., H. Fischer, and H. O. Sjogren.** 1988. Binding of staphylococcal enterotoxin A to accessory cells is a requirement for its ability to activate human T cells. *J. Immunol.* **140:**2484–2488.

14. **Chatila, T., and R. S. Geha.** 1993. Signal transduction by microbial superantigens via MHC class II molecules. *Immunol. Rev.* **131:**43–59.

15. **Chatila, T., N. Wood, J. Parsonnet, and R. S. Geha.** 1988. Toxic shock syndrome toxin-1 induces inositol phospholipid turnover, protein kinase C translocation, and calcium mobilization in human T cells. *J. Immunol.* **140:**1250–1255.

16. **Chen, J. Y., Y. Qiao, K. L. Komisar, W. B. Baze, I. C. Hsu, and J. Tseng.** 1994. Increased susceptibility to staphylococcal enterotoxin B intoxication in mice primed with actinomycin D. *Infect. Immun.* **62:**4626–4631.

17. **Chesney, P. J., P. J. Davis, W. K. Purdy, P. J. Wand, and R. W. Chesney.** 1981. Clinical manifestations of toxic shock syndrome. *JAMA* **246:**741–748.

18. **Chintagumpala, M. M., J. A. Mollick, and R. R. Rich.** 1991. Staphylococcal toxins bind to different sites on HLA-DR. *J. Immunol.* **147:**3876–3882.

19. **Choi, Y., B. Kotzin, L. Hernon, J. Callahan, P. Marrack, and J. Kappler.** 1989. Interaction of *Staphylococcus aureus* toxin "superantigens" with human T cells. *Proc. Natl. Acad. Sci. USA* **86:**8941–8945.

20. **Darenberg, J., B. Soderquist, B. H. Normark, and A. Norrby-Teglund.** 2004. Differences in potency of intravenous polyspecific immunoglobulin G against streptococcal and staphylococcal superantigens: implications for therapy of toxic shock syndrome. *Clin. Infect. Dis.* **38:**836–842.

21. **DaSilva, L., B. Welcher, R. Ulrich, M. Aman, C. David, and S. Bavari.** 2002. Humanlike immune response of human leukocyte antigen-DR3 transgenic mice to staphylococcal enterotoxins: a novel model for superantigen vaccines. *J. Infect. Dis.* **185:**1754–1760.

22. **Fischer, H., M. Dohlsten, U. Andersson, G. Hedlund, P. Ericsson, J. Hansson, and H. O. Sjogren.** 1990. Production of TNF-α and TNF-β by staphylococcal enterotoxin A activated human T cells. *J. Immunol.* **144:**4663–4668.

23. **Florquin, S., Z. Amraoui, D. Abramowicz, and M. Goldman.** 1994. Systemic release and protective role of IL-10 in staphylococcal enterotoxin B-induced shock in mice. *J. Immunol.* **153:**2618–2623.

24. **Fraser, J., V. Arcus, P. Kong, E. Baker, and T. Proft.** 2000. Superantigens—powerful modifiers of the immune system. *Mol. Med. Today* **6:**125–132.

25. **Fraser, J., M. Newton, and A. Weiss.** 1992. CD28 and T-cell antigen receptor signal transduction coordinately regulates interleukin 2 gene expression in response to superantigen stimulation. *J. Exp. Med.* **175:**1131–1134.

26. **Geller-Hong, E., M. Möllhoff, P. R. Shiflett, and G. Gupta.** 2004. Design of chimeric receptor mimics with different TcRVβ isoforms: type-specific inhibition of superantigen pathogenesis. *J. Biol. Chem.* **279:**5676–5684.

27. **Hale, M. L., S. B. Margolin, T. Krakauer, C. J. Roy, and B. G. Stiles.** 2002. Pirfenidone blocks in vitro and in vivo effects of staphylococcal enterotoxin B. *Infect. Immun.* **70:**2989–2994.

28. **Hamad, A. R., P. Marrack, and J. W. Kappler.** 1997. Transcytosis of staphylococcal superantigen toxins. *J. Exp. Med.* **185:**1447–1454.

29. **Herman, A., G. Croteau, R. P. Sekaly, J. Kappler, and P. Marrack.** 1990. HLA-DR alleles differ in their ability to present staphylococcal enterotoxins to T cells. *J. Exp. Med.* **172:**709–712.

30. **Herrmann, T., R. S. Acolla, and H. R. MacDonald.** 1989. Different staphylococcal enterotoxins bind preferentially to distinct MHC class II isotypes. *Eur. J. Immunol.* **19:**2171–2174.

31. **Hewitt, C., J. Lamb, J. Hayball, M. Hill, M. Owen, and R. O'Hehir.** 1992. MHC Independent clonal T cell anergy by direct interaction of staphylococcal enterotoxin B with the T-cell antigen receptor. *J. Exp. Med.* **175:**1493–1499.

32. **Hodoval, L. F., E. L. Morris, G. J. Crawley, and W. R. Beisel.** 1968. Pathogenesis of lethal shock after intravenous staphylococcal enterotoxin B in monkeys. *Appl. Microbiol.* **16:**187–192.

33. **Holmberg, S. D., and P. A. Blake.** 1984. Staphylococcal food poisoning in the United States. New facts and old misconceptions. *JAMA* **251:**487–489.

34. **Hudson, K. R., R. E. Tiedemann, R. G. Urban, S. C. Lowe, J. L. Strominger, and J. D. Fraser.** 1995. Staphylococcal enterotoxin A has two cooperative binding sites on major histocompatibility complex class II. *J. Exp. Med.* **182:**711–720.

35. **Jo, D., D. Liu, S. Yao, R. D. Collins, and J. Hawiger.** 2005. Intracellular protein therapy with SOCS3 inhibits inflammation and apoptosis. *Nat. Med.* **11:**892–898.

36. **Jupin, C., S. Anderson, C. Damais, J. E. Alouf, and M. Parant.** 1988. Toxic shock syndrome toxin 1 as an inducer of human tumor necrosis factors and gamma interferon. *J. Exp. Med.* **167:**752–761.

37. **Kappler, J. W., A. Herman, J. Clements, and P. Marrack.** 1992. Mutations defining functional regions of the superantigen staphylococcal enterotoxin B. *J. Exp. Med.* **175:**387–396.

38. **Kotb, M.** 1995. Bacterial pyrogenic exotoxins as superantigens. *Clin. Microbiol. Rev.* **8:**411–426.

39. **Kotzin, B. L., D. Y. M. Leung, J. Kappler, and P. Marrack.** 1993. Superantigens and their potential role in human disease. *Adv. Immunol.* **54:**99–166.

40. **Krakauer, T.** 1994. Costimulatory receptors for the superantigen staphylococcal enterotoxin B on human vascular endothelial cells and T cells. *J. Leukoc. Biol.* **56:**458–463.

41. **Krakauer, T.** 1994. A sensitive ELISA for measuring the adhesion of leukocytic cells to human endothelial cells. *J. Immunol. Methods* **177:**207–213.

42. **Krakauer, T.** 1995. Inhibition of toxic shock syndrome toxin-induced cytokine production and T cell activation by interleukin 10, interleukin 4, and dexamethasone. *J. Infect. Dis.* **172:**988–992.

43. **Krakauer, T.** 1999. Immune response to staphylococcal superantigens. *Immunol. Res.* **20:**163–173.

44. **Krakauer, T.** 1999. The induction of CC chemokines in human peripheral blood mononuclear cells by staphylococcal exotoxins and its prevention by pentoxifylline. *J. Leukoc. Biol.* **66:**158–164.

45. **Krakauer, T.** 2001. Suppression of endotoxin- and staphylococcal exotoxin-induced cytokines and chemokines by a phospholipase C inhibitor in human peripheral blood mononuclear cells. *Clin. Diagn. Lab. Immunol.* **8:**449–453.

46. **Krakauer, T.** 2002. Stimulant-dependent modulation of cytokines and chemokines by airway epithelial cells: cross-talk between pulmonary epithelial and peripheral blood mononuclear cells. *Clin. Diagn. Lab. Immunol.* **9:**126–131.

47. **Krakauer, T.** 2004. Caspase inhibitors attenuate superantigen-induced inflammatory cytokines, chemokines and T-cell proliferation. *Clin. Diagn. Lab. Immunol.* **11:**621–624.

48. **Krakauer, T.** 2004. Molecular therapeutic targets in inflammation: cyclooxygenase and NF-κB. *Curr. Drug Targets Inflamm. Allergy* **3:**317–324.

49. **Krakauer, T., and M. Buckley.** 2003. Doxycycline is anti-inflammatory and inhibits staphylococcal exotoxin-induced cytokines and chemokines. *Antimicrob. Agents Chemother.* **47:**3630–3633.

50. **Krakauer, T., and M. Buckley.** Dexamethasone attenuates staphylococcal enterotoxin B-induced hypothermic response and protects mice from superantigen-induced toxic shock. *Antimicrob. Agents Chemother.,* in press.

51. **Krakauer, T., B. Q. Li, and H. A. Young.** 2001. The flavonoid baicalin inhibits staphylococcal superantigen-induced inflammatory cytokine and chemokine production in human peripheral blood mononuclear cells. *FEBS Lett.* **500:**50–55.

52. **Krakauer, T., L. Pitt, and R. E. Hunt.** 1997. Detection of IL-6 and IL-2 in serum of rhesus monkeys exposed to a nonlethal dose of staphylococcal enterotoxin B. *Mil. Med.* **162:**612–615.

53. **Krakauer, T., and B. G. Stiles.** 1999. Pentoxifylline inhibits staphylococcal superantigen induced toxic shock and cytokine release. *Clin. Diagn. Lab. Immunol.* **6:**594–598.

54. **Krakauer, T., J. Vilcek, and J. J. Oppenheim.** 1998. Proinflammatory cytokines: TNF and IL-1 families, chemokines, TGFβ and others, p. 775–811. *In* W. Paul (ed.), *Fundamental Immunology,* 4th ed. Lippincott-Raven Press, Philadelphia, Pa.

55. **LaSalle, J. M., F. Toneguzzo, M. Saadeh, D. E. Golan, R. Taber, and D. A. Hafler.** 1993. T cell presentation of antigen requires cell to cell contact for proliferation and anergy induction. *J. Immunol.* **151:**649–657.

56. **LeClaire, R. D., W. Kell, S. Bavari, T. Smith, and R. E. Hunt.** 1996. Protective effects of niacinamide in staphylococcal enterotoxin B induced toxicity. *Toxicology* **107:**69–81.

57. **Linsley, P. S., and J. A. Ledbetter.** 1993. The role of the CD28 receptor during T cell responses to antigen. *Annu. Rev. Immunol.* **11:**191–212.

58. **Liu, D., X. Y. Liu, D. Robinson, C. Burnett, C. Jackson, L. Seele, R. A. Veach, S. Downs, R. D. Collins, D. W. Ballard, and J. Hawiger.** 2004. Suppression of staphylococcal enterotoxin B-induced toxicity by a nuclear import inhibitor. *J. Biol. Chem.* **279:**19239–19246.

59. **Marrack, P., and J. Kappler.** 1990. The staphylococcal enterotoxins and their relatives. *Science* **248:**705–709.

60. **Matthys, P., T. Mitera, H. Heremans, J. Van Damme, and A. Billiau.** 1995. Anti-gamma interferon and anti-interleukin-6 antibodies affect staphylococcal enterotoxin B-induced weight loss, hypoglycemia, and cytokine release in D-galactosamine-sensitized and unsensitized mice. *Infect. Immun.* **63:**1158–1164.

61. **Mattix, M. E., R. E. Hunt, C. L. Wilhelmsen, A. J. Johnson, and W. B. Baze.** 1995. Aerosolized staphylococcal enterotoxin B-induced pulmonary lesions in rhesus monkeys (*Macaca mulatta*). *Toxicol. Pathol.* **23:**262–268.

62. **Mattsson, E., H. Herwald, and A. Egsten.** 2003. Superantigens from *Staphylococcus aureus* induce procoagulant activity and monocyte tissue factor expression in whole blood and mononuclear cells via IL-1β. *J. Thromb. Haemost.* **1:**2569–2575.

63. **McCormack, J. E., J. E. Callahan, J. Kappler, and P. C. Marrack.** 1993. Profound deletion of mature T cells in vivo by chronic exposure to endogenous superantigen. *J. Immunol.* **150:**3785–3792.

64. **McCormick, J. K., J. M. Yarwood, and P. M. Schlievert.** 2001. Toxic shock syndrome and bacterial superantigens: an update. *Annu. Rev. Microbiol.* **55:**77–104.

65. **McKay, D. M.** 2001. Bacterial superantigens: provocateurs of gut dysfunction and inflammation? *Trends Immunol.* **22:**497–501.

66. **Mehindate, K., R. al-Daccak, F. Damdoumi, and W. Mourad.** 1996. Synergistic effect between CD40 and class II signals overcomes the requirement for class II dimerization in superantigen-induced cytokine gene expression. *Eur. J. Immunol.* **26:**2075–2080.

67. **Meissner, H. C., and D. Y. M. Leung.** 2000. Superantigens, conventional antigens and the etiology of Kawasaki syndrome. *Pediatr. Infect. Dis. J.* **19:**91–94.
68. **Meissner, H. C., and D. Y. M. Leung.** 2003. Kawasaki Syndrome: where are the answers. *Pediatrics* **112:**672–676.
69. **Miethke, T., C. Wahl, K. Heeg, B. Echtenacher, P. H. Krammer, and H. Wagner.** 1992. T cell-mediated lethal shock triggered in mice by the superantigen staphylococcal enterotoxin B: critical role of tumor necrosis factor. *J. Exp. Med.* **175:**91–98.
70. **Miethke, T., C. Wahl, K. Heeg, B. Echtenacher, P. H. Krammer, and H. Wagner.** 1993. Superantigen mediated shock: a cytokine release syndrome. *Immunobiology* **189:**270–284.
71. **Miller, C., J. Ragheb, and R. Schwartz.** 1999. Anergy and cytokine-mediated suppression as distinct superantigen-induced tolerance mechanisms in vivo. *J. Exp. Med.* **190:**53–64.
72. **Mollick, J. A., M. Chintagumpala, R. G. Cook, and R. R. Rich.** 1991. Staphylococcal exotoxin activation of T cells. Role of exotoxin-MHC class II binding affinity and class II isotype. *J. Immunol.* **146:**463–468.
73. **Monday, S. R., and G. A. Bohach.** 1999. Properties of *Staphylococcus aureus* enterotoxins and toxic shock syndrome toxin-1, p. 589–610. *In* J. E. Alouf and J. H. Freer (ed.), *The Comprehensive Sourcebook of Bacterial Protein Toxins.* Academic Press, London.
74. **Mourad, W., K. Mehindate, T. Schall, and S. McColl.** 1992. Engagement of MHC class II molecules by superantigen induces inflammatory cytokine gene expression in human rheumatoid fibroblast-like synoviocytes. *J. Exp. Med.* **175:**613–616.
75. **Neumann, B., B. Engelhardt, H. Wagner, and B. Holzmann.** 1997. Induction of acute inflammatory lung injury by staphylococcal enterotoxin B. *J. Immunol.* **158:**1862–1871.
76. **Norrby-Teglund, A., S. Chatellier, D. E. Low, A. McGeer, K. Green, and M. Kotb.** 2000. Host variation in cytokine responses to superantigens determines the severity of invasive group A streptococcal infection. *Eur. J. Immunol.* **30:**3247–3255.
77. **Origuchi, T., K. Eguchi, Y. Kawabe, I. Yamashita, A. Mizokami, H. Ida, and S. Nagataki.** 1995. Increased levels of serum IgM antibody to staphylococcal enterotoxin B in patients with rheumatoid arthritis. *Ann. Rheum. Dis.* **54:**713–732.
78. **Ou, L. S., E. Goleva, C. Hall, and L. Y. Leung.** 2004. T regulatory cells in atopic dermatitis and subversion of their activity by superantigens. *J. Clin. Allergy Immunol.* **113:**756–763.
79. **Papageorgiou, A. C., and K. R. Acharya.** 2000. Microbial superantigens: from structure to function. *Trends Microbiol.* **8:**369–375.
80. **Parsonnet, J.** 1989. Mediators in the pathogenesis of toxic shock syndrome: overview. *Rev. Infect. Dis.* **11:**S263–S269.
81. **Pless, D. D., G. Ruthel, E. K. Reinke, R. G. Ulrich, and S. Bavari.** 2005. Persistence of zinc-binding bacterial superantigens at the surface of antigen-presenting cells contributes to the extreme potency of these superantigens as T-cell activators. *Infect. Immun.* **73:**5358–5366.
82. **Proft, T., and J. D. Fraser.** 2003. Bacterial superantigens. *Clin. Exp. Immunol.* **133:**299–306.
83. **Proft, T., S. Sriskandan, L. Yang, and J. D. Fraser.** 2003. Superantigens and streptococcal toxic shock syndrome. *Emerg. Infect. Dis.* **9:**1211–1218.
84. **Rajagopalan, G., M. M. Sen, and C. S. David.** 2004. In vitro and in vivo evaluation of staphylococcal superantigen peptide antagonists. *Infect. Immun.* **72:**6733–6737.
85. **Saha, B., B. Jaklic, D. M. Harlan, G. S. Gray, C. H. June, and R. Abe.** 1996. Toxic shock syndrome toxin-1 induced death is prevented by CTLA4Ig. *J. Immunol.* **157:**3869–3875.
86. **Sarawar, S. R., M. A. Blackman, and P. C. Doherty.** 1994. Superantigen shock in mice with an inapparent viral infection. *J. Infect. Dis.* **170:**1189–1194.
87. **Scheuber, P. H., C. Denzlinger, D. Wilker, G. Beck, D. Keppler, and D. K. Hammer.** 1987. Staphylococcal enterotoxin B as a nonimmunological mast cell stimulus in primates: the role of endogenous cysteinyl leukotrienes. *Int. Arch. Allergy Appl. Immunol.* **82:**289–291.
88. **Scholl, P., R. Sekaly, A. Diez, L. Glimcher, and R. Geha.** 1990. Binding of toxic shock syndrome toxin-1 to murine major histocompatibility complex class II molecules. *Eur. J. Immunol.* **20:**1911–1916.
89. **Scholl, P. R., N. Trede, T. A. Chatila, and R. S. Geha.** 1992. Role of protein tyrosine phosphorylation in monokine induction by the staphylococcal superantigen toxic shock syndrome toxin-1. *J. Immunol.* **148:**2237–2241.
90. **Schwab, J. H., R. R. Brown, S. K. Anderle, and P. M. Schlievert.** 1993. Superantigen can reactivate bacterial cell wall-induced arthritis. *J. Immunol.* **150:**4131–4138.

91. **See, R. H., and A. W. Chow.** 1992. Staphylococcal toxic shock syndrome toxin 1-induced tumor necrosis factor alpha and interleukin-1β secretion by human peripheral blood monocytes and T lymphocytes is differentially suppressed by protein kinase inhibitors. *Infect. Immun.* **60:**3456–3459.

92. **See, R. H., W. W. Kum, A. H. Chang, S. H. Goh, and A. W. Chow.** 1992. Induction of tumor necrosis factor and interleukin-1 by purified staphylococcal toxic shock syndrome toxin 1 requires the presence of both monocytes and T lymphocytes. *Infect. Immun.* **60:**2612–2618.

93. **Spiekermann, G. M., and C. Nagler-Anderson.** 1998. Oral adminstration of the bacterial superantigen staphylococcal enterotoxin B induces activation and cytokine production by T cells in murine gut-associated lymphoid tissue. *J. Immunol.* **161:**5825–5831.

94. **Sriskandan, S., M. Unnikrishnan, T. Krausz, H. Dewchand, S. Van Noorden, J. Cohen, and D. M. Altmann.** 2001. Enhanced susceptibility to superantigen-associated streptococcal sepsis in human leukocyte antigen-DQ transgenic mice. *J. Infect. Dis.* **184:**166–173.

95. **Stiles, B. G., S. Bavari, T. Krakauer, and R. G. Ulrich.** 1993. Toxicity of staphylococcal enterotoxins potentiated by lipopolysaccharide: major histocompatibility complex class II molecule dependency and cytokine release. *Infect. Immun.* **61:**5333–5338.

96. **Sugiyama, H., E. M. McKissic, M. S. Bergdoll, and B. Heller.** 1964. Enhancement of bacterial endotoxin lethality by staphylococcal enterotoxin. *J. Infect. Dis.* **4:**111–118.

97. **Sundstedt, A., L. Hoiden, A. Rosendahl, T. Kalland, N. van Rooijen, and M. Dohlsten.** 1997. Immunoregulatory role of IL-10 during superantigen-induced-hyporesponsiveness in vivo. *J. Immunol.* **158:**180–186.

98. **Tak, P. P., and G. S. Firestein,** 2001. NFκB: a key role in inflammatory diseases. *J. Clin. Invest.* **107:**7–11.

99. **Tessier, P. A., P. H. Naccache, K.R. Diener, R. P. Gladue, K. S. Neote, I. Clark-Lewis, and S. R. McColl.** 1998. Induction of acute inflammation in vivo by staphylococcal superantigens. II. Critical role for chemokines, ICAM-1, and TNF-alpha. *J. Immunol.* **161:**1204–1211.

100. **Thibodeau, J., I. Cloutier, P. M. Lavoie, N. Labrecque, W. Mourad, T. Jardetzky, and R. P. Sekaly.** 1994. Subsets of HLA-DR1 molecules defined by SEB and TSST-1 binding. *Science* **266:**1874–1878.

101. **Tiedemann, R. E., and J. D. Fraser.** 1996. Cross-linking of MHC class II molecules by staphylococcal enterotoxin A is essential for antigen-presenting cell and T cell activation. *J. Immunol.* **157:**3958–3966.

102. **Trede, N. S., R. S. Geha, and T. Chatila.** 1991. Transcriptional activation of IL-1 beta and tumor necrosis factor-alpha genes by MHC class II ligands. *J. Immunol.* **146:**2310–2315.

103. **Tschaikowsky, K. J., J. Schmidt, and M. Meisner.** 1999. Modulation of mouse endotoxin shock by inhibition of phosphatidylcholine-specific phospholipase C. *J. Pharmacol. Exp. Ther.* **285:**800–804.

104. **Ulrich, R. G., S. Bavari, and M. A. Olson.** 1995. Staphylococcal enterotoxins A and B share a common structural motif for binding class II major histocompatibility complex molecules. *Nat. Struct. Biol.* **2:**554–560.

105. **Visvanathan, K., A. Charles, J. Bannan, P. Pugach, K. Kashfi, and J. B. Zabriskie.** 2001. Inhibition of bacterial superantigens by peptides and antibodies. *Infect. Immun.* **69:**875–884.

106. **Yarovinsky, T. O., M. P. Mohning, M. A. Bradford, M. M. Monick, and G. W. Hunninghake.** 2005. Increased sensitivity to staphylococcal enterotoxin B following adenoviral infection. *Infect. Immun.* **73:**3375–3381.

107. **Yarwood, J. M., D. Y. Leung, and P. M. Schlievert.** 2000. Evidence for the involvement of bacterial superantigens in psoriasis, atopic dermatitis, and Kawasaki syndrome. *FEMS Microbiol. Lett.* **192:**1–7.

108. **Zhang, W. J., S. Sarawar, P. Nguyen, K. Daly, J. E. Rehg, P. C. Doherty, D. L. Woodland, and M. A. Blackman.** 1996. Lethal synergism between influenza infection and staphylococcal enterotoxin B in mice. *J. Immunol.* **157:**5049–5060.

109. **Zhao, Y.-X., A. Abdelnour, T. Kalland, and A. Tarkowski.** 1995. Overexpression of the T-cell receptor Vb3 in transgenic mice increases mortality during infection by enterotoxin A-producing *Staphylococcus aureus. Infect. Immun.* **63:**4463–4469.

Chapter 16

Countermeasures against Superantigens: Structure-Based Design of Bispecific Receptor Mimics

Goutam Gupta and Meghan Kunkel

INTRODUCTION

Superantigens (SAgs) are a family of highly potent immunostimulatory proteins produced by bacteria or viruses. The family includes many proteins that may be unrelated by sequence or structure and yet share the ability to bypass the mechanisms of conventional antigen processing and trigger excessive activation of T cells. The advantages gained by microbes through SAg production are not well understood. Since they cause massive activation of the host immune system SAgs might prolong survival by promoting local inflammation and thereby increase blood and nutrient supply (13). The massive lymphokine release by the activated cells within hours and the excessive T-cell proliferation in 2 to 3 days could ultimately lead to an immunosuppressive state and favor the microbe. However, there is a general agreement that the primary function of the SAgs is to debilitate the host immune system to facilitate the onset and progression of disease (9).

SAg-BASED DISEASE

Human diseases caused by microbes that utilize SAgs as their major virulence factors are characterized by fever and shock. The *Staphylococcus aureus* enterotoxins A-1 are thought to be the causative agents in 33% of all food-poisoning cases (3) and are the most frequent cause of hospital-acquired infections (4). Dangerous toxic shock syndrome is mediated by the *S. aureus* toxin TSST-1 and occurs when *S. aureus* infects surgical wounds or injury sites. In chronic conditions such as inflammatory skin disease, *S. aureus* SAgs are implicated in the onset of disease by disrupting normal immune activity. Also, SAgs have been proposed to promote autoimmune and immunodeficiency diseases such as multiple sclerosis and HIV infection by continually weakening the host immune response (10, 18).

Goutam Gupta and Meghan Kunkel • Los Alamos National Laboratory, Bioscience Division, Los Alamos, NM 87545.

PREVENTION AND THERAPY

Presently, the treatment of superantigen-mediated infections is limited to the administration of antibiotics and handling of the state of shock. However, the development of multiple antibiotic-resistant, superantigen-producing bacterial strains calls for alternative treatments. Novel SAg vaccines and therapies, including the production of neutralizing antibodies, inhibitory peptide/receptor molecules, blockage of superantigen gene transcription, and small molecule inhibitors, are currently being developed and tested. One promising avenue for the development of new SAg therapies is through structure-based drug design.

STRUCTURE-BASED DRUG DESIGN

For the past ten years, combinatorial chemistry and diversity-based high-throughput screening were the approaches of choice for lead drug identification while computational methods were employed predominantly in drug optimization activities. Due to the availability of a large number of three-dimensional structures of protein targets and protein-ligand complexes, structure-based drug design has become a logical strategy for lead generation as well as for optimization. Structure-based design has become an integral part of modern drug discovery and is rooted in a firm understanding of molecular recognition in protein-ligand complexes. Structural studies over the past 10 years have provided a great deal of information regarding the complex interactions of SAgs with host molecules and therefore have paved the way for the structure-based design of protein therapeutics.

SAgs VERSUS CONVENTIONAL ANTIGENS

One of the key insights garnered from structural studies of SAgs is the manner in which they interact with the immune system. Conventional antigens are phagocytosed by antigen-presenting cells (APCs) and are processed into discrete peptides. The peptides form a complex with the major histocompatibility complex (MHC) class II receptor and travel through the secretory pathway to be displayed on the cell surface. T cells will only respond if their surface receptors CD4 recognize the specific peptide on the class II molecule. Thus, only a tiny fraction of the host's T-cell repertoire ($<0.01\%$) is activated through this mechanism. SAgs, however, are not processed into peptides and instead they bind as intact proteins to the receptor complex formed by the MHC class II receptors on APCs and the T-cell receptor (TCR) on T cells. This alternative mode of SAg binding causes massive cytokine release and T-cell proliferation. Monocytes, macrophages, B cells, and natural killer cells can act as APCs in SAg pathogenesis (17).

The binding of the SAg to a class II molecule occurs outside the conventional antigen binding groove (see Color Plate 16). The complex of superantigen and MHC class II interacts directly with the variable region of the β-chain of the T-cell receptor (TCRVβ). Thus, any T cell with the appropriate Vβ element can be stimulated, whereas antigen specificity is required in conventional antigen binding. Since the number of different Vβ regions in the human T-cell repertoire is restricted to less than 50 and since most superantigens can bind more than one, up to 25% of an individual's T cells may be stimulated by superantigens, resulting in massive detrimental cytokine release, including interleukin 2 (IL-2), gamma interferon (IFN-γ), IL-1β, and tumor necrosis factor alpha (TNF-α) (17).

PROTOTYPE SAgs

The exotoxins produced by *S. aureus* and *Streptococcus pyogenes* are SAg prototypes and are the best characterized structurally. *S. aureus* can express two different types of toxin with superantigen activity, enterotoxins (SEs), of which there are more than 10 serotypes (A, B, C1–3, D, E, G, H, I, J, K, L, and M), and toxic shock syndrome toxin (TSST-1). *S. pyogenes* produces pyrogenic exotoxins (Spes) A1–4, C, G, H, I, J, L, and M, the streptococcal superantigen (SSA), and the streptococcal mitogenic exotoxin (SMEZ) 1 and 2. These SAgs can be divided into three genetic subfamilies: (i) SpeC, SpeJ, SpeG, and SMEZ1; (ii) SEC1-3, SEB, SSA, SpeA, and SEG; (iii) SEA, SEE, SED, SEH, SEI, SEJ, SEK, and SEL, with two subfamilies containing SpeH and TSST-1 (19).

SAg STRUCTURE

The SAgs of *S. aureus* and *S. pyogenes* share a common architecture despite their significant difference in sequence. SAgs are globular proteins of 22 to 29 kDa, composed of two domains, amino- and carboxy-terminal, that are separated by a long, solvent-accessible α-helix spanning the center of the molecule (see Color Plate 17). The amino-terminal domain consists of a concave β-barrel, which has an α-helix at one end. This domain resembles the oligosaccharide/oligonucleotide binding (OB) fold present in other protein families. However, no such functions have been attributed to SAgs. The OB fold has been proposed to represent an ancient motif that contains a stable binding face capable of accommodating high sequence and function variability (15). Most SAgs have been observed to use three unique interfaces to interact with MHC class II molecules, and two of these sites are found in the amino-terminal domain. The carboxy-terminal domain comprises a four-stranded β-sheet flanked by the long α-helix. This domain has high sequence similarity to immunoglobulin-binding motifs (5, 20). The third MHC class II interface is found in the carboxy-terminal domain. The TCR-binding site is located in a shallow cavity between the two domains. The SAg residues involved in DRα1 and TCRVβ binding span a distance that cannot be covered by a single Fab fragment of an antibody. Each epitope contains noncontiguous amino acids and therefore can be recognized only when presented in the context of the native superantigen structure.

SAgs IN COMPLEX WITH MHC CLASS II AND T-CELL RECEPTORS

The crystal structures of bipartite complexes reveal important features of superantigen-receptor interactions. First, neither superantigen nor MHC class II or TCR undergoes significant structural changes upon complex formation. Second, the key residues of superantigen and MHC class II/TCR are identified including the nature of the pairwise interactions (i.e., hydrophobic, electrostatic, water-mediated, etc.) as well as the structures of the interacting epitopes. It appears superantigens are able to cross-link MHC class II molecules and

TCRs by a variety of subtly different ways through the use of various structural regions within each toxin (2).

MHC CLASS II STRUCTURE

Each MHC class II molecule consists of an extracellular peptide-binding cleft followed by a pair of immunoglobulin-like domains, the α- and β-chains, and is anchored to the cell by transmembrane and cytoplasmic domains. The amino-terminal α1 and β1 segments of the chains interact to form the peptide-binding cleft (see Color Plate 16). The most studied are MHC class II members, i.e., human leukocyte antigens (HLA) DP, DQ, and DR. HLA-DR molecules all possess two independent binding sites for bacterial SAgs. The conserved α-domain contains a low-affinity site ($K_d \sim 10^{-5}$ M), and the polymorphic β-chain contains a zinc-dependent high-affinity site ($K_d \sim 10^{-7}$ M). Not all MHC molecules necessarily share these sites. Some SAgs bind exclusively to the low-affinity site, such as SEB and TSST-1. These SAgs bind the α1 domain of the DR, and make contact only with the two amino-terminal interfaces of the SAg. Other SAgs bind only to the high-affinity site, e.g., SpeC and SEH, while some bind to both sites, e.g., SEA. In complexes of SAgs with the high-affinity site, the SAg contacts the α-helix of the β1 domain of the class II molecule (17).

T-CELL RECEPTOR STRUCTURE

The T-cell receptor is a transmembrane heterodimer, composed of α- and β-chains. Each chain is composed of constant (C) and variable (V) regions. The amino-terminal Vα and Vβ segments of the chains interact to form the peptide-binding cleft (see Color Plate 16). Each superantigen is associated with a characteristic Vβ profile, i.e., SAgs specifically expand T cells bearing a specific subset of TCRVβs (7). About 60 different Vβ elements of human TCRs have been identified. Structural variation in the Vβ domains is mainly restricted to its three complementarity-determining region (CDR) loops. The affinities for SAg-TCRVβ interactions are relatively low, with a K_d in the range of 10^{-4} to 10^{-6} M (11), and this is similar to the affinities for MHC/peptide-TCRVβ interactions.

RATIONALE FOR THERAPY BY CHIMERIC RECEPTOR MIMICS

Based on the wealth of structural information available, we proposed an alternative SAg therapy using structure-based design. This approach involves the use of receptor mimics, or decoy molecules, that prevent the binding of bacterial toxins to their specific receptors on the surface of human host cells. We hypothesized that the structural requirements for toxin-receptor binding could be exploited in the structure-based design of a toxin-specific ligand that can compete with cell surface receptors. The strategy for the construction of such a receptor mimic was to incorporate the structural elements of the receptor required only for toxin binding and not for the binding of the natural ligand. Thus, the designed receptor mimics are expected to inhibit only the binding of toxins to the host cell receptors and not the binding of the natural ligands to the same host cell receptors. We combined experimental and theoretical approaches to examine the inhibitory properties of chimeric proteins designed to block *S. aureus* SAgs.

We tested our hypothesis using *Staphylococcus* enterotoxins B (SEB), C3 (SEC3), and TSST-1 as model toxins. Structural data available for these toxins included crystal structures of SEB complexed with HLA-DRα1 (1SEB), SEB complexed with TCRVβ (1SBB), SEC3 complexed with TCRVβ (1JCK), TSST-1 (2TSS), and HLA-DRα1-peptide complexed with TCR (1FYT). Since DRα1 and TCRVβ are the only two receptor-binding domains required for the pathogenesis of these model toxins, we envisioned that a DRα1-linker-TCRVβ chimera should be an efficient receptor mimic of the cell surface-bound MHC class II-TCR complex. Like the native MHC class II-TCR complex, such a chimera should also target two nonoverlapping sites on a SAg. As a result, this bispecific chimera should act as a decoy and prevent SAg from binding to the target APC and T cell, and thereby inhibit SAg-induced cytokine production and T-cell proliferation. The DRα1-linker-TCRVβ chimera (a bispecific ligand) should also show a higher affinity for SAg binding than the individual DRα1 and TCRVβ ligands because the presence of two different binding modules in the same molecule should facilitate the synergy of the two binding events. That is, the covalent linkage should provide spatial proximity of each of the ligands to the SAg. Thus, the binding of DRα1 to SAg should increase the local concentration of TCRVβ and its level of binding to SAg and vice versa.

DESIGN OF CHIMERAS

A set of DRα1 sequences was analyzed computationally for stable folding and optimal contacts with the target SAgs. The best candidate sequence was used to make up the DRα1 portion of all three chimeras (6, 12). Our DRα1 model in all complexes corresponds to the observed fold in the single crystal of SEB-MHC class II complex (1SEB).

Three different TCRVβ sequences were selected because of their preferential binding to the toxins: human (h) TCRVβ3.0 for the SEB-specific chimera (15), human (h) TCRVβ2.0 for the TSST-specific chimera, and a mouse (m) analog of TCRVβ8.2 for the SEC3-specific chimera. A mutagenized variant of the single-chain TCR, a Vβ8.2/Vβ3.1 fusion protein (mL2.1/A52V), has been shown to yield a 1,000-fold increased binding affinity to SEC3 (8). A truncated TCRVβ8.2 part of the Vβ8.2/Vβ3.1 fusion protein was used to construct a SEC3 specific chimera. A homology model of hTCRVβ3.0 was constructed using the closely related TCRVβ fold in the crystal structure of SEB-TCR complex. Similarly, the TCRVβ fold in the crystal structure of SEC3-TCR complex was used to build a homology model of mTCRVβ8.3. Homology modeling was also used to obtain the structure of the hTCRVβ2.0 sequence.

The designed DRα1 and TCRVβ sequences were covalently joined by the linker sequence, (GSTAPPA)$_2$, a linker sequence derived from the human tandem repeat protein mucin and shown to be flexible and nonantigenic, to obtain the chimera. The length and amino acid sequence of the linker were designed to allow the simultaneous binding of these two subdomains to SAg, without steric hindrance of the native folding of the individual DRα1 and TCRVβ (6, 12).

A restrained molecular dynamics (MD) simulated annealing was performed for the chimera-SAg complexes such that the backbone (φ and ψ) conformations of DRα1, TCRVβ, and SAg and the SAg-DRα1 and SAg-TCRVβ contacts were kept close to those of their native MHC class II-SAg and TCR-SAg complexes (6, 12).

CHIMERIC PROTEINS EXHIBIT TYPE-SPECIFIC INHIBITION
OF IL-2 RELEASE AND CELL PROLIFERATION

The designed chimera genes were cloned into pET 32B (SEBc) or pRSETc (SEC3c and TSST-1c) bacterial expression vectors. The chimeras were then subcloned into AD 494 cells or BL21 cells, respectively, and expressed as thioredoxin-His fusion proteins containing N-terminal enterokinase domains. They were purified on TALON metal-affinity resin (6, 12).

IL-2 release and T-cell proliferation assays in donor-matched peripheral blood mononuclear cells and dendritic cells were used to measure the efficacy of the chimeric proteins. ELISAs were performed to measure SAg-induced IL-2 release in the presence of each chimeric protein to determine whether the different chimeras specifically inhibited the cytokine release induced by the SAg against which the chimera was designed. The Vialight cell proliferation assay was used to measure cellular ATP. The TSST-1 and SEC3 chimeras inhibited IL-2 release in a SAg type-specific manner, when compared with cells stimulated with SAg alone. SEB chimera IL-2 release assays could not be carried out reliably due to the extreme sensitivity of the donor cells to the SEB toxin. In the cell proliferation assays, $20\times$ concentration of SEBc showed 30% inhibition. At $20\times$ concentration, TSST-1c and SEC3c inhibited T-cell proliferation by 40% (6).

The inhibitory activity exhibited by the three receptor mimics indicates that the native DRα1 and TCRVβ folds are maintained, and that the TCRVβ domains do, indeed, impart SAg specificity to the chimeras. The chimeras are able to distinguish not only two distantly related SAg family members, SEB and TSST-1, but also the more closely related SEB and SEC3.

MOLECULAR MODELING OF CHIMERAS ELUCIDATES
DETAILS OF THE INTERACTION

After demonstrating the successful inhibition of the three chimeras, we performed molecular modeling on the SAg-chimera complexes based on available biochemical and crystallographic data to understand the structural basis of the type-specific inhibition, especially the role of various pairwise contacts between SAg and DRα1, SAg and TCRVβ, and the role of the (GSTAPPA)$_2$ linker in determining binding and specificity. With this information, we compared the inhibitory properties of SEBc, SEC3c, and TSST-1c.

The spatial position and orientations of DRα1 and TCRVβ in the chimeras with respect to the superantigens were derived mainly from the crystal structures of bipartite complexes such as SEB-MHC class II (1SEB), SEB-TCR (1SBB), and SEC3-TCR (1JCK) by superposition of the toxins. In the case of the TSST-1 complex, conserved structural features of the toxins such as the long central α-helix were chosen to orient the superantigen in the complex. The MHC and TCR components were positioned relative to TSST-1 by using information from literature. The superantigen-chimera complex was minimized locally in vacuum without any constraints using the AMBER 4.1 force field (16); the parm94 parameter set was applied with a dielectric constant of 80 to a gradient limit of $<10^{-2}$ kcal/mol Å^2 (14).

From our molecular modeling studies, we show that the three SAgs contact the DRα1 domain in a similar manner (see Color Plate 18), although there are slight differences in the relative orientation between SAg and DRα1. The major differences in specificity occur

at the contact regions between the Vβ domains and SAgs, as expected from our original design of using different TCRVβ isoforms to impart specificity to our chimeras. That SEB/SEBc and SEC3/SEC3c complexes share similar contact residue profiles but differ from TSST-1/TSST-1-c is also not surprising, given that TSST-1 shares only ~28% homology with other SAg family members, compared with ~60% homology between SEB and SEC3. However, there are also observable differences in the SEB/SEBc and SEC3/SEC3c complexes. These differences include the loop region between α3/β10, in which Phe-177 in SEB contacts CDR2 of the Vβ3 domain, whereas Phe-176 and Asn-177 of SEC3 contact HV4 of the Vβ8.2 domain. In addition, only SEC3 maintains simultaneous DRα1 and Vβ contacts at D209/Q210 and interactions with the linker in the loop region between β2/β3. These differences most likely contribute to the ability of SEBc and SEC3c to specifically inhibit their respective chimeras despite the relatively high level of homology between SEB and SEC3 (14).

Because SEC3c exhibited the highest relative level of type-specific inhibition in both IL-2 release and T-cell proliferation compared with the other chimeras, it was of interest to examine whether the observed inhibition was due to the specific choice of Vβ isoform in the SEC3c. A truncated version of the mouse Vβ8.2 isoform originally obtained by screening a mutagenized library of Vβ8.2 variants using yeast display and flow cytometry sorting was used for this chimera. This Vβ8.2 variant displayed a K_d of 7 nM for binding to SEC3, which is ~1,000-fold lower than for the original Vβ8.2 isoform. The mutagenized Vβ8.2 isoform in SEC3c was truncated and contains seven of the nine mutations in the original mL2.1/A52V mutant, since the additional two mutations lay outside our consensus Vβ domain used for SEBc and TSST-1c. While the truncated Vβ8.2 isoform in SEC3c may not display exactly the same binding properties of its full-length counterpart, we examined how the seven mutations changed the residue contact profile with SEC3 using molecular modeling. The calculated relative interaction energy for the native V8.2 sequence is higher (~ +3.5 kcal/mol) upon complex formation than the mutagenized, truncated Vβ8.2 sequence, indicating that the Vβ8.2 sequence in SEC3c yields a more stable complex and most likely enhanced the inhibitory properties of SEC3c (14).

USING MOLECULAR MODELING TO IMPROVE AFFINITY OF THE CHIMERAS FOR SAgs

After we demonstrated the type-specific inhibitory properties of our chimeras in cell culture studies, we predicted that affinity enhancement of the chimeras to increase binding affinity for the different SAgs would produce a more effective inhibitor, especially for the practical implementation of the chimeras in therapy. Production of chimeras with a much higher binding affinity to SAg compared with the K_d ~μM displayed by SAg binding to the MHC class II and T-cell receptors would more effectively prevent SAgs from binding their receptor targets and forming an immune synapse to activate immune cells. Since the TCRVβ domain imparts SAg binding specificity, affinity enhancement of the TCRVβ domain may yield receptor mimics with more enhanced inhibitory properties against a given SAg. The mutagenesis of the Vβ8.2 isoform to increase binding affinity for SEC3 by ~1,000-fold strongly supports this strategy as being particularly effective. The type specificity displayed by the different chimeras can be explained on the basis of structure specificity and depends on the choice of unique TCRVβ isoforms.

Backbone interactions play a significant role in SAg binding. This may imply that a large subset of Vβ isoforms adopt similar folds and all of them can bind the same SAg through the common backbone interaction pattern. In the rational design of specific chimeras, it is possible to enhance the binding affinity by introducing new side-chain-stabilizing interactions while retaining the backbone interaction. We decided to apply modeling studies of the SAg/chimera complexes to identify site-specific mutations that would increase the stability of the interaction.

We applied two strategies to analyze the pairwise contacts between superantigen and specific chimera: (i) intermolecular contacts were identified by computing distances between residues of DRα1, TCRVβ, or linker to the superantigen within a 4Å cutoff; (ii) changes in solvent accessibility per residue were computed for the free toxin and chimera and the toxin-chimera complex. A threshold of 3% change of the solvent-accessible surface per residue was applied to define contacts between the free superantigen and the chimera due to complex formation. In principle, each contact interface is stabilized by three main contributions: (i) enthalpy gain from pairwise interactions; (ii) change in free energy due to transfer of amino acids involved in pairwise interactions from aqueous to nonaqueous environment of the contact interface between superantigen and chimera; and (iii) entropy loss due to freezing of the side-chain motion in the contact interface. Contribution iii may not be mutually exclusive of contribution ii. Interaction energies between the toxin and the chimera were estimated from contributions from the force-field energies (enthalpic contribution) and estimates of free energies due to transfer of various amino acids from aqueous to hydrophobic environment and the corresponding change in the accessible surface area. Based on the analysis of the pairwise contacts between the toxin and the specific chimera, mutations were suggested to improve the affinity of the chimeric proteins toward the superantigens (14).

Most similarities are observed for contacts between the superantigens and DRα1 of the chimeric protein, whereas most of the differences are observed for the TCRVβ contacts. The structural differences in binding impart the specificity in the complex formation. The sequence similarity of SEB and SEC3 and their dissimilarity to TSST-1 (1) are also reflected by the binding specificity of these toxins. SEB contacts bear much greater similarities to SEC3 than to TSST-1. In addition, careful analyses of pairwise interactions at the contact interfaces formed by loop1, loop2, and α-helix of DRα and CDR1, CDR2, and HV4 of TCRVβ, and the targeted superantigen, reveal specific mutations that are likely to improve the binding affinity of the chimera.

A simple empirical approach was used to estimate whether an amino acid substitution on any of the six binding epitopes as well as in the linker region of a chimera has a stabilizing effect. Based on this criterion, we expect that mutations such as N15E, I72T, S147Y, and K150Q should have a stabilizing effect on the SEB chimera, whereas substitutions such as G323S (linker) and K371Y (CDR2) destabilize the complex. For the SEC3-chimera complex, we expect the following mutations to have stabilizing effects: E279T, E285I, F293Q, and I302N within DRα, P328N and G331V of the linker, and N375T, E377Q, and P390N within TCRVβ. G372V, G372T, and G374V substitutions in the CDR2 region of TCRVβ are expected to destabilize the SEC3-chimera complex. Mutations Y13K, K75E, A161S, and I182N should have a stabilizing effect on the TSST-1 chimera. Most of the other substitutions indicated a destabilizing effect in the TSST-1-chimera complex (14).

CONCLUSIONS AND FUTURE WORK

Our approach, which employs the use of a chimeric protein to block the initial step of SAg pathogenesis, namely the ligation of APC and T cells, has several unique features. The synergistic binding of the constituent DRα1 and TCRVβ domains to the SAgs was made possible by our choice of a flexible linker that allows the chimeric protein to simultaneously interact with two functional sites on the SAg, which are too far apart to be spanned by a single antibody. Therefore, the fact that the chimera can block the two functional sites on SAg simultaneously would make the chimera a superior inhibitor to an antibody that can block only one of the two functional sites. This is supported by the observation that an antibody that binds to SEB with high affinity (K_d ~nM), but only partially covers the DRα1 binding site on SEB, is a poor inhibitor of pathogenesis.

The observation that the DRα1-linker-TCRVβ chimeras are effective against several SAgs is significant in terms of their practical use against *S. aureus* infections. During the onset of *S. aureus*-based diseases such as food poisoning or systemic shock, multiple superantigens are released in the body to cause productive infection. While antibiotics can potentially kill the whole bacterium and stop the release of all superantigens, the emergence of antibiotic-resistant *S. aureus* strains necessitates the development of alternative measures to protect against the released superantigens, the primary causative agents of infection. Therefore, our therapeutic approach, based on the concept of using rationally designed receptor mimics that can be effective inhibitors against multiple superantigens, may prove to be a viable strategy against antibiotic-resistant *S. aureus*. Our finding that the DRα1-linker-TCRVβ receptor mimics are effective against different SAgs is a strong validation of our hypothesis.

Development of more effective inhibitors against individual SAgs or chimeras that bind to multiple SAgs would be prime candidates to use in assaying therapeutic efficacy in whole animal studies. SEB and TSST-1 chimeras, incorporating site-specific mutations identified through molecular modeling, are currently being produced for in vitro testing.

Acknowledgments. We acknowledge Elizabeth Hong-Geller, Patrick Shirtleff, and Margit Molhoff for their published work that has been cited in this chapter.

REFERENCES

1. **Arcus, V. L., T. Proft, J. A. Sigrell, H. M. Baker, J. D. Fraser, and E. N. Baker.** 2000. Conservation and variation in superantigen structure and activity highlighted by the three-dimensional structures of two new superantigens from *Streptococcus pyogenes*. *J. Mol. Biol.* **299**(1):157–168

2. **Baker, M. D., and K. R. Acharya.** 2004. Superantigens: structure-function relationships. *Int. J. Med. Microbiol.* **293**(7–8):529–537.

3. **Chesney P. J., M. S. Bergdoll, J. P. Davis, and J. M. Vergeront.** 1984. The disease spectrum, epidemiology, and etiology of toxic-shock syndrome. *Annu. Rev. Microbiol.* **38**:315–338.

4. **Emori, T. G., and R. P. Gaynes.** 1993. An overview of nosocomial infections, including the role of the microbiology laboratory. *Clin. Microbiol. Rev.* **6**(4):428–442.

5. **Gronenborn, A. M., and G. M. Clore.** 1993. Identification of the contact surface of a streptococcal protein G domain complexed with a human Fc fragment. *J. Mol. Biol.* **233**(3):331–335.

6. **Hong-Geller, E., M. Möllhoff, P. R. Shiflett, and G. Gupta.** 2004. Design of chimeric receptor mimics with different TcRVβ isoforms. *J. Biol. Chem.* **279**:5676–5684.

7. **Kappler, J., B. Kotzin, L. Herron, E. W. Gelfand, R. D. Bigler, A. Boylston, S. Carrel, D. N. Posnett, Y. Choi, and P. Marrack.** 1989. V beta-specific stimulation of human T cells by staphylococcal toxins. *Science* **244**:811–813.

8. **Kieke, M. C., E. Sundberg, E. V. Shusta, R. A. Mariuzza, K. D. Wittrup, and D. M. Kranz.** 2001. High affinity T cell receptors from yeast display libraries block T cell activation by superantigens. *J. Mol. Biol.* **307**(5):1305–1315.

9. **Kotzin, B. L., D. Y. Leung, J. Kappler, and P. Marrack.** 1993. Superantigens and their potential role in human disease. *Adv. Immunol.* **54**:99–166.

10. **Laurence, J., A. S. Hodtsev, and D. N. Posnett.** 1992. Superantigen implicated in dependence of HIV-1 replication in T cells on TCR V beta expression. *Nature* **358**(6383):255–259.

11. **Leder, L., A. Llera, P. M. Lavoie, M. I. Lebedeva, H. Li, R. P. Sekaly, G. A. Bohach, P. J. Gahr, P. M. Schlievert, K. Karjalainen, and R. A. Mariuzza.** 1998. A mutational analysis of the binding of staphylococcal enterotoxins B and C3 to the T cell receptor beta chain and major histocompatibility complex class II. *J. Exp. Med.* **187**(6):823–833.

12. **Lehnert, N. M., D. L. Allen, B. L. Allen, P. Catasti, P. R. Shiflett, M. Chen, B. E. Lehnert, and G. Gupta.** 2001. Structure-based design of a bispecific receptor mimic that inhibits T cell responses to a superantigen. *Biochemistry* **40**:4222–4228.

13. **Marrack, P., and J. Kapler.** 1990. The staphylococcal enterotoxins and their relatives. *Science* **248**:705–711.

14. **Möllhoff, M., H. B. Vander Zanden, P. R. Shiflett, and G. Gupta.** 2005. Modeling of receptor mimics that inhibit superantigen pathogenesis. *J. Mol. Recognit.* **18**:73–83.

15. **Murzin, A. G.** 1993. Can homologous proteins evolve different enzymatic activities? *Trends Biochem. Sci.* **18**(11):403–405.

16. **Pearlman, D. A., D. A. Case, J. W. Caldwell, W. S. Ross, T. E. Cheatham, S. DeBolt, D. Ferguson, G. Seibel, and P. Kollman.** 1995. AMBER, a package of computer programs for applying molecular mechanics, normal mode analysis, molecular dynamics and free energy calculations to simulate the structural and energetic properties of molecules. *Com. Phys. Comm.* **91**(1):1–41.

17. **Petersson, K., G. Forsberg, and B. Walse.** 2004. Interplay between superantigens and immunoreceptors. *Scand. J. Immunol.* **59**(4):345–355.

18. **Schiffenbauer, J., H. M. Johnson, E. J. Butfiloski, L. Wegrzyn, and J. M. Soos.** 1993. Staphylococcal enterotoxins can reactivate experimental allergic encephalomyelitis. *Proc. Natl. Acad. Sci. USA* **90**(18):8543–8546.

19. **Sundberg, E. J., Y. Li, and R. A. Mariuzza.** 2002. So many ways of getting in the way: diversity in the molecular architecture of superantigen-dependent T-cell signaling complexes. *Curr. Opin. Immunol.* **14**(1):36–44.

20. **Wikstrom, M., T. Drakenberg, S. Forsen, U. Sjobring, and L. Bjorck.** 1994. Three-dimensional solution structure of an immunoglobulin light chain-binding domain of protein L. Comparison with the IgG-binding domains of protein G. *Biochemistry* **33**(47):14011–14017.

INDEX